Drugs and Addictive Behaviour

In this completely revised and updated third edition of his highly successful book, Hamid Ghodse presents a comprehensive overview of substance misuse and dependence. There is a particular emphasis on practical, evidence-based approaches to the assessment and management of a wide range of drug-related problems in a variety of clinical settings, and he has written an entirely new chapter on alcohol abuse. He defines all the terms, and describes the effects of substance misuse on a patient's life. Epidemiology, and international prevention and drug control policies are covered to address the global nature of the problem, and the appendix provides a series of clinical intervention tools, among them a Substance Misuse Assessment Questionnaire.

This will be essential reading for all clinicians and other professionals dealing with addiction, from counsellors and social workers to policy makers.

Hamid Ghodse is Professor and Director of the Centre for Addiction Studies at St George's Hospital Medical School in London. He is also the Director of the Board of International Affairs of the Royal College of Psychiatrists and member of the Expert Advisory Panel of WHO on Alcohol and Drug Dependence. He has been six times president of the UN International Narcotics Control Board.

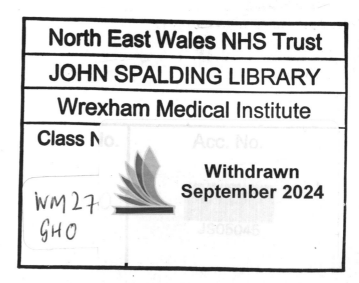

Drugs
and Addictive
Behaviour

A Guide to Treatment

Third edition

Hamid Ghodse

CBE (Hon.) MD PhD FFPHM FRCP FRCPE FRCPsych
Professor and Director, Centre for Addiction Studies
Department of Addictive Behaviour and Psychological Medicine
St George's Hospital Medical School, University of London
Honorary Consultant Psychiatrist
South West London and St George's Mental Health Trust

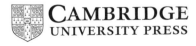

CAMBRIDGE
UNIVERSITY PRESS

PUBLISHED BY THE PRESS SYNDICATE OF THE UNIVERSITY OF CAMBRIDGE
The Pitt Building, Trumpington Street, Cambridge, United Kingdom

CAMBRIDGE UNIVERSITY PRESS
The Edinburgh Building, Cambridge CB2 2RU, UK
40 West 20th Street, New York NY 10011-4211, USA
477 Williamstown Road, Port Melbourne, VIC 3207, Australia
Ruiz de Alarcón 13, 28014 Madrid, Spain
Dock House, The Waterfront, Cape Town 8001, South Africa

http://www.cambridge.org

First published 1989
Second edition 1995
Third edition 2002

Printed in the United Kingdom at the University Press, Cambridge

Typeface Minion 10.5/14pt   *System* Poltype® [v n]

A catalogue record for this book is available from the British Library

Library of Congress Cataloguing in Publication data

Ghodse, Hamid.
Drugs and addictive behaviour : a guide to treatment / Hamid Ghodse. – 3rd ed.
  p.   cm.
Includes bibliographical references and index.
ISBN 0 521 00001 7 (pb)   0 521 81354 9 (hb)
1. Substance abuse – Treatment.   I. Title.
RC564.G39 2002   616.86'06–dc21   2001043440

ISBN 0 521 00001 7 paperback
ISBN 0 521 81354 9 hardback

When you can cure by regimen,
avoid having recourse to medicine;
and when you can effect a cure
by means of a single medicine,
avoid using a compound one.

Razi (Rhazes)
Persia, AD 850–922

To Barbara, Amir-Hossein, Nassrin and Ali-Reza

Contents

Preface

Although the structure of the third edition of this book remains unchanged, there has been significant updating and revision throughout. Every attempt has been made to retain the straightforward approach adopted in the first and second editions, so that the contents are easily accessible to a wide audience and the emphasis, throughout, has been on practical approaches so that the book is genuinely 'a guide to treatment'.

Two major changes have been made. Firstly a separate chapter has been included on Alcohol (Chapter 4). Obviously, a short chapter can only touch on a few of the major issues of this very complex subject. However, this makes the text more comprehensive and emphasizes the close links between dependence on alcohol and other substances. The other major change has been the inclusion of references in the text, in line with the need for evidence-based practice. However, the book remains an authoritative text, extensively based on wide experience.

In view of the increasing globalization of drug use and misuse, a wide range of international statistics have been included in Chapter 2 and the international bodies involved in drug control are described in Chapter 12. The Guiding Principles on Demand Reduction adopted by the Special Session of the General Assembly of the United Nations in 1998 emphasize the importance of prevention, treatment and rehabilitation which are all covered in various sections of this book. Some aspects of the book relate primarily to UK practice, but every attempt has been made to make it useful to practitioners world-wide. Reflecting changes in this field over the past few years, sections dealing with HIV and hepatitis C in relation to substance misuse have been extensively revised.

It is impossible to acknowledge all the sources of inspiration and information on which I have drawn while writing this book, but first of all, and above all, I must thank my patients – *all* the patients with drug problems whom I have met over the last 25 years and more. They are the *raison d'être* of the book and the experience I have gained with them and from them is central to it.

Additional material has been drawn from the work of the world-wide community of scientists and researchers in the field, and the World Health Organization, the United Nations, the UN Drug Control Programme, the International Narcotics Control Board, NIDA and Interpol have all been valuable sources of information.

I thank, sincerely, my colleagues Jan Annan, John Corkery, Paul Davis, Colin Drummond, Nek Oyefeso, Mike Pollard and Gill Tregenza for their generous help. I would also like to thank Richard Barling and Pauline Graham of Cambridge University Press for their support and unfailing patience. For administrative support, I thank Kate Borrett and Rosie Chick. Health care students, both undergraduate and postgraduate, of all disciplines, have contributed through their interest and enthusiasm and their enlightening discussions. I also thank the World Health Organization and the American Psychiatric Association for permission to reprint parts of ICD-10 and DSM-III-R and DSM-IV.

Hamid Ghodse

Introduction

Drug use of one sort or another has occurred for a very long time – probably ever since the time that early humans, eating plants that grew around them, found that some plants had medicinal properties and that some made them feel different. Since that time, drug use has been part of the human lifestyle, with different societies using different 'natural' intoxicants depending on the indigenous flora. A few of these drugs have become familiar to many, beyond the confines of their original use. Opium, alcohol and cannabis spring immediately to mind; they have been used for centuries and are still widely used today. So too is coffee, which although it is bought in packets and jars as a food, fits all five definitions of the word 'drug' given in Chapter 1.

Coffee is indigenous to Ethiopia where it was first consumed by chewing the beans or infusing the leaves. It was certainly known to the Arabs in the sixth century and its medicinal properties were described by the Persian physicians, Razi (or Rhazes; 850–922) and Ibn-sina (or Avicenna; 980–1037). In the four-teenth century the technique of roasting and grinding coffee beans was developed and only then did coffee drinking become prevalent. By this time, the cultivation and use of coffee had spread to Arabia where its popularity was enhanced because the use of alcohol had been banned by the Koran. Coffee was used medicinally as well as for religious purposes, particularly by the Dervishes to keep themselves awake during long religious rituals. With the increasing popularity of coffee, coffee houses were established which soon became meeting places for intellectuals. The use of coffee in its social setting of the coffee house spread through the Arab world and to Turkey, Persia and beyond. There were many attempts, in different countries, to close down the coffee houses which were seen as centres of sedition and dissent, and to ban the use of coffee altogether. All of these attempts at prohibition eventually failed and coffee was then heavily taxed so that coffee houses became valuable sources of revenue for the authorities. During the seven-teenth century, coffee drinking spread to England and other parts of Europe. As in Arabia, it was first used medicinally, and in particular as a cure for drunkenness which was then rife. Coffee houses soon opened and again became important social, political and business centres, attracting opposition, almost from the start, from brewers and others with vested interests in the sale of alcohol. Taxes were imposed and provided considerable revenue, but despite this, attempts were made in England to close the coffee houses that were once again seen as centres of radicalism and political dissent. As in Arabia these attempts failed and heavier taxes were imposed instead. Gradually in the latter part of the eighteenth century, the clientele of the coffee houses started to join clubs and the heyday of coffee houses was over, this change being accelerated by the importation of tea by the British East India Company and the acceptance of tea (which also contains caffeine) as the national drink.

From this necessarily brief history of coffee it is possible to identify certain themes that crop up repeatedly when modern drugs of abuse and dependence are considered. For example, many of these drugs were first used, like coffee, for medicinal purposes even though they are now considered to have minimal or no therapeutic value; alcohol, tobacco, cannabis and LSD (lysergic acid diethylamide) all fit into this category. In the case of the first three drugs, all of which have a long history, it is easy to imagine them as the 'wonder drugs' of their time, being prescribed enthusiastically for a variety of conditions. Modern sophisticated research produces many such drugs, and many have psychoactive properties. Some of these have already repeated the cycle from apparently safe therapeutic agent to drug of misuse or dependence, and undoubtedly more will do so in the future. Apart from their medicinal value, many drugs (e.g. opium, cannabis, cocaine and mescaline) have been used, as coffee was, in religious rituals, and the use of alcohol in this way continues today in two of the world's three monotheistic religions. It is of interest that the third and youngest religion, Islam, bans its use altogether.

A third way in which drugs are used is for social and recreational purposes and it was this use of coffee that provoked so much controversy and opposition, just as it does today for the other drugs. All of the 'old' drugs (those with a long history, e.g. opium, cannabis and alcohol) were used in this way and drug use was often the whole reason for a group coming together; the drug became the very substance of communication, the dynamic of the group activity. Alcohol continues in this role today, in public houses, night clubs, cocktail parties and so on, and for some drugs, notably cannabis and other psychedelic drugs, taken specifically by those interested in mysticism and exploration of the inner world, the setting in which the drug is taken and the shared group experiences remain important. As far as illicit drug use is concerned, the very fact that the drug is forbidden encourages the formation of a group (and often of a whole subculture) concerned, among other things, with obtaining the drug and concealing its use from the authorities.

The story of coffee also illustrates the significance of technological innovation in drug use. Only when the techniques of roasting and grinding the coffee beans became prevalent, did the use of coffee become popular and spread widely and become perceived as problematic. Similarly the use of alcohol was profoundly affected by Razi's discovery of the process of distillation, which made it easier to transport alcohol and to become drunk. Later the identification of the active alkaloids of opium and the subsequent development of the process of acetylation, by which morphine is converted to heroin, changed the whole pattern of opiate use, not only in the West where this discovery was made, but also in the East, where the parent drug originated. The extraction of cocaine from the leaf of the coca plant and more recently, the ability to prepare pure cocaine 'free-base' ('crack') have had equally profound effects, and now the process has gone one stage further, with new 'designer' drugs being manufactured for the sole purpose of abuse.

It is often assumed that the spread of drug use from one country to another is a new problem brought about by modern, rapid means of transport. The story of coffee, or indeed of any of the 'old' drugs, suggests that this is not so. For centuries there has been travel not only from one country to another, but also from one continent to another, and humans on their travels have taken drugs with them. There is no doubt, however, that modern methods of travel and communication have had a profound effect on drug use and abuse because the physical transportation of drugs is so much easier and speedier. In addition, the rapid movement of large numbers of people means that many more people are exposed to the drug-taking practices of another culture. This exposure is increased still further by the effect of the media, so that no drug or drug-taking practice can remain localized. They are bound to spread and in so doing there is usually a loss of the traditional constraints upon drug use imposed by the family and society as a whole. This means that new drugs and new ways of taking them gain acceptance much more easily than when drug use was under strict, local, sociocultural control.

Despite traditional methods of control, the drug scene has never been static. Five hundred years ago in Arabia the use of coffee superseded that of alcohol; this was partly because of the prohibition of alcohol by the Koran, but also occurred because of the availability of coffee. In England too, coffee drinking in the seventeenth century reduced the popularity of alcohol, but in turn gave way to tea. Similar changes in the pattern and fashions of drug use have occurred in the past and continue today, the availability of the particular drug often playing a crucial role.

Governments have long been concerned in controlling drug availability. Centuries ago, in Arabia, there were attempts at prohibiting coffee and when these failed, high taxes were imposed, ostensibly to discourage its use. However, this resulted in such high revenues that it then became economically almost impossible to pursue definitive policies to reduce coffee consumption. This cycle of events was repeated when coffee drinking spread to England and has also occurred with alcohol and tobacco – both of which now occupy entrenched positions within the economy of most countries.

Many other parallels can be drawn between what has happened to coffee in the past and what is happening to many drugs of abuse and dependence today. Recognition of this fact is not a counsel of despair. It is not meant to imply that heroin will ever be available on the shelves of the supermarket, as coffee is today. But the generality of the themes that have emerged over centuries of drug use does suggest that problems of drug abuse and of dependence on different types of drugs have similarities that transcend substance-specific problems. This in turn suggests that it is the nature of drug abuse and dependence that is important rather than the specific drug that is causing concern at that particular time. However threatening, however modern, however unique present problems appear, it is undoubtedly true that their similarities to what has arisen before are more striking than differences which are more likely to be quantitative than qualitative.

Unfortunately, this quantitative difference, the enormous scale of modern drug abuse and drug dependence, has caused particular problems. Nowadays, so many people have drug-related problems that their care can no longer be left to a small band of interested specialists. All health care professionals come into contact with drug abusers and drug-dependent individuals, as do probation officers and the police and others involved with the law, as well as those concerned with welfare services. All of these people require a basic understanding of the problems of drug abuse and dependence if their interventions are to be effective, and this book attempts to convey the general knowledge about drug abuse and dependence that is essential for that understanding.

In addition to general knowledge, however, there is a need for clear and practical advice on what to do in particular situations. Despite a wealth of research literature and a plethora of weighty tomes on drug dependence, it is difficult to find such advice. This book attempts to fill that gap, with chapters on how to assess individuals with drug-related problems and how to go about helping them. Although the emphasis is first on general measures of intervention, specific treatment programmes are also described so that the nonspecialist, armed with a general understanding of the nature of the problem, is able to make intelligent decisions and to initiate treatment. Here the emphasis is on flexibility and a variety of treatment options are described and discussed, from acupuncture to intravenous heroin maintenance. Obviously it is not possible to cover every eventuality but many problems and problematic situations are included, such as the management of an intoxicated, psychotic patient in the accident and emergency department; the care of children of drug-abusing parents; the question of whether drug-dependent individuals are eligible for driving licences; the management of drug-abusing health care professionals, and so on.

Although drug-dependent individuals and drug abusers need help and it is essential that there are sufficient trained people to provide it, local responses to particular individual drug problems will never be enough. The final chapters of the book therefore examine the problem from a wider perspective, describing and explaining national and international control measures. Most important of all, perhaps, is the chapter on prevention which emphasizes the personal responsibility of every individual to develop more thoughtful attitudes towards drug taking.

In a book of this size it is only possible to cover a small fraction of the topics related to drug abuse and drug dependence. For example, problems associated with tobacco are not included at all. This omission is not intended to imply that because use of tobacco is widespread and socially acceptable, dependence on it is unimportant. Rather the magnitude and complexity of this legal recreational drug is such that it cannot be adequately dealt with in one small general book such as this. Similarly, although alcohol has been included for the first time in this edition, it can only be dealt with at a very simplistic level, in the space of a single chapter. The interested reader should consult one of the many specialist books on these very important aspects of substance misuse.

The choice of topics covered by this book has been influenced by their practical relevance, but sufficient background information has been included to enable understanding of basic principles. It is hoped that it will encourage those who are inexperienced and unfamiliar with the field to become involved. In the past, many professionals have taken avoiding action when faced by a drug-abusing or drug-dependent individual, preferring to shunt the person off to another agency. They often justified their action by the belief that nothing could be done to help the person anyway, but such responses usually concealed underlying anxiety about their own ability to respond effectively. It is hoped that this book, by explaining some of the basic facts and practical approaches in a simple and straightforward way, will demonstrate that many substance-dependent individuals can be helped, and encourage more professionals to become involved in helping them.

Drugs, addiction and behaviour

What is a 'drug'?

There are several possible definitions of a drug, as the examples below will show, but all have their limitations.

'A substance which, when injected into a rat, produces a scientific paper' – facetious, certainly, but probably accurate.

'A substance used as a medicine in the treatment of diagnosed mental or physical illness'. This definition is based on the shifting sands of therapeutic efficacy; coffee, cannabis and tobacco were used in times gone by for their medicinal properties and, accordingly, would then have been classified as drugs. Nowadays, however, all would escape that definition, a decision that would make most people uneasy, certainly as far as cannabis is concerned, and perhaps for tobacco and coffee too.

'Any chemical substance, other than a food, that affects the structure of a living thing'. This too is unsatisfactory because there are a few substances generally considered to be drugs which are also consumed as foods. Alcohol is the obvious example, but there are others: some mushrooms would be 'food' while others would be drugs; caffeine, obtained in coffee jars from the supermarket, is perceived as a food, whereas in tablet form from the chemist, it is considered a drug.

A drug is 'any substance, other than those required for the maintenance of normal health, which, when taken into the living organism, may modify one or more of its functions'.[1] This very broad definition was developed by the World Health Organization (WHO), and had the advantage of being used and understood internationally.

Definitions change with time however and, more recently, the WHO has developed a 'Lexicon of alcohol and drug terms'[2] which acknowledges that 'drug' is a term of varied usage. In medicine it refers to any substance with the potential to prevent or cure disease or enhance physical or mental welfare and in pharmacology to any agent that alters the biochemical or physiological processes of tissues or organisms. Hence a drug is a 'substance that is, or could be, listed in a pharmacopoeia'. In common usage, however, the Lexicon recognizes that 'drug' often refers specifically to psychoactive drugs, which are separately defined as 'substances that, when ingested, affect mental processes, i.e. cognition or affect'. 'Psychotropic drug' is used as an alternative and equivalent term for the whole class of substances, licit and illicit, with which drug policy is concerned. Both terms have the advantage of being descriptive and neutral.

Most of this book will, in fact, be concerned with psychoactive substances, their effects and the problems related to their use. However, nonpsychoactive substances may, on occasion, give rise to very similar problems. This is of theoretical, if not numerical, importance because it emphasizes the point that the drug-related problems with which this book deals, are not solely due to the particular properties of psychoactive drugs, but are also due to qualities of the individual concerned and of society. It is also worth noting that, nowadays, 'substance' (meaning psychoactive substance) is often used as synonymous with 'drug'.

What is drug misuse?

At first it seems easy to define misuse: 'To use or employ wrongly or improperly', according to the *Shorter Oxford English Dictionary*. However, when 'misuse' refers to drug misuse, definitions again become elusive. The term carries implications, according to the drug concerned, of social unacceptability, of illegality or of harmfulness. Sometimes it seems to mean that the drug is being used without medical approval, sometimes that it is being used excessively. Because of such ambiguities, and because the term suggests value judgements that say more about the attitudes of the observer than they do about the way in which the drug is taken, it is often avoided altogether. The term 'drug use' is substituted, qualified by an appropriate adjective, such as illegal drug use, unsanctioned use (when the use of a particular drug is not sanctioned by society or a group within society), hazardous use (probably leading to harmful consequences for the user), dysfunctional use (leading to impaired social or psychological functioning), non-medical drug use (not in accordance with recommended medical practice), etc. Obviously this format begs the question of what constitutes misuse, but it can give a more precise picture of the way in which a particular drug is taken.

The terms 'recreational' use and 'casual' use are comparative newcomers to the vocabulary and reflect new patterns of drug use and new attitudes towards this. Both imply the infrequent use of small amounts of drugs, which the user often claims carries little risk. The former acknowledges an hedonistic motive, with drugs being taken purely for their pleasurable effects; casual drug use emphasizes that use is occasional, rather than regular, and therefore offers a reassurance that the user is not dependent. However, as serious adverse effects may occur even with small doses, taken only occasionally, these terms may lull users into a false sense of security.

Drug abuse; harmful use

Drug abuse is an alternative phrase, although it too is often used imprecisely and is considered by many to be value laden. It has the advantage of an international (WHO) definition, utilized in the international conventions for drug control: 'Persistent or sporadic excessive use inconsistent with or unrelated to acceptable medical practice'.[1] This is an uncomfortable definition for those who smoke tobacco and for many of those who drink alcohol, forcing them to face up to the nature of their own drug-taking behaviour. It also emphasizes the close relationship between socially acceptable drug-taking behaviour and the range of drug-related problems with which this book is largely concerned.

More recently, the WHO Expert Committee on Drug Dependence introduced the term 'harmful use': a pattern of psychoactive drug use that causes damage to health, either mental or physical. The Committee also noted that the harmful use of a drug by an individual often has adverse effects on the drug user's family, the community and society in general.[3]

Drug dependence

The difficulties of defining the essential characteristics of drug dependence are illustrated by the changes that have taken place in the last 30 years. At one time, drug addiction and drug habituation were recognized as separate entities, with the former being more severe than the latter and distinguished on such grounds as the intensity of desire to take the drug, the tendency to increase the dose and the detrimental effect on the individual and/or society. Thus some drugs were described as habituating and others as addictive, and one individual might be considered addicted to a drug whereas another was merely habituated to the same drug. Such terms were impractical, particularly for international application and a new term, drug dependence, was introduced: 'a state, psychic and sometimes also physical, resulting from the interaction between a living organism and a drug, characterized by behavioural and other responses that always include a compulsion to take the drug on a continuous or periodic basis in order to experience psychic effects, and sometimes to avoid the discomfort of its absence. Tolerance may or may not be present'.[1]

Within this definition are two components of very different importance: psychological dependence, without which the state of dependence cannot be said to exist, and physical dependence which may or may not be present. Thus an individual may be dependent on a drug without manifesting any physical dependence and, conversely, an individual taking drugs that cause physical but not psychological dependence, is correctly described as physically dependent, but not as drug dependent.

However, in practice, physical and psychological dependence are often so closely linked that it can be difficult make the distinction. Therefore, in line with the approach adopted in The ICD-10 Classification of Mental and Behavioural Disorders[4] (see Chapter 5), the WHO's Expert Committee developed the following, more modern definition for drug dependence:

A cluster of physiological, behavioural and cognitive phenomena of variable intensity in which the use of a psychoactive drug (or drugs) takes on a high priority. The necessary descriptive characteristics are preoccupation with a desire to obtain and take the drug and persistent drug-taking behaviour. Determinants and the problematic consequences of drug dependence may be biological, psychological, or social, and usually interact.[3]

It can now be appreciated that drug abuse or harmful use may occur without causing physical or psychological dependence. LSD, for example, is a common and dangerous drug of abuse, but does not induce physical or psychological dependence; indeed the sporadic abuse of most drugs is not likely to cause dependence.

Psychological dependence

It will be perceived that at the core of the definition of drug dependence lies psychic or psychological dependence upon the drug. This is a 'feeling of satisfaction and a psychic drive that requires periodic or continuous administration of the drug to produce pleasure or to avoid discomfort'.[5] This precise but dry definition conveys nothing of what it is like to be severely psychologically dependent upon a drug. Eloquently described by those experiencing it as 'the drug calling to them' or as 'always a little geyser in there, hammering away at you to take it', the psychic drive to obtain and to take the drug is often dismissed by those who have not experienced it as a manifestation of 'weak will' or as evidence of a lack of motivation to stop. Nothing could be further from the truth; psychological dependence is an overriding compulsion to take the drug even in the certain knowledge that it is harmful and whatever the consequences of the method of obtaining it.

Craving and drug-seeking behaviour

Craving is a fundamental component of psychological dependence and implies a constant preoccupation with the drug with intrusive thoughts and obsessive thinking about everything to do with it – particularly its desired effects and the need to obtain it. This in turn may be translated into action in the form of drug-seeking behaviour which may involve literally searching for drugs, different activities, both legal and illegal, to obtain money to buy them, identifying the source of supply, purchasing, etc. When craving is severe, drug-seeking behaviour dominates daily activity.

Physical dependence and the withdrawal syndrome

Physical dependence is 'an adaptive state manifested by intense physical disturbances when the drug is withdrawn'.[5] Many, but not all drugs cause physical dependence and of those that do, not all are drugs of abuse. Chlorpromazine, for example, causes physical dependence but is not usually abused. The development of physical dependence depends on the drug being administered regularly, in sufficient dosage over a period of time; the necessary dose and duration of administration depend on the particular drug and may also vary from person to person.

In the condition of physical dependence, the body becomes so 'used' or accustomed or adapted to the drug that there is little, if any, evidence that the person concerned is taking it. However, sudden drug withdrawal is followed by a specific array of symptoms and signs collectively known as the withdrawal or abstinence syndrome. The nature of the withdrawal syndrome is characteristic of each drug type, and the symptoms and signs tend to be opposite in nature to the effects of the drug when it is acutely administered. Thus, physical dependence on a stimulant drug such as amphetamine is manifested by drowsiness, apathy and depression when drug administration ceases, whereas physical dependence on a sedative drug such as a barbiturate leads to a very different type of withdrawal syndrome with hallucinations and convulsions as evidence of stimulation in certain parts of the brain. However, as sudden drug withdrawal is intensely stressful for a physically dependent individual, all the body's responses to stress are called into play and the clinical picture becomes blurred by the activity of the autonomic (involuntary) nervous system.

Although partial symptomatic relief of some of the manifestations of the withdrawal syndrome is possible using a variety of measures, the condition can be treated effectively only by administration of the drug concerned, or one of similar type. Thus, the symptoms of the opiate withdrawal syndrome are relieved only by opiates, of the amphetamine withdrawal syndrome only by amphetamines and so on. Many of the common drugs of abuse cause physical dependence and it can be readily understood that the unpleasant nature of the withdrawal syndrome – or fear of it – can increase the intensity of drug-seeking behaviour because of the need to avoid or relieve withdrawal discomfort. Sometimes, the physiological changes may be of sufficient severity to require medical treatment.

Because physical dependence is sometimes confused with the more general term of drug dependence, the WHO Expert Committee decided to focus on the phenomenon of abstinence and to use the term 'withdrawal syndrome', which is described in terms of its consequences:

After the repeated administration of certain dependence-producing drugs, e.g. opioids, barbiturates and alcohol, abstinence can increase the intensity of drug-seeking behaviour because of the need to avoid or relieve withdrawal discomfort and/or produce physiological changes of sufficient severity to require medical treatment.[3]

The withdrawal syndromes associated with particular drug types are described in Chapter 3.

Tolerance

Tolerance is 'a reduction in the sensitivity to a drug following its repeated administration in which increased doses are required to produce the same magnitude of effect previously produced by a smaller dose'.[3] Many drugs, including some that are abused, induce tolerance, and therefore those who take them regularly can consume, without intoxication, far larger doses than can be tolerated by those without prior exposure. For tolerance to develop and to be maintained, the drug must be taken regularly and in sufficient dosage. If drug administration is interrupted for any reason, tolerance is lost and the high dose that was previously tolerated without adverse effect becomes as toxic as it is for the drug-naive individual. This situation arises not infrequently when a drug-dependent individual resumes drug taking after a period of abstinence – in hospital or in prison for example – and the high dose of drug that he or she had previously been taking regularly and safely may then have fatal consequences.

Tolerance does not necessarily develop equally or at the same rate to all the effects of a drug. For example, a very high degree of tolerance develops to the actions of opiates that cause analgesia, mental clouding and respiratory depression (slow and shallow breathing) so that these effects of opiates are not apparent even when the individual is consuming a very high daily dose – as long as that dose level has been reached gradually. However, little or no tolerance develops to the action of opiates on the pupil of the eye or on the bowel so that the same individual usually displays a typically constricted pupil and suffers from constipation.

Although tolerance to most of the effects of opiates is apparently open-ended (the dose can be gradually increased to any level), this is not true for all drugs. A barbiturate-tolerant individual, for example, can take a dose of barbiturate that would render a nontolerant individual comatose; there comes a point, however, when a further increase of dose will lead to severe toxicity or death even for someone who is barbiturate tolerant. In this case tolerance can be said to have reached a 'ceiling'. Tolerance is not completely drug specific. If an individual has become tolerant to the effects of heroin, for example, he or she can take large doses of any other opiate (but not of other classes of drugs). If heroin is withdrawn, the resulting abstinence syndrome can be relieved by the administration of any opiate (but not by any other type of drug). This phenomenon is known as cross-tolerance.

Mechanisms of tolerance

Tolerance can develop in different ways. Pharmacokinetic tolerance arises when changes in the metabolism or distribution of the drug following repeated administration affect its concentration in the blood and consequently its effect upon target cells. For example, tolerance to barbiturates is partly due to the induction (switching on) of special enzymes in the liver (hepatic microsomal enzymes) by the barbiturates themselves. These enzymes then metabolize (break down) the barbiturates, which can therefore be said to speed their own destruction. An increased dose is then needed to maintain the original effect.

Tolerance that is due to changes in specific receptors (see Chapter 2) is classified as psychodynamic tolerance. This reflects either a change in receptor density, or an altered response to neurotransmitters, or a change in the availability of the neurotransmitters themselves.

Tolerance can also be 'learned', that is, the individual learns to cope with the effects of the drug, so that they are less apparent. The most obvious example is the way in which an alcoholic learns to recognize the motor impairment associated with intoxication and how best to overcome it and disguise it by altered behaviour (e.g. walking or driving more slowly). This sort of learned behavioural tolerance only has limited effectiveness.[6]

Relationship between tolerance and physical dependence

The nature of the relationship between tolerance and physical dependence is not clear. Some of the drugs to which tolerance develops also cause physical dependence and the drugs of abuse and dependence with which this book is mostly concerned are in this group. For these drugs, physical dependence, with unpleasant symptoms on drug withdrawal leads to the need to take the drug regularly. This is, of course, a necessary condition for tolerance to develop, which in turn leads to escalating doses, greater physical dependence and so on. Because of this parallel development it has been suggested that a common mechanism is responsible for both phenomena. This hypothesis probably emerged because the drugs which have been studied the longest and most intensively are the opiates, drugs to which open-ended tolerance develops rapidly and on which physical dependence is severe and easily recognizable. Similarly tolerance develops to some of the effects of alcohol, barbiturates, benzodiazepines and other sedatives, and physical dependence on these drugs is again well known. From observations such as these grew the belief that tolerance and physical dependence are both manifestations of a single, as yet unknown neural mechanism. However, tolerance is a very general phenomenon, observed with many drugs. It is after all very common in medical practice to start with a small dose of a drug and to increase it gradually as the patient becomes tolerant of the side effects, and physical dependence does not develop in every situation in which tolerance develops.

Perhaps the best way to understand the relationship between tolerance and physical dependence is to say that the existence of tolerance, by permitting the administration of large doses of the drug, enables or enhances the development of severe physical dependence, if the drug has a dependence-producing liability as well. Undoubtedly, the two conditions, of tolerance and physical dependence, occur after chronic administration of a wide range of drugs (including tricyclic antidepressants, phenothiazines and anticholinergics) that are not self-administered by animals or usually abused by humans. This serves to emphasize the point that neither tolerance nor physical dependence, separately or together, are sufficient to cause a true state of dependence on a drug. For that, the psychological element, the inner compulsion, must always be present.[5]

Types of drug dependence

The definition of drug dependence used in this chapter is broad-based and embraces dependence on a very wide range of drugs, some of which are used medically (e.g. opiates, sedative hypnotics) while others (khat, hallucinogens, cannabis) are not. It is perhaps not surprising that the characteristics of the dependent state vary according to the type of drug. Some drugs cause marked physical dependence with a correspondingly severe withdrawal syndrome, others cause less physical dependence but profound psychological dependence. The extent to which tolerance develops also varies with different classes of drugs. Caffeine, consumed as it is by most people in tea or coffee, produces a limited degree of psychological dependence sometimes manifested as 'I can't get going in the morning without my cup of tea', and a mild state of physical dependence with headaches on drug withdrawal. This degree of dependence is not particularly harmful either to the individual or to society, although it should be noted that a more severe degree of dependence on caffeine (often in cola-type drinks) may sometimes arise.

However, several classes of dependence-producing drugs affect the central nervous system profoundly, producing stimulation or depression and disturbances in perception, mood, thinking, behaviour or motor function. The use of these

Table 1.1. Drugs recognized by the Tenth Revision of the International Classification of Diseases (ICD-10)

Alcohol

Opioids: including naturally occurring opiates (e.g. opium, morphine, codeine), synthetic or semisynthetic opiates (e.g. methadone, pethidine, dipipanone, dextromoramide) and opiate agonist-antagonists (e.g. pentazocine, buprenorphine)

Cannabinoids: preparations of *Cannabis sativa* (e.g. marijuana, ganja, hashish)

Sedative hypnotics: including barbiturates, nonbarbiturate sedatives (e.g. chloral, methaqualone, glutethimide, meprobamate) and benzodiazepines

Cocaine

Other stimulants: including amphetamines and similar stimulants (e.g. methylphenidate, phenmetrazine), anorectic agents (e.g. diethylpropion, phentermine), khat (preparations of *Catha edulis)* and hallucinogenic stimulants (e.g. MDMA (Ecstasy), MDA, MDE)

Hallucinogens: including LSD, mescaline, psilocybin

Tobacco

Volatile solvents: including substances such as toluene, acetone, carbon tetrachloride

Multiple drug use and other psychoactive substances

drugs may produce individual, public health and social problems and is, therefore, a justifiable cause for concern.

There is no wholly satisfactory way of classifying drugs of abuse and dependence because drugs with similar pharmacological effects may produce quite different types of dependence. Cannabis, for example, has both sedative and hallucinogenic effects but the pattern of its abuse, by millions of people world-wide, is quite different to the abuse of barbiturates or benzodiazepines which are sedatives, and LSD which is a hallucinogen.

The Tenth Revision of the International Classification of Diseases (ICD-10)[4] recognizes the psychoactive drugs or drug classes listed in Table 1.1, the self-administration of which may produce mental and behavioural disorders, including dependence (see Chapter 5).

Abuse and dependence on a wide range of other drugs also occurs. For example, abuse of minor analgesics, such as aspirin and compound analgesics, is so widespread that it has been estimated that there may be as many as a quarter of a million analgesic abusers in the UK alone. This problem is frequently ignored in studies of drug abuse and dependence, firstly because it involves drugs over which there are no legal controls (or only very limited ones) and which may be easily obtained from outlets such as newsagents, supermarkets and even slot-machines, as well as from pharmacists. Secondly, it is easy to dismiss it as uninformed self-medication by a group ignorant of the dangers of excessive use of these drugs. In many ways, however, those who abuse minor analgesics (and other drugs not included on the above list) resemble those who abuse illicit or restricted drugs: they often deny their drug-taking and may go to considerable lengths to conceal it; they often admit that they take the drugs for the feeling of well-being that they induce and, in the case of aspirin, specifically to experience the dangerous state of salicylism (aspirin intoxication) that they find pleasurable. Above all, they are psychologically dependent on these drugs: showing craving, drug-seeking behaviour and an inability to stop taking them.[7]

In addition to the drugs already discussed, there are many other drugs each of which is abused by few people who may then become dependent on them. Some, such as the antiparkinsonian anticholinergic drugs, may be taken for their psychic effects. Others, such as purgatives or anticoagulants may be taken to produce fictitious disease, those who abuse them often concealing this fact, and seeking and apparently enjoying repeated, intensive medical investigation and care. Finally, some drugs prescribed for somatic disease may be taken excessively, primarily to avoid unpleasant withdrawal symptoms although eventually a true dependent state may develop. For example, increasing doses of ergotamine, prescribed for migraine, may be consumed to avoid withdrawal headaches, and increasing doses of steroids may be taken to avoid unpleasant psychological effects on drug withdrawal. The family, friends and colleagues of doctors, as well as doctors themselves, may be vulnerable to this type of drug abuse if their powers of persuasion overcome normal professional prescribing practices.

These, much less common types of drug dependence have been introduced into the discussion because their existence illustrates and emphasizes a very important point: that abuse and dependence do not only occur with 'dangerous' psychoactive drugs. In other words, dependence is not just a manifestation of a specific drug effect, but is a behaviour profoundly influenced by the individual personality and the environment, as well as by the specific drugs that are available. As a behaviour, drug dependence is similar to compulsive gambling and compulsive eating, and what all have in common is an overwhelming psychic drive to behave in a certain way. A better understanding of this compulsion and of the nature of intrusive thought will enable us to reach out towards a better understanding of drug dependence and a whole range of similar human behaviours.

Causes of drug dependence

The cause or causes of drug dependence are not known. More specifically, it is not known why some people but not others in the same situation start experimenting with drugs, or why some, but not others, then continue to take them and, finally, why some but not all become dependent on drugs.

When seeking causes it is easy to limit the scenario to that of the local problems which receive so much publicity: poverty, unemployment, break-up of local communities, drug pushers, organized crime, breakdown of parental authority. These often-repeated phrases spring to mind and they may well be contributory factors, as far as the European and North American drug scene is involved, in the ever increasing number of people abusing or dependent on drugs – but they are not the causes of drug dependence.

It must never be forgotten that drug dependence is not a new phenomenon; the use of drugs is probably as old as man himself and dependence has been recognized for thousands of years. It occurs in every culture and any theory of drug dependence should be sufficiently general to encompass the vast range of dependent behaviour that exists today; for example, the young drug abuser, taking a wide range of drugs, the housewife dependent on benzodiazepines, the adolescent sniffing glue, the Middle Eastern opium smoker, a Jamaican cannabis smoker, the American free-basing cocaine, the Yemeni khat chewer, the mystic seeking truth with LSD, the doctor injecting himself with pethidine, to describe just a few. These many different scenarios of psychoactive drug consumption can be summarized in four categories which are not mutually exclusive: traditional/cultural, medical/therapeutic, social/recreational and occupational/functional. For example, drug consumption may start with a prescription for a diagnosed condition but may continue illegally; or stimulant drugs, taken initially to promote alertness when studying, may be continued purely for recreational purposes.

It is perhaps not surprising, therefore, that there are almost as many theories about dependence and its causes as there are types of dependence behaviour. While recognizing that very different situations may share hidden commonalities, it is fair to comment that many theories seem to say more about the viewpoint of the investigator than about the dependent state they attempt to describe, and as such they are not helpful in getting to grips with the phenomenon of drug dependence. Specifically, although many research studies explore features of personality, family history and environment that occur more or less frequently in those who abuse drugs than in those who do not, any such correlations do not necessarily indicate causality although a variety of models of drug dependence have been developed that do indeed explain correlative factors in a causal mechanism. Within a diversity of approaches and different models, three factors – the drug, the individual and society – interact to lead to a variety of drug-related behaviours; none of them alone is sufficient to cause drug dependence/abuse and their relative importance varies in different circumstances.

The drug

The availability of the drug is obviously a prerequisite for abuse and dependence, and the rapid transport methods of the modern world ensure that most drugs are obtainable everywhere. Transportation of drugs is not, of course, a recent occurrence – opium was moved halfway round the world centuries ago – but modern communications have greatly increased the speed and volume of this traffic. It is easy to be misled by reports in the media of vast quantities of illicit drugs coming into developed countries and to believe that the traffic is entirely one way. Going in the opposite direction, however, are equally vast quantities of alcohol and manufactured drugs which pose problems of their own to the countries that import them, and which are as vital to the economies of the exporting countries as the highly profitable cash crops of illicit drugs are to their producers.

In addition to the availability of a drug, the form in which it is available is very important. Modern chemical techniques permit the extraction of highly purified and very potent forms of drugs at source, making them easier to transport and smuggle, and because of their greater potency, much more efficient at causing dependence. For example, one can only conjecture how long it would take a South American Indian to chew sufficient coca leaves to obtain the same dose of cocaine as that in a single vial of 'crack', the purified version of cocaine currently in vogue in the USA and Europe; and it is unlikely that the Indian ever achieves blood levels (or nervous system levels) of cocaine sufficient to cause serious dependence. Again, this is nothing new: the ability to distil alcohol must have had equally dramatic effects when it was first discovered. Similarly, it can be understood that the invention and dispersal of the syringe and needle has had a profound effect upon drug abuse and dependence, by virtue of the ability to deliver large doses of dependence-producing drugs straight into the bloodstream and thence to the brain.

Although a few people become dependent upon apparently extraordinary drugs, such as laxatives, most drug dependence is concerned with just a few types of psychoactive substances. The question arises therefore as to how these drugs produce dependence. What is it that they have in common? It is immediately apparent that they have very different chemical and pharmacological properties and affect different parts of the central nervous system and different neurotransmitter systems within it. For example, cocaine and amphetamine are central nervous stimulants while opiates and sedative hypnotic drugs are depressants. Although the effects of cocaine and amphetamine are in some ways remarkably similar, there is no cross-tolerance so that the abstinence syndrome of one is not relieved by the other. Cocaine too has local anaesthetic properties, which amphetamine does not, but other local anaesthetic drugs do not cause dependence. Equally obvious pharmacological differences exist between the different classes of abused drugs, but the one factor that all drugs with a strong dependence potential share is a rewarding or reinforcing property. This is best demonstrated in a laboratory situation where an animal (usually a rat or a monkey) obtains a dose of a drug, such as cocaine, by pressing a lever. Thereafter the animal will press the lever repeatedly to obtain more cocaine and, as it receives more, will press the lever more and more rapidly. In other words, cocaine increases – or reinforces – behaviour resulting in its own administration, and is said to be a primary reinforcer and to have primary reinforcing properties.[8,9] Not all drugs possess this property; those that do and which are administered by animals in a laboratory situation are the same as those commonly abused by humans. They include stimulants (amphetamine, cocaine), opiates, sedative hypnotics, alcohol and some, but not all, hallucinogens (e.g. phencyclidine). Of these, cocaine and heroin stand out as the most powerful reinforcers, as defined by the rapidity of acquisition of self-administration.

It is not known why drugs with such different pharmacological properties should share the property of primary reinforcement, and the underlying neural mechanisms are not fully understood. They are, however, the subject of intense research, and it has been suggested that reinforcement works by centrally activating endogenous reward circuits which evolved, not for the sake of cocaine or opiates, but to reward behaviour such as obtaining food, water, warmth and shelter – all essential to survival. It has been found, for example, that stimulating particular sites in the brain via electrodes is positively reinforcing, particularly at the lateral hypothalamic level of the medial mid-brain bundle and in the ventral tegmentum. Several lines of evidence suggest that dopaminergic neural pathways within the brain are implicated within this ventral tegmental reward system, with the main site of action being the nucleus accumbens. Dependence-producing drugs, it is suggested, activate this reward system, 'switching on' the circuits at different points. Stimulants and cocaine, for example, lead to a functional increase in the levels of dopamine and other neurotransmitters within the nucleus accumbens, while opiates and alcohol increase the activity of cells in the ventral tegmental area.[10,11]

It seems, therefore, that psychological dependence, which is central to any concept of drug dependence, is the real-life manifestation of the reinforcing property of a drug, demonstrable by laboratory animals. Of course, there is a difference between a rat or monkey pressing a lever to get a dose of drug and an individual's overwhelming craving for it. There are, however, certain similarities between the two conditions: the monkey will press the lever thousands of times just to get a dose of a powerfully reinforcing drug and, given unlimited access to it, may stop eating food and drinking water altogether, and will increase its intake of drug to the point of starvation, dehydration, severe toxicity and death. There are obvious parallels with human drug-seeking behaviour so intense that it disrupts all normal activities and sometimes so self-destructive that the individual dies as a consequence.

It should therefore be understood that the reinforcing drug does not necessarily produce a pleasurable state and, if it does, it is not exclusively the pleasurable state that leads to drug-seeking behaviour. In other words, the monkey, or the human, is not just (if at all) taking the drug for enjoyment, but because it (or he or she) has to. Many drugs of abuse also cause physical dependence and the rigours of the abstinence syndrome, or fear of it, are another reason for continuing to take the drug. Although many opiate-dependent individuals claim that this is why they cannot stop taking opiates, it is not the only reason. Even if they are provided with sufficient opiate to prevent the onset of withdrawal symptoms, drug-seeking behaviour often persists – a manifestation of the powerful reinforcing properties of opiates.

Psychological dependence on a drug can therefore be presented as a direct effect of a drug; some drugs cause psychological dependence, some do not. If those that do are abused they are likely to cause dependence, the 'drive to take the drug on a continuous or periodic basis to experience psychic effects'. Some drugs of abuse, particularly cocaine and heroin, cause intense psychological dependence; others (e.g., cannabis) are much less potent in this respect.

The people who take drugs also vary tremendously in their response to drugs, from those who are very sensitive to a particular drug, requiring only a small dose to experience its effects, to those who require a large dose. This is true for all classes of drugs and is particularly apparent in the case of psychoactive substances where the suggested therapeutic dose range may be very wide. It does not seem surprising, therefore, that a drug that is known to cause psychological dependence may do so rapidly in some individuals and slowly or negligibly in others, and it is possible to reconcile apparently conflicting accounts of 'being hooked after the first dose' with stories of long-term, occasional, noncompulsive use of the same drug.

The individual

The underlying reason for such differing vulnerabilities is very interesting, or would be if it were understood. There have been many attempts to define the psychological characteristics of a dependence-prone personality and even to demonstrate that certain personality types develop substance-specific dependence, in other words, that alcoholics are a different 'type' from those dependent on heroin, who in turn are different from those dependent on cocaine.

Many studies have shown that there is indeed an increased incidence of personality disorder among drug addicts and that there is a higher incidence of drug abuse among those with personality disorder than in those without. Therefore, while it is fair to conclude that there is an epidemiological association between drug abuse and personality disorder, no deductions can be made about causality. Most studies have compared drug-dependent with nondependent individuals and it would be just as reasonable to conclude that prolonged drug-taking had affected the results of personality testing as to assume that personality disorder had caused the drug dependence. Thus, behaviour such as crime or prostitution, often perceived as maladaptive behaviour and an evidence of underlying personality disorder, may in fact be highly adaptive behaviour, carried out in an attempt to get money to support an ever-growing irresistible drug habit.

Another problem is that any one study usually concentrates on a particular, highly selected subgroup of drug-dependent subjects, such as those in prison or in hospital, who are probably unrepresentative of the drug-dependent population as a whole. In addition, institutionalization and other factors may affect the results of personality testing. Clearly, what is needed is knowledge of the personality before drug-taking started, but prospective personality testing, with a waiting period to see who later becomes a drug abuser, is very difficult to carry out. Retrospective personality assessment, by asking about early relationships, school records, truancy, employment, etc., before drug abuse started is notoriously difficult to assess and very unreliable.

Bearing all these limitations in mind, the conclusion of many investigators is that drug-dependent individuals have 'personality disorders' in excess of their prevalence in the general population, and the terms often used to describe them include 'immature', 'unable to delay gratification', 'difficulty forming stable relationships', 'low self-esteem and confidence', 'high anxiety', 'low assertiveness', 'impassivity', 'rebelliousness', 'tendency towards hypochondria' and so on.[12–14]

In psychoanalytic terms it has been suggested that psychoactive drugs, with their near-instant effect on the brain, attract those who cannot delay gratification and reward in the normal, adult fashion and who seek immediate, infantile gratification, thus avoiding the challenges of adulthood. In Freudian terms this represents 'deficient ego functioning' and this theory permits dependence to be seen as a character trait in some individuals who use drugs to protect themselves from life, in all its rawness, with which they cannot cope.

However, the notion that 'addicts' are, in some way 'weak' and unable to cope with life without the 'support' of drugs, is not borne out in practice. For example, a now classic study carried out in the 1960s in New York showed that heroin addicts successfully completed very challenging activities (obtaining money, procuring drugs, avoiding the police) on a daily basis. Indeed the researchers concluded that the addict, far from attempting to escape from life, was seeking to escape from the monotony of existence through an 'exacting, challenging, adventurous and rewarding' career, suggesting that this contributed, at least in part, to the continuation of addiction.[15]

Taking the psychoanalytic approach further, some researchers believe that the specific drug abused by an individual depends on 'the developmental state to which the user wishes to regress and that when an individual finds an agent that chemically facilitates his pre-existing mode of conflict solution, it becomes the drug of choice'.[16] Specifically, it has been suggested that individuals who respond passively to stress are more likely to become dependent on opioids because their effects reinforce withdrawal, while those who react actively will tend to use stimulants.[17] Such theories are difficult to reconcile with a modern, polydrug scene and it is also difficult to recognize a modern illegal opioid user as a passive and withdrawn individual.[15]

Those who abuse drugs undoubtedly do so for many different reasons both stated and unconscious. It is a behaviour that often starts in adolescence or young adulthood and there can be many contributory factors including curiosity and a range of social and personal reasons.[18] Disregard of conventional social expectations, personal independence and a corresponding willingness to participate in deviant activities have also been identified as characteristics of those exhibiting problem behaviour, including drug abuse. Although much emphasis is sometimes placed on peer pressure as a reason for drug abuse, it is worth noting that as more children do not take illicit drugs than do so, one would expect peer group pressure to be exerted against drug-taking, rather than for it. However, this may be confounded if the friends that form the peer group are selected on the basis of their drug-taking or related behaviour. Undoubtedly, peer networks can provide opportunities for drug use and support this behaviour.[19]

The importance of peer networks in an adolescent's life may of course reflect the support or lack of support that the child is receiving at home and the importance of the parent–child relationship as a protective factor against the use of drugs has been identified in several studies.[20,21] Factors such as family disruption, criminality and drug abuse of parents and siblings have all been identified as important predisposing factors for drug abuse later on, as have inadequate or ineffective parental supervision and enforcement of rules. However, it appears that a violent family environment is particularly associated with drug use behaviour in the children.[22] Family breakdown (divorce, separation) is less important, providing that the family environment is one in which problems are discussed and parents are interested in their children.

While satisfactory family relationships and climate, and emotional support to adolescents are influences that appear to delay or diminish initiation into drug use, they can only be developed over a long period of time and attempts to make up for their absence by measures such as a sharp increase in parental control of the adolescent's behaviour may lead to increased rather than diminished drug abuse. Within the family, parental use of drugs may also influence their children's drug-taking behaviour. However, it is difficult to disentangle the nature of this influence. For example, if parent and child both drink heavily, does the latter do so because of an inherited predisposition, or to relieve the stress of living with a heavy drinker, or as a copied behaviour; or is there an interplay of all three factors?

While acknowledging that curiosity about drugs may be an important factor in initiating drug abuse, it cannot account for the continued use of drugs over many years. Similarly, peer pressure to be part of a group with shared experience diminishes over time. Then, there tends to be a shift away from drug-taking as a social activity towards more solitary use and this may indicate the onset of a more dependent pattern of use, with the consumption of larger quantities of the drug and with attention being focused on its effects rather than the social experience.

Adolescent drug abuse is of particular importance not only because of the potential for drug-induced harm in a young person but also because taking drugs in childhood and adolescence is a strong predictor for drug use in adulthood. Such observations have led to theories about a 'gateway effect' or 'escalation hypothesis' which suggests that using one drug, such as cannabis, leads on to the consumption of more dangerous drugs and specifically those with a higher dependence liability. However, although most heroin users have previously taken cannabis, only a small proportion of those who use cannabis ever try opioids and the evidence for any gateway effect of cannabis is, at best, conflicting. However a number of longitudinal studies have shown that the early onset of smoking tobacco and drinking alcohol is associated with the later use of cannabis so that the risk of progression to cannabis and perhaps other drugs is greater among smokers and drinkers than in those who never smoked or drank alcohol.[23,24] There is also an almost four-fold increase in the likelihood of problems with cigarettes and a more than doubling of the odds of alcohol and marijuana problems when there has been early marijuana use.[25]

Other reasons for the initiation of drug abuse may be of greater importance at different ages and in different cultures. For example, the consumption of sedatives and tranquillizers by older people may begin as self-medication, or as treatment prescribed by a doctor for anxiety or insomnia. Drugs may be taken to overcome hunger or fatigue, to enhance sexual performance or for religious purposes, as an aid to meditation or to induce mystical states.

The reasons for continuing to use a drug may or may not be the same as those that led to its original consumption. If, for example, the anxiety-provoking situation that made tranquillizers necessary persists, it is not surprising if their use continues. If drug use which started out of curiosity leads to acceptance within an attractive peer group, it too is likely to continue. Again, if drug use produces feelings of ease and relaxation or provides escape from immediate problems, there is every reason to expect it to persist. It is obvious, therefore, that in addition to the primary reinforcing properties of the drug itself, nonpharmacological consequences may be rewarding and thus function as reinforcers too. In other words, repetitive and persistent drug-taking can be seen as a learned behaviour, and more specifically as an operant behaviour, established and maintained by its own consequences. For a drug that induces physical dependence, the instant relief of the symptoms of withdrawal brought about by drug administration is instantly rewarding and it can be argued that in this case drug-taking is under the control of aversive stimuli and is continued to avoid the unpleasant experience of the abstinence syndrome. Environmental stimuli associated with drug-taking may also assume importance in the maintenance of drug-taking behaviour. For intravenous drug abusers, for example, the syringe and needle may become secondary reinforcers because of their association with the rewards of the drug itself; measures aimed at the extinction of such secondary reinforcers may make a significant contribution to the treatment of drug dependence.

The importance of the individual personality interacting with the effect of the drug is emphasized and illustrated by two descriptions of somewhat different types of drug-taking behaviour. The first is the individual prescribed opiates for severe pain; if the prescriptions continue for some time, the patient becomes physically dependent on opiates and, were they to be suddenly stopped, the symptoms and signs of the withdrawal syndrome would be manifest. In practice, this rarely if ever occurs because the most common situation for prolonged prescription of opiates is in terminal disease and prescription continues until death. Usually, therefore, neither doctor nor patient is aware of the existence of physical dependence. It is interesting that tolerance does not always develop, or at any rate, not to the level that is common with recreational use, and continuing escalation of dose is rarely necessary to control pain. It is also puzzling that there is usually no evidence of psychological dependence either – no craving, or demands for drugs or for increasing doses, although this behaviour is common in 'recreational' opiate-dependent individuals even when they are receiving a regular prescription. These observations show that opiates, despite their powerful reinforcing properties, do not necessarily or always cause dependence. Psychological dependence does develop in some individuals treated with opiates, usually those being treated for chronic pain, often of indeterminate origin. Such patients are described as 'therapeutic addicts' and although they may be regarded as the innocent 'victims' of medical treatment, their behaviour is similar in many ways to that of the much more common nontherapeutic addicts.

The second example is of those who are dependent on 'unusual' drugs, which do not have primary reinforcing properties and which are not abused by animals in a laboratory situation. The personality of the people who do abuse them seems to be the 'cause' of the behaviour in this case, rather than any innate property of the drug.

It is, of course, of considerable interest to know whether individual factors contributing to drug dependence can be inherited. Most research has focused on alcohol abuse which, it has been noted, tends to 'run in families' and the question then arises as to whether this is due to 'nature' or 'nurture'. The finding in many studies is that alcoholism in the biological family predicts alcoholism in children reared away from home while the converse is not true. This suggests an inherited, and therefore genetic, basis for at least some types of alcoholism which is supported by the observation of a higher concordance rate for alcoholism in identical twins than in fraternal twins. Nevertheless, even among identical twins there is not 100% concordance, suggesting that more than one gene and/or environmental factors are also involved.[26] Biological research on the enzyme aldehyde dehydrogenase which metabolizes alcohol in the liver has demonstrated that some individuals possess it only as an inactive variant; consumption of alcohol then leads on to an accumulation of acetaldehyde and an unpleasant, toxic reaction 5–10 minutes after ingestion which discourages further consumption. There is a low incidence of alcoholism among this population, supporting genetic theories for the basis of alcoholism.[27] It must be remembered, however, that this is a quite specific example and cannot be extrapolated to a general theory on hereditary factors in drug dependence.

The discovery within the body of endogenous receptor systems for a number of psychoactive substances has revived interest in a link between drug dependency and genetic predisposition. It is possible, for example, that drug-dependent individuals have some sort of genetic weakness which is compensated for by the administration of specific drugs. It has also been suggested that there might be a neurochemical substrate for the observed personality differences in drug-dependent individuals and that this may be the basis of links with other types of compulsive behaviour, including gambling and eating disorders.[28] However, there is as yet little evidence to support such theories. A variation on this theme, similarly unproven, is that anhedonia – an inability to experience pleasure in the usual way, which is said to be associated with opiate addiction – could be related to a genetic disorder and thus predispose the affected individual to seeking drug-induced pleasure. Again, it has not been possible to establish whether anhedonia antedates dependence or is a consequence of it.[29]

Society

What then of society? What is the role of society in the triple interaction that leads to drug abuse behaviour? It is quite understandable that environmental factors should be blamed for drug abuse, particularly when its prevalence starts to rise sharply, and in Western urban society poverty and unemployment are the usual candidates for blame. They may indeed be relevant, although it must be remembered that not everyone in a particular environment – however deprived – abuses or becomes dependent on drugs. Equally, there are frequent stories which often receive even greater attention in the media, of abuse and dependence among the affluent, educated, employed, etc. Ultimately, of course, environmental factors such as these are local and inapplicable to general and global theories of drug abuse. Undoubtedly, however, society does play a significant role in the development and control of drug-abuse problems and there are various sociological theories of addiction, seeking to find causes in the way that individuals interact with society as a whole. However, no theory provides a satisfactory explanation for the wide range of addictive behaviours that exists. Instead, they tend to focus on causes of addiction in urban, deprived youth. The important theory of 'anomie',[30] for example, describes the goals of society and the prevailing culture, the norms to achieve the goals, and the 'institutionalized means' which is the distribution of opportunities available for achieving the goals. If there is marked disjunction between these factors, the resultant social strain can be dealt with in various ways. One way is to reject the goals and to 'retreat' from the inevitable conflict. Alternatively, goals such as status and influence may be achieved by illegal methods. According to this theory, drug use becomes a way of life in its own right, giving the user a sense of identity and a clearer role.

When considering such theories, it is worth remembering that psychoactive substances have been known and available to humans for thousands of years. For most of that time their use was geographically restricted and under societal constraints, and (with the exception of distilled alcohol) the drugs themselves were available only as crude plant products which contained only small quantities of the active drug.

Within the last few decades several changes have taken place simultaneously, which together have had a profound influence on drug-taking behaviour. Firstly, as already mentioned, highly potent psychoactive substances are widely available way beyond their societies of origin and therefore without the cultural traditions that might naturally restrict their use and abuse. In the case of manufactured psychoactive drugs, these are of such recent origin that cultural traditions controlling their use are as yet rudimentary or nonexistent. More important, however, than availability is a general attitude to drugs and drug-taking, an attitude which has become so widespread that it can probably be described as truly global. For example, in nearly all countries, two drugs – alcohol and tobacco – are recognized as legal, recreational drugs, and even though the former is prohibited in Islamic countries, few people would care to guarantee that it is not consumed there. Of course, there is nothing new about this situation, both alcohol and tobacco have been widely used for centuries, but what has been happening over those centuries is their gradual absorption into the fabric of society. They have become incorporated into every aspect of daily life: they are widely advertised, they are seen being consumed on films and television, they are present at sports events. The cost of an average 'habit' of these drugs forms part of the cost of living index. Revenue from their taxation is so enormous that few governments would care to do without it. They affect the employment of millions. Consumption of these two drugs is therefore, by any standard, perceived as 'normal' and ordinary.

More recently, over decades rather than centuries, many other psychoactive substances have been attaining a similar status. A vast number of psychoactive drugs are now manufactured for the treatment of psychiatric illness, and indeed they are so effective that many patients who would once have been confined to mental hospitals for life can now live within the community. Much of the fear of mental illness has been allayed and there is less stigma attached to it. It has become correspondingly easier for people to admit to symptoms of mental stress, knowing that effective and acceptable treatment is available. Often these symptoms are attributable not to illness, but to personal and interpersonal problems, and whereas they would once have been dealt with or suffered within the community, pharmacological solutions are now sought and provided. Gradually, these manufactured drugs are being incorporated into daily life, in the same way as tobacco and alcohol, although not yet to the same extent. Already, however, they are shared and borrowed like cigarettes ('can you lend me a sleeping pill?'); they are taken like alcohol, and sometimes together with alcohol, to achieve a relaxed mental state; they are mentioned casually in books and on television. Everyone by now knows what Valium and Prozac are. The pharmaceutical industry that manufactures them makes significant contributions to employment and the economy. Many of these drugs, like alcohol and tobacco, cause psychological dependence and the widespread abuse of many drugs in the form of drug overdoses, has, at times, appeared virtually endemic in some places.[31]

Thus we find ourselves in a society that is drug orientated to a degree previously unknown, at a time when very pure and potent forms of drugs, such as heroin and cocaine with a severe dependence liability, are widely available. When seen in this context, the illicit use of drugs by young people who have grown up surrounded by drug-taking behaviour – albeit legal drug taking – is perhaps an understandable, if undesirable behaviour. It is further reinforced by the influence of the peer group, which may be another important determinant among the young who are normally introduced to drug-taking by friends. Participating in this activity permits entry to a group and the drug-taking in turn reinforces the identity of the group, becoming a ritualized behaviour. Furthermore, as a drug becomes freely available and acceptable in society, those using it heavily and becoming dependent on it are less likely to show evidence of pre-existing personality disorders. These psychologically 'normal' individuals are often able to stop their drug use if their sociocultural environment alters, and the drug is no longer available and acceptable. In other words, the more normal drug-taking becomes, the more normal are the drug abusers.

Clearly it is a much smaller step into drug abuse and dependence now than it was when psychoactive drugs were medicines that were unfamiliar to the general population and taken, if at all, only for the treatment of specified illness. It is this total background acceptance of drug-taking behaviour that is the most significant change that has taken place in society in recent years and it has set the scene for new problems of abuse and dependence.

Drug dependence in the UK – and elsewhere

In the midst of current concern about drug-related problems and of endless dialogue about what should or should not be 'done' about them, it is interesting and valuable to consider the historical background to the present situation in the UK. Interesting because it increases our understanding about how present policies have evolved, and useful because of the possibility of learning from previous experience. This chapter considers the epidemiology of substance misuse in the UK and globally, and reviews the policies of countries that have adopted different approaches from the UK.

Drug dependence in the UK

It is perhaps surprising to learn that opium was widely used in Britain during most of the nineteenth century; so widely used, so ordinary that it aroused little interest or concern. It was available in a variety of patent medicines, obtainable from any sort of shop without any legal restriction, and crude opium was sold for eating or smoking.[1] The first attempts to restrict its sale were probably more for the sake of pharmacists trying to obtain a monopoly of this profitable trade, than because of concern about the effects of opiates. Medical interest in the topic became keener with the introduction of the hypodermic syringe and the concept of 'morphinomania' emerged. Despite an awareness of the addictive properties of opiates no prescription was necessary to obtain opium or its preparations. These could be purchased from a pharmacist by anyone known or personally introduced to the pharmacist, as long as the Poisons Register was signed.[2]

Growing international concern about opiate use led to the First Opium Convention in The Hague in 1912 and Britain, as one of the signatories, agreed to the principle of adopting controls over opium, morphine and cocaine. However, no legislation was passed until concern about the use of cocaine by members of the armed forces led to the Defence of the Realm Regulations (1916), which made it an offence to give or sell cocaine to soldiers. Subsequently the Regulations were changed so that only authorized people (members of the medical profession and those receiving a prescription) were allowed to be in possession of cocaine.

After the First World War, the 1920 and 1923 Dangerous Drugs Acts were passed and for the first time a doctor's prescription was necessary to obtain opium and its derivatives and cocaine. In the first year of operation there were only 67 prosecutions of which 58 were for cocaine, and in 1927 there were only two cocaine prosecutions out of a total of 60. Thus it was possible for Britain to say with pride – and some complacency – that drug addiction was not prevalent.[3]

The birth of the 'British system'

The problem then arose about whether the prescription of opiates to addicts constituted legitimate medical treatment. In the USA, for example, the 1914 Harrison Act had decided that it did not; the right of doctors to prescribe opiates was severely restricted and prescribing to regular users was illegal unless it was part of an attempt to cure (detoxify) the habit.

In the UK the Ministry of Health set up a committee to examine this question. The Rolleston Committee as it came to be known after its chairman, Sir Humphrey Rolleston, was composed of members of the medical profession anxious no doubt to safeguard their valued clinical freedom to prescribe whatever they thought fit for any patient for whom they considered it necessary. At the time that the committee was deliberating, many addicts, probably the majority, were either members of the medical or nursing professions ('professional' addicts), who had easy access to drugs, or those who had become addicted during the course of treatment with opiates ('therapeutic' addicts). There were also a few non-therapeutic addicts in London, obtaining their heroin largely by trips to the continent. In general these people were of 'good' social standing and did not form any sort of criminal network. It is not surprising that the equally respectable members of the Rolleston Committee did not perceive these addicts as criminals and thought that they should continue to be treated as patients. The report[4] therefore recommended that heroin could be prescribed to addicts if, after every effort had been made to cure them, complete withdrawal produced serious symptoms which could not be satisfactorily treated, or if the patient, while capable of leading a useful and normal life so long as he/she took the drug of addiction, ceased to be able to do so if it were withdrawn. In other words, maintenance – the legal supply of a daily dose of opiate to an opiate-dependent individual – was permitted.

With the Rolleston Report arose the so-called British system for dealing with addiction. A system was never planned or even visualized, but the idea that addicts were patients and not criminals and could receive drugs on prescription contrasted sharply with the situation in the USA. There, where opiate maintenance had been banned, drug addiction increased rapidly and was associated with major crime, while in the UK the drug scene remained small and stable. This was attributed, complacently, to the correctness of the British approach which was promoted into a 'system'.

From about 1950, however, it became apparent that there was an increasing interest in drugs by young people. This was shown by the sharply increasing number of prosecutions for cannabis offences. At first this largely involved West End jazz clubs in London and seamen, but it spread from different seaports to many parts of the country. At this time too, occurred the first serious cases of drug trafficking involving heroin, cocaine and morphine stolen from pharmacies.[3]

An awareness of the changing drug scene prompted the Ministry of Health to convene an Interdepartmental Committee on Drug Addiction, chaired by Sir Russell Brain. As a result of enquiries made in 1958–59, the Brain Committee came to the conclusion that the problem of addiction was static and that no special measures needed to be taken. This first report[5] was soon overtaken by events as the number of heroin addicts known to the Home Office began to increase rapidly, approximately doubling every 2 years, from 94 in 1960 to 175 in 1962 and to 342 in 1964.[3] At this time, it should be emphasized, there was no compulsory notification of addicts to the Home Office and statistics were compiled from an inspection of pharmacists' records and from doctors, police, prisons and hospitals.

An important cause of the increasing number of addicts identified in the early 1960s was overprescribing of heroin and cocaine by a few doctors who soon achieved notoriety and who provided surplus heroin for addicts to peddle on the black market. If it seems an exaggeration to claim that overprescribing could precipitate such a crisis, it should be noted that one doctor alone prescribed 600 000 tablets, equivalent to 6 kg of heroin, in the course of 1 year. Even today in a much larger drug scene a seizure of 6 kg of pure heroin would be regarded as a major haul. As a result of this situation, Canadian addicts came to Britain because of the ease with which they could obtain heroin here: as a group of experienced drug users with a large daily habit, they brought with them knowledge and experience of an organized black market and undoubtedly contributed to its organization in the UK.[6–8]

The Dangerous Drugs Act 1967

By 1964 it was apparent that the situation was worsening rapidly and the Brain Committee was hurriedly reconvened. Its second report,[9] published in 1965, formed the basis of the Dangerous Drugs Act of 1967. Its most important features were:

- Compulsory notification of addicts to the Home Office;
- The limitation of the right to prescribe heroin and cocaine to addicts to those doctors holding a special licence from the Home Office;
- The setting up of special clinics to treat drug addicts.

Central to the recommendations of the Brain Committee was the belief that the

British system of legal prescription of drugs to addicts had been responsible for the fairly low and static addiction figures between 1926 and 1960. Undercutting the legal supplier had apparently prevented the development of an organized criminal black market, whereas in the USA where drugs were not prescribed there was a highly organized black market and the prevalence of addiction had increased rapidly. The comfortable situation in Britain seemed to have changed only because of irresponsible prescribing by some doctors and it was believed that the resumption of 'sensible' prescribing policies would restore the status quo. To prevent this problem recurring only specially licensed doctors, usually working in the new treatment clinics, would be allowed to prescribe to addicts and the compulsory notification of addicts would permit ongoing monitoring of the situation.

In retrospect this interpretation of the rising addiction rate was an oversimplification. It is far more likely that between 1926 and 1960, because of the prevailing social conditions and the generally low availability of drugs, Britain had only a small addiction problem which could be satisfactorily managed by the policy of legal prescription. However, by the early 1960s social changes had accelerated and the demand for drugs grew and unscrupulous doctors took advantage of the liberal system to respond to this demand.

Home Office statistics show that the total number of known addicts increased rapidly between 1961 and 1967. The numbers taking morphine and pethidine, many of whom were therapeutic addicts, remained more or less static and the big increase was due almost entirely to an increased number of young nontherapeutic, recreational heroin and cocaine users.[10]

At the end of 1967 and during 1968, the new treatment clinics recommended by the 1967 Act started to open. They were faced with a large number of patients who could no longer obtain heroin and cocaine from general practitioners (GPs) who did not have the necessary licence to prescribe to them. The addicts, many of whom had drug habits too large to support on the black market, had no choice but to present to the clinics. This brought to light many who were previously unknown and this accounts for the increase in the number of known addicts from 1729 in 1967 to 2782 in 1968.[3] The overall total fell in 1969 to 2661, suggesting that the sharp increase was probably due to the introduction of statutory notification in July 1968 and this view is supported by the fact that the number of new addicts fell from 1476 in 1967, to 1030 in 1968 and to 711 in 1969.

Originally it was believed that somehow the clinics would prescribe just the 'right' amount of drug for each patient, sufficient to prevent them supplementing it from the black market, but with no surplus to sell. However, the initial response of the clinics, most of whose staff lacked experience, was very much an emergency response. Initially, prescriptions were often for the drug and dose that the patient had been receiving from their GP, and daily doses of heroin of 300–400 mg were not unusual; cocaine was also prescribed to some patients.

With growing experience, the requirements of individual patients were assessed more critically, the doses prescribed became smaller and the price of black market heroin rose sharply – a clear indication of its reduced availability. Heroin withdrawal was attempted by methadone substitution, a change that was strongly resisted by many patients who preferred heroin, and it was not uncommon for part of the maintenance dose of opiate to be prescribed as heroin and part as methadone. By the end of the 1960s new patients were presenting with primary methadone dependence, confirming the continuing diversion of prescribed drugs to the black market. This accelerated the trend away from prescribing injectable drugs which had, and still have, a high black market value, in favour of the less desirable oral preparation – in practice, oral methadone.

Polydrug abuse

The changes in opiate abuse and dependence that occurred during the 1960s did not occur in isolation, but were only a part, albeit a very important part, of the growing drug scene. The increasing interest of young people in cannabis has already been mentioned and this interest has persisted. Nowadays, although it is difficult to obtain accurate data about the prevalence of cannabis use, smoking cannabis seems to be commonplace behaviour with one study demonstrating that 30–40% of 15- to 16-year-olds have tried it.[11] Among university students it was found that about 60% had some experience of cannabis and 20% reported regular use (at least weekly).[12]

Lysergic acid diethylamide (LSD) also became popular, particularly during the 1960s, and especially among those interested in mysticism and exploration of the inner world. Its use was part of the hippie culture at that time and was much in evidence at pop music festivals. Since then it has become an integral part of the clubbing scene, involving large numbers of adolescents and young adults.

More important than the hallucinogens, however, was the explosion that took place in the use and abuse of prescribed psychoactive drugs. Since the 1950s more and more have been (and continue to be) synthesized and prescribed for symptoms such as anxiety, insomnia and depression – symptoms which everyone experiences at one time or another and which may be due to real psychiatric illness or to personal or interpersonal problems. These drugs contributed substantially to a pool (a lake?, an ocean?) of easily available psychoactive substances. The sheer scale of their increased availability in the 1970s may not be readily appreciated but in 1975, for example, it was estimated that there were 47 500 000 prescriptions for these psychotropic drugs in the UK, an increase of 8% over the previous 5 years.[13,14]

The disadvantages and side effects of some of the drugs became apparent only gradually. Many were found to have a dependence liability. Barbiturates, for example, were first introduced into clinical practice in 1903, but nearly 50 years elapsed before dependence on them was described. In the early 1960s, therefore, when about 50 000 000 prescriptions were being issued annually for barbiturate hypnotics,[14] it seems likely that there must have been a good number of people who had become dependent on their nightly drug. At that time, a 'typical' barbiturate-dependent individual was a middle-aged woman obtaining her drugs on prescription from her GP, probably with neither of them recognizing or acknowledging her dependence status.

Amphetamines, too, caused problems: first introduced for the treatment of asthma and as a nasal decongestant, they became popular by virtue of their stimulant and appetite-suppressant properties. Although amphetamine dependence had been identified as a problem in the late 1950s and its serious consequences had been described,[15] amphetamines still constituted about 2.5% of all prescriptions issued in the NHS in the 1960s.[14] Middle-aged women receiving amphetamine on prescription for the treatment of depression or obesity again formed a sizeable proportion of the dependent population. Since then other new drugs, both sedative (meprobamate, methaqualone, benzodiazepines, etc.) and stimulant (e.g. methylphenidate, phenmetrazine), have been introduced, often with confident claims that they lack the dependence-producing properties of their predecessors. The passage of time all too often revealed their abuse potential with reports of escalating dose, drug-seeking behaviour and characteristic withdrawal syndromes. These drugs have been widely prescribed as a medicopharmacological response to a variety of problems. Often this response involves more than one drug – one psychoactive drug for insomnia, another for symptoms of anxiety, and perhaps another for depressive symptoms, to give an extreme example. As the pool of psychoactive drugs increased, their use in incidents of self-poisoning increased too, a problem which became one of epidemic or even endemic proportions. In this form of drug abuse too it was possible to detect the trend towards multiple drug use.

At a time when many young people were becoming interested in drugs and their effects, this ever-growing pool of psychoactive substances did not remain untapped. Illicit drug-taking, using exactly these drugs, became very common and for many youngsters it was and is a convivial social activity and part of their general leisure behaviour. Drugs are taken like alcohol, purely for their psychic effects and indeed are often taken together with alcohol as a cheap way of becoming intoxicated. Polydrug abuse (i.e., the abuse of more than one drug at a time), in a search for heightened and different effects has become part of this recreational activity despite its risks. During the 1960s, for example, amphetamines became an important part of the multiple drugs scene, often being taken in conjunction with barbiturates. The majority of young abusers started their illicit use at weekends and this gradually spread through the week to counteract the withdrawal, depression and irritability induced by amphetamines. Such was the concern about the scale of abuse of amphetamines that there was a voluntary ban on its prescription by many doctors.

Those who abused or were dependent on opiates did not remain aloof from the more ordinary psychoactive drugs. For them multiple drug abuse was not a new phenomenon. Before the clinics opened, many heroin-using individuals had also used cocaine, often administering it in the same syringe to counteract the sedative effect of the opiate. When the right to prescribe cocaine to addicts was restricted, some doctors prescribed methylamphetamine as a substitute; an epidemic of methylamphetamine abuse was curtailed only when the drug was withdrawn from retail pharmacies.[16]

Following the establishment of the drug-dependence treatment clinics, it became apparent that multiple drug use by their patients was very common. The adoption by the clinics of a frugal prescribing policy prevented, or at any rate reduced, overspill to the black market which for a time suffered a shortage of heroin and cocaine. Their scarcity, coupled with the wealth of other psychoactive drugs available, contributed to the addicts' willingness to experiment. In particular, it became common in the 1970s for barbiturates and other drugs manufactured for oral use to be crushed and injected, a highly dangerous practice that can cause serious systemic and local complications. Indeed, a significant proportion of addicts known to the Home Office because they were dependent on a notifiable drug died not from this drug but from barbiturate abuse.[17] It should be emphasized, however, that it was not just opiate-dependent individuals who were involved in barbiturate and polydrug abuse – many young people abused a variety of drugs including opiates and barbiturates and became dependent on one or more of them.

Such were the problems caused by barbiturate abuse that there was a general trend towards prescribing newer and apparently safer sedative hypnotics instead. This trend was accelerated by the Campaign for the Use and Restriction of Barbiturates (CURB) and the number of prescriptions for barbiturates fell sharply. Their place in therapeutics was taken over by the benzodiazepines, which were widely prescribed for their anxiolytic and hypnotic properties. Once again, however, an apparently safe group of drugs was found to have dependence and abuse potential and again, like the barbiturates before them, it took years for the significance of this observation to be fully appreciated.

The Misuse of Drugs Act 1971, was the response to the increasingly complex and rapidly changing drug scene. It replaced earlier legislation and provided a more rational and comprehensive framework for all aspects of drug control. It is discussed in more detail in Chapter 12.

The 1980s

Initial complacency that problems of opiate dependence had been satisfactorily dealt with by setting up the clinics was soon threatened by the new complexity of drug-abuse problems. The clinics became increasingly irrelevant to the totality of drug abuse in the whole community, offering treatment only to those dependent on opiates while excluding those not physically dependent on opiates but who were still abusing the same range of drugs. However, the clinics set up to deal with opiate (and cocaine) dependence were overstretched and did not have sufficient resources to deal with a huge number of other drug problems. An unforeseen difficulty was that instead of the majority of patients being rapidly withdrawn from opiates as originally envisaged, many remained on long-term oral methadone maintenance and often continued to attend the clinics for years. Long waiting lists developed at some clinics and some drug abusers preferred to approach, often privately, nonclinic doctors. As these doctors were not licensed to prescribe heroin, they often prescribed other opiates such as dipipanone or dextromoramide, and stimulants such as methylphenidate.

Although manufactured for oral use, dipipanone and dextromoramide tablets were crushed and injected in a search for heightened effect and some were sold on the black market. This was reflected in an increasing number of cases of primary dependence on them and by the early 1980s the situation was reminiscent of the mid-1960s, before the clinics opened. For this reason, the prescription of dipipanone, which was causing the most problems, was made subject to the same restrictions as heroin and cocaine. Following the introduction of stricter controls, the number of deaths involving dipipanone fell from 93 in 1982 to 13 in 1986.[10]

There were calls to extend the licensing restrictions to more drugs, but the relative importance of prescribed opiates in causing dependence declined in the face of a flood of illicit heroin, often of a high degree of purity, reaching the UK from different parts of the world – South-East Asia, the Middle East and the Indian Subcontinent. Its price on the black market became as low, relatively, as it had been in the 1960s, reflecting its easy availability.[18,19] Instead of injecting, it became common for it to be taken by 'chasing the dragon': a small amount is heated in a spoon or on a piece of foil and the resultant fumes are inhaled. This method attracts many who dislike, at least at first, the idea of injecting themselves and who believe that inhaling heroin is somehow less addictive. Perhaps for this reason, the number of heroin-dependent individuals increased very rapidly and inevitably a proportion of them became injectors, with all the attendant hazards. This, coupled with the increased abuse of cocaine and fears of large-scale importation of 'crack' (a very pure and potent form of cocaine), again concentrated attention on the 'traditional' drugs of dependence, heroin and cocaine. Anxiety was exacerbated because, historically, both heroin and cocaine had been drugs that were frequently injected. In the face of the impending AIDS (acquired immune deficiency syn-drome) epidemic, the existence of a large population of drug injectors, who habitually share syringes and needles, raised the spectre of AIDS being transmitted into the general population by drug abusers. These fears diverted public attention away from the more mundane problems of abuse of prescribed psychoactive drugs. Nevertheless, they remained a constant backdrop to the changing drug scene and important because of the millions of people who had become inadver-tently dependent during the course of treatment.

The fear of an AIDS epidemic had other consequences too. Specialists in public health medicine took the lead in initiating action to prevent it and, in an environment of near-panic and with very little knowledge about addictions and their treatment, introduced new measures which, almost without exception, focused on the communicable disease component of the problem and ignored their consequences for the treatment of addictions. Thus the emphasis on 'harm reduction' (see Chapter 7) for the apparent sake of public health, undermined the effective treatment of individual addicts and often became an end in itself.

Faced with an escalating problem and inadequate treatment facilities, a different approach had to be developed and a report from the Advisory Council on the Misuse of Drugs, *Treatment and Rehabilitation*, was published in 1982,[20] recom-mending a new framework for services, with an emphasis on Community Drug Teams (CDTs), based in each health authority (see below). District Drug Advisory Committees were also established in each health authority, involving representa-tion from CDTs, voluntary organizations, social services, probation service, police, pharmacies, general practice and specialist treatment services. This multi-disciplinary, multiprofessional group monitored problem drug misuse in the local patch, sharing intelligence and working together to improve services and develop future strategies.

At the same time, more funding was made available to tackle what was now perceived as a serious problem. Because no one knew or could decide on the best approach, small amounts of short-term funding were given to a large number of new initiatives in both the statutory and voluntary sectors with the specific aim of encouraging a diversity of services. However, the consequent proliferation of different services, often run on a shoe-string from year to year, led to fragmenta-tion and made it difficult for patients/families/carers to find their way round the system. Increasingly there was an emphasis on harm reduction, with easier access to methadone replacement therapy and syringe exchange schemes.

The new scale of the problem made it increasingly apparent that substance misuse could no longer be left only to specialist services and that *all* doctors would need to know how to respond. 'Guidelines on Good Clinical Practice' were therefore issued by the Department of Health[21] and have since been revised.[22] They make it clear that 'Every doctor should address the general health needs of his patients who misuse drugs, including straightforward treatments for drug dependence such as methadone withdrawal from opioids'.

The 1990s

The last decade of the century saw the development of a national strategy: 'Tackling Drugs Together: a Strategy for England 1995–8'[23] with a firm commitment to law enforcement, accessible treatment and effective education and prevention. Under the new strategy, the local and Regional Drug Advisory Committees disappeared, to be replaced by Drug Action Teams and Drug Reference Groups. The former includes the heads of key local services such as the health authority, local authority, social services, education, police, probation and prisons, while the Reference Group is made up of local people with relevant expertise who can advise the Drug Action Team.

In the 1980s and 1990s, a few high-level intergovernmental conferences were convened as the problems of drug abuse and trafficking became more pronounced and needed action. The international response to the problem of drug abuse during the 1990s put greater emphasis on demand reduction and correspondingly a more comprehensive response to the situation was developed in the UK. This included treatment services in prisons, arrest referral schemes, Drug Testing and Treatment Orders (DTTO) and a recommendation for special drug courts, similar to those in the USA.

Following the appointment in 1998 of the first Anti-Drugs Coordinator in the UK, modelled on the Drug Czar in the USA, a further drug strategy was published: 'Tackling Drugs Together to Build a Better Britain: the Government's ten year strategy for tackling drug misuse'.[24] This reiterated the key objectives of the earlier strategy:

- To help young people resist drug misuse in order to achieve their full potential in society;
- To protect communities from drug-related antisocial and criminal behaviour;
- To enable people with drug problems to overcome them and live healthy, crime-free lives;
- To stifle the availability of drugs on the street.

By including all potential areas of prevention and intervention: health, law enforcement, education, social services, voluntary services, the strategy ensured the active involvement of many different government departments. Gone are the days when substance misuse was managed only as a health issue. In the more recent reorganization, the Central National Coordinating Office has been moved to the Home Office and a National Treatment Agency has been established to enhance treatment.

The Clinical Guidelines have also been updated[22] and, in line with the modern approach towards care pathways, clarifies the level of care that is expected of generalists and specialists. In addition, in an ambitious approach to performance monitoring, there are now clear targets for improvement, such as reducing the number of people under the age of 25 years who use heroin and crack cocaine by 25% over 5 years; increasing the number in treatment by 66% and so on. However, at this stage it is not clear how performance in such a complex area can be accurately monitored, particularly because the Home Office's Addicts Index has been discontinued and the Regional Substance Misuse Databases which replaced it contain only anonymized data.

Guidelines for the clinical management of substance misuse detainees in police custody were developed in 1994[25] and revised in 2000[26] (see Chapter 9).

Drug policy in other countries

Despite the changes outlined above, drug policy in the UK has remained firmly based on principles of prevention and treatment and the associated legal framework has similarly remained largely unchanged with pressure for legalization or 'decriminalization' firmly resisted, at least until now. Since the advent of human immunodeficiency virus (HIV)/AIDS, harm reduction has been practised within this framework. Elsewhere in the world, quite different approaches have been adopted and it is important to note that, although parties to the United Nations Conventions on Narcotic Drugs (1961), Psychotropic Drugs (1971) and Illicit Trafficking (1988) (see Chapter 12) are required to meet certain broad obligations, there is considerable scope for difference in how they do so, particularly in relation to how possession offences are managed. For example, the possession of drugs for personal use is an administrative issue in Italy and Spain and in the Netherlands no action is taken against the possession of small quantities of cannabis or even the sale of small quantities from 'coffee shops' (see below). In contrast the UK is unique in the way that it classifies drugs according to their relative harmfulness and then links the penalties for possession and sale to this classification (see Chapter 12). Despite these different approaches to possession, it appears that, within western Europe, there is a convergence in legislation against trafficking. An overview of some other countries' practices is given below.

The Netherlands

In the Netherlands, the primary focus has been on harm reduction and, in pursuit of this principle, the government decided to control drug markets according to the perceived risk of different drugs. The risks associated with cannabis use, for example, are perceived as socially acceptable and therefore an attempt has been made to separate the cannabis market from those of the more dangerous cocaine and heroin. Because the Netherlands is a signatory of the International Conventions, cannabis trafficking remains illegal but is not a priority for law enforcement agencies, which concentrate instead on cocaine and heroin. Under this system, a network of 'coffee houses' was permitted that could sell cannabis, albeit in small amounts ($<30\,g$), to those aged 16 years and over, and was regulated, inasmuch as no cocaine or heroin was allowed on the premises. However, neighbouring European countries complained of an increase in 'drug tourism' and there was an increase in the domestic consumption of cannabis. This, together with fears about organized crime using this relaxed approach to hide trafficking in more dangerous drugs, led to the reintroduction of stricter controls. The number of 'coffee shops' has been reduced by 50% and sales are limited to 5 g. Furthermore, they are not allowed to advertise, to sell to minors, to sell 'hard' drugs or to be a nuisance in their neighbourhoods. Finally, it should be noted that, as part of the approach to 'normalizing' drug problems, there is also an extensive programme of methadone maintenance and drug users are helped to re-establish themselves within 'normal' society. Dealing in more dangerous drugs is not tolerated and lengthy prison sentences can be imposed.

United States of America

The USA is always cited as an example of a country that tried total prohibition as an approach to substance misuse – and then abandoned it! This was, of course, in the 1920s and early 1930s when the manufacture, sale or transportation of 'intoxicating liquors' was banned as well as their importation or exportation (rather than possession or consumption per se). During the 14-year period of prohibition, alcohol consumption fell (by one third to a half) but did not cease and there was a corresponding reduction in the incidence of cirrhosis of the liver in men. However, organized crime, corruption and violence increased and there was a high incidence of morbidity and mortality related to the consumption of domestically produced spirits and industrial alcohol. It is difficult to draw conclusions from these findings that are applicable to illicit substance misuse in the twenty-first century but both those who are in favour of 'decriminalization' of drugs that are currently illicit, and those who are against it, cite American experience in relation to the prohibition of alcohol in support of their position.

In contrast to previous attitudes towards alcohol, there is now ongoing controversy in the USA about the decriminalization of cannabis with 11 states adopting this course of action in 1970, making it a civil offence punishable by a fine. Most of these states did not report increased consumption in comparison with states that did not decriminalize – although the findings were perhaps obscured by a generally more relaxed attitude towards enforcement. However, in Alaska 12- to

17-year-olds were found to be smoking at twice the national average after de-criminalization, highlighting the way in which local factors can influence the outcome of legislation.[27]

Generally, however, at federal level and in spite of moves towards decriminaliz-ation in some parts of the country, the USA has maintained an uncompromising stance against substance misuse, and continues to refer to the 'war' against drugs with a strong emphasis on law enforcement. The importance of treatment, including the prescription of opioids to dependent individuals, is also acknowl-edged.

A comprehensive and long-term drug strategy ranging from effective law enforcement to prevention, treatment and education is in place. The USA expends huge resources combating drug trafficking and abuse, spending more than any other nation on various aspects of addictions including treatment and education. Over the last couple of decades policies on drug issues have been high on the agenda with a great deal of interest on the part of the public, government and politicians. A large amount continues to be spent on research in this field.

Switzerland

In contrast to the USA, Switzerland, for the last two decades, has tried out new and radical approaches to substance misuse. Liberal and relaxed responses to open cannabis dealing in particular parts of Zurich was followed by an influx of heroin dealers and a rapid spread of HIV/AIDS infection. This prompted the designation of Platzspitz as a 'needle park' where a range of voluntary and statutory agencies provided medical and social services to those who were substance dependent. Far from containing the problem within one defined area, it started increasing, as more and more users moved in to benefit from the easily available drugs and other services – a situation reminiscent of that pertaining in the UK in the 1960s. Health and social problems increased, as did crime rates, leading to the introduction of a range of harm reduction measures including low-threshold methadone and the distribution of free syringes, which did lead to a reduction in the rate of HIV infection. Eventually, however, the rate of violent crime and drug overdoses became so high that the park was closed, and other services were substituted, not just in one place, but more widely throughout Zurich. Unfortunately, the open drug scene did not disappear but transferred elsewhere, where the recurrence of unacceptable levels of antisocial behaviour led to stricter law enforcement and the closure of this area too. These stricter policies, which aim to reduce the public nuisance component of substance misuse, have been combined with some very radical approaches to harm reduction including the distribution of injectable opiates (heroin, morphine and injectable methadone) to addicts, under medical supervision, up to three times a day. These drugs are often prescribed in very large doses, sometimes in combination, as happened in the UK and Sweden in the 1960s. The whole experiment is being evaluated by an expert group convened by the World Health Organization. The Swiss Government has also provided special 'shooting galleries' where known drug-dependent individuals may go to self-inject although, strictly speaking, such provision may contravene International Drug Control Conventions.

Germany

Liberal approaches akin to those described for the Netherlands and Switzerland have also been adopted in Germany where offences involving the possession, purchase and sale of small quantities of cannabis are not prosecuted in the courts, even though they remain illegal. However, the different states in Germany have adopted very different margins for the personal use of cannabis which vary from 6 g to 30 g. Some German towns also provide 'shooting galleries' and there is a sizeable body of opinion in favour of the decriminalization of cannabis.

Sweden

Sweden has had a consistent drug policy for many years. Possession of heroin or cocaine even in very small quantities is punishable by law and drug legislation is strictly adhered to. There are comprehensive treatment and rehabilitation services in place. Harm reduction and syringe exchange schemes are considered to convey an ambiguous message and although some methadone-assisted rehabilitation programmes exist, their extent is more limited than in other European programmes and generally drug policies are not liberal.

Australia

The Australian approach to the management of substance abuse is similar to that adopted in many European countries, with the overall objective of the National Drug Strategy being to minimize the harmful effects of drugs. Treatment provision is comprehensive and various 'harm reduction' activities are advocated. The Government evaluates drug policy at regular intervals and the possession and use of small amounts of cannabis has been decriminalized in some territories.

Pakistan

Various activities relating to demand reduction attained more importance during the 1990s and a few hundred treatment centres have been established throughout the country in response to the growing problem of heroin injection.

Like other Asian countries, drug laws are strict and are rigorously enforced. At the same time, prevention, treatment and rehabilitation activities have been enhanced in recent years. The use of traditional herbal medicines for the treatment of drug dependence continues.

Around the world, the range of treatment services offered to drug abusers is varied and extensive. Self-referral and voluntary treatment is common in Africa whereas compulsory treatment is more common in Malaysia, Japan and Bangladesh. Buddhist temples in Thailand and elsewhere have developed their own model of treatment involving herbal medicines and religious ceremonies. The Russian Federation and some other CIS states have large hospital-based residential treatment services. Scandinavian countries, China and Sri Lanka have both compulsory and voluntary components to their treatment services. Many countries have provision based within the criminal justice system to provide the option of treatment rather than a custodial sentence.

Organization of treatment services in the UK

Primary health care

Individuals resident in the UK are entitled to free medical care under the National Health Service (NHS). Most register with a local GP, the primary health care physician, whom they consult free of charge whenever they wish. The GP maintains a record of such consultations and of the treatment that is prescribed and, if necessary, may refer the patient for a specialist opinion. Reports from specialists together with results of laboratory investigations are retained by the GP who thus maintains a comprehensive record of the patient's health and treatment status. This record is passed on if the patient transfers to the care of another GP, for example, on moving house.

A drug-related problem, such as drug dependence, is therefore just one among a huge range of problems for which the GP may be consulted. In practice, some GPs do not 'like' drug-dependent individuals and may refuse to accept them as patients; in other cases a GP may refuse to see a particular patient who has been especially troublesome in the past. In this situation a patient may apply to the local Health Authority who will then allocate the patient to a GP.

The management of a patient with a drug-related problem lies with the GP. Usually, patients with serious problems are referred to a specialized Drug Dependence Treatment Unit (DDTU). However, the explosion of drug-related problems in recent years, involving opiates as well as a wide range of psychotropic drugs, has led to a realization that GPs should become more involved in the management of these patients. There have been considerable efforts to offer additional training to interested GPs and attempts are being made on the part of the specialized treatment centres to reach out into the community and to work from local venues in conjunction with GPs. It is hoped in this way to be able to offer a prompter and more appropriate response to more patients presenting with drug-related problems so that an opportunity for intervention while the patient is motivated is not lost. This involvement by specialist drug workers in primary-care settings has the advantage that GPs who are supported in this way feel more confident about managing complex cases themselves and, with greater experience, gain in knowledge and skill.[28–30] It is hoped that this approach will be enhanced by the recent formation of Primary Care Trusts (PCTs) which bring groups of GPs together to work in a more coordinated way to improve the health of the local community.

Some patients prefer to consult a medical practitioner privately, paying for the consultation and the full cost of any prescribed drugs. Drug-dependent individuals sometimes do this to obtain larger supplies of the drug(s) of dependence and may then sell some of it to finance the cost of the consultation and prescription. It is also not unknown for such patients to attend and/or register with more than one GP, perhaps using an alias in an attempt to obtain several prescriptions. It is in fact an offence to make a false statement to obtain a prescription, or to obtain a prescription for controlled drugs from one doctor without disclosing that another doctor has also prescribed controlled drugs for the same patient.

Drug Dependence Treatment Units (DDTUs)

The DDTUs were set up in 1967 to deal with the growing problem of heroin (and cocaine) abuse. At that time most clinics were in or near London usually in or attached to a general hospital, but as the drug-abuse problem has grown numerically and spread geographically, other clinics have opened. In its 1982 report on Treatment and Rehabilitation,[20] the Advisory Council on the Misuse of Drugs recommended that each of the Regional Health Authorities should establish a multidisciplinary Regional Drug Problem Team, with an identifiable base, usually a designated treatment clinic or another existing specialist service. This would ensure a geographical spread of specialist services within the UK. If a specialized unit is not available, a general psychiatrist may take responsibility for patients with drug-related problems, either because of personal interest in this area or in response to the pressure of referrals.

DDTUs are multidisciplinary units under the overall charge of the consultant psychiatrist, who is usually licensed by the Home Office to prescribe heroin and cocaine to addicts if this is appropriate. The number and disciplines of supporting staff, which may include junior doctors, nurses, social workers, clinical psychologists and clerical administrative staff, vary from clinic to clinic and this may significantly affect the orientation of the clinic.

As it is usually the nurse who has first contact with prospective patients it is his or her responsibility to adequately engage them in assessment and treatment. The nurse is also responsible for maintaining a high standard of clinical nursing care and, in particular, for preventing the spread of infection between patients and from patient to staff.

The social worker assesses the patients' social functioning, social networks (including family involvement) and accommodation. He or she can offer help with social problems, such as housing, welfare rights and financial difficulties, and can liaise with outside agencies, such as the probation service, with which the patient may have been in contact. The social worker may work with the family of a patient and also has a statutory responsibility for the interests and safety of the children of drug-abusing parents. He or she has a particular role in advising and supporting patients who are considering undertaking a period of residential rehabilitation following drug withdrawal.

The psychologist uses an established repertoire of techniques from cognitive/behavioural and other branches of psychology, either as the sole form of treatment or in conjunction with other interventions, to meet identified treatment or management goals. For example, relaxation training, anxiety and anger management, desensitization, social skill training and cognitive restructuring are some of the special techniques available to psychologists in the treatment of drug-related and other problems. Similarly psychologists working in collaboration with community and voluntary agencies can deploy psychological processes to facilitate rehabilitation.

Patients referred to a DDTU will be assessed by different members of the multidisciplinary team. Findings and opinions are shared at a team meeting and a management plan is worked out. Although individual team members may each have a case load of patients for whom they are specially responsible, all patients are under the care of the consultant psychiatrist in charge of the unit, and only the medical staff can prescribe medication for the patients. Although they may be licensed to prescribe heroin and cocaine to those dependent upon them, cocaine prescription has virtually ceased, and heroin is prescribed less often than before, and rarely to new patients.

Patients may be referred to the local clinic by their GP or another doctor, or by a social worker, probation officer or other agency. Some drug-dependent individuals refer themselves, often because a fellow addict is or has been a patient, although some units insist on a formal referral letter from another doctor.

Because the specialist units were initially set up to deal with opiate (and cocaine) abuse, this has always been their primary responsibility. Permanently understaffed and under-resourced they have, in the past, been unwilling and unable to deal with other types of drug abuse and dependence. However, the modern trend towards viewing substance abuse as a whole, rather than in terms of individual drugs, is bringing about changes in the role of the specialist units and their policies. Many units will now see patients with other drug-abuse problems, such as solvent sniffing or sedative hypnotic dependence, if the GP feels that these patients have particular problems that require specialist intervention. These sessions are usually separate from those attended by opiate-dependent individuals. This, coupled with a strategy of greater community involvement will, it is hoped, enable the DDTUs to be perceived as a more ordinary place to seek help for all types of drug-related problems, rather than as the 'end of the road' for long-term opiate-dependent individuals.

Community Drug Teams (CDTs)

The changing nature of substance dependence in the UK, and in particular the ever-growing number of people who misuse drugs and the problems that have developed in relation to AIDS, have led to changes in the way that services are provided for these individuals. While the importance of hospital-based, specialist DDTUs is undisputed, there is also an acknowledged need for Community Drug Teams (CDTs) which have now been established in many areas.

Although the structure and activities of different CDTs may vary, they are usually multidisciplinary with input from a variety of professionals, such as psychologist, nurse, social worker, etc. Their purpose is to extend the specialist expertise of the hospital-based unit into the community so that more patients can benefit from this expertise, and to improve the quality of care by broadening the range of available treatment options and enabling patients to be seen in the setting most appropriate to their particular circumstances. To achieve this, CDTs may participate in a number of different and complementary activities:

- Providing a telephone advisory service to encourage those who may not other-wise approach any agency for help, to make contact through a confidential and anonymous service;
- Providing clinical services in community-based settings thereby engaging those individuals who, for one reason or another, do not wish to attend hospital, or for whom treatment in the community may be a more appropriate intervention;
- Increasing services for drug misusers by providing training for other professional groups who can then offer more appropriate support for their clients who are misusing drugs;
- Monitoring the extent and nature of drug misuse in the local area and evaluating existing services;
- Preparing and maintaining a directory of local services for drug misusers for them and their families and also for all workers involved with this client group, so that, when onward referral is necessary, it is appropriate to the needs of the individual concerned.

In-patient units

In-patient facilities specifically for the treatment of drug dependence are very limited, although when the clinics opened it was envisaged that in-patient care would be an important component of treatment. It was hoped that regular attendance at the out-patient clinic would lead to a therapeutic relationship between the clinic staff and the patient, who would then feel able to accept in-patient detoxification and long-term rehabilitation. In practice, in-patient units have not played a numerically important role in the management of drug dependence although it is not clear if this is due to reluctance on the part of the patients, the availability and quality of facilities, or a belief on the part of doctors that out-patient withdrawal is preferable.

Because most DDTUs do not have their own in-patient unit, those that do have this facility extend its use to patients from other areas. In-patient care may therefore necessitate patients being treated in a hospital at some distance from home and by staff whom they do not know. This is more helpful if effective arrangements for after-care are made prior to admission, because a brief period of in-patient treatment on its own is unlikely to bring about lasting change in long-term problems such as drug dependence.

Patients may be admitted to hospital for assessment of a drug-abuse problem, for stabilization of the dose of their drugs, for detoxification, for treatment of the complications of drug abuse, or for a general sorting out of the chaos brought about by their lifestyle. They may remain in hospital for weeks to months for rehabilitation which may be on or off drugs.

Rehabilitation and after-care

Drug withdrawal is only the first phase of a treatment programme, which must be completed by a much longer-term response known as rehabilitation: the process of integrating the drug abuser into society so that he/she can cope without drugs and can be restored to the best possible level of functioning. Sometimes, however, it has to be accepted that an individual cannot cope without drugs and rehabilitation has to take place in the context of continuing, although controlled, drug use.

In the UK 'treatment', usually meaning drug withdrawal, is the responsibility of the NHS while rehabilitation is the statutory responsibility of social service departments. This administrative dichotomy has reinforced the separation of the two components of the treatment process, which ideally should occur concurrently with long-term counselling, psychotherapy and social work support, starting as soon as the drug-dependent individual presents for treatment. In practice, and perhaps because drug withdrawal is the easier component of the package as far as provision of services is concerned, much more emphasis has been placed on

facilities for drug withdrawal and much less on long-term facilities for rehabilitation and after-care.

Religious and other charitable organizations have perceived these deficiencies in
services for rehabilitation and have set out over many years to remedy them. In
doing so they have gained skills and experience that now cannot be matched by
statutory services, so that the Government's role in the provision of rehabilitation
has largely become confined to providing funding for the work of the voluntary
agencies. The Standing Conference on Drug Abuse (SCODA), a voluntary body
funded by the Department of Health and Social Security (DHSS), acted as a
coordinating body for all voluntary services dealing with drug abusers until April
2000 when it merged with the Institute for the Study of Drug Dependence (ISDD)
to form 'Drug Scope'.

Because rehabilitation services have developed from the activities of voluntary
organizations, they have done so in an unplanned and often haphazard fashion
according to local needs, local interests, local skills and available funding, rather
than in a comprehensive country-wide plan. A number of residential establish-
ments exist, most of which insist that prospective entrants must be 'off' drugs
before admission. They try to detach residents from their previous environment
and to teach them to lead their life without recourse to drugs. In recent years, the
voluntary agencies have increasingly extended their activities outside the field of
rehabilitation and now offer a variety of services for drug abusers at any stage of a
drug-taking career. These include day centres, walk-in counselling services, telephone advisory services, self-help groups and parents' support groups in all parts
of the country.

Arrest referral schemes

Because of the high incidence of drug-related crime, drug users frequently come
into contact with the criminal justice system. This offers a window of opportunity
for intervention at a time when the drug user may be particularly receptive to
offers of help. As the title suggests, arrest referral schemes operate at the earliest
stage of contact with the criminal justice system – at the point of arrest. The
schemes vary from the police officer issuing a card containing information on how
and where the arrestee can seek help for their drug problem, to drug workers
attending or being assigned to police stations or courts so that help and advice is
immediately available 'face-to-face'. Early evaluation shows that almost half of
those seen have not had previous contact with drug agencies, despite a long history
of criminality. Follow-up studies suggest that 6–8 months after referral, a quarter
reported not using illicit drugs and over half had stopped self-injecting.[31] It is
therefore planned that face-to-face arrest referral schemes should be extended to
all police custody suites.

Drug Treatment and Testing Orders

A recent innovation in the criminal justice system is the introduction and application of Drug Treatment and Testing Orders (DTTOs) as an alternative to custody for those who have been found guilty of drug-related offences. Under such an order, the offender can be referred for treatment by the court but remains under the supervision of the probation service who submit progress reports to the court. In the absence of demonstrable improvement, the order may be revoked and a custodial sentence imposed. It is hoped that the desire to avoid imprisonment may increase motivation and full participation in an effective treatment programme; however, full evaluation of their effectiveness is not yet available.[32]

Prison medical service

Many people admitted to prison either on remand or as convicted prisoners may be dependent on drugs or have a drug-related problem.[33–35] In fact, their dependent state may come to light for the first time in this situation, which would seem to be an excellent opportunity for intervention and treatment. Prison medical officers are experienced at dealing with drug withdrawal and may admit drug-dependent prisoners to the prison hospital temporarily, so that dose reduction can be supervised more closely. Until recently there were no special treatment facilities for drug-dependent patients in prisons so that, after drug withdrawal and the achievement of abstinence, the essential components of rehabilitation were lacking. Compulsory 'treatment' in prison, consisting only of detoxification, therefore had little long-term effect after the prisoner was released. However, as part of the UK government's anti-drugs strategy (1998), 'Tackling Drugs To Build a Better Britain',[24] the framework for drug interventions for prisoners is developing an integrated Counselling, Assessment, Referral, Advice and Throughcare Service (CARATS) within and across the prison service. CARATS will provide a range of easily accessible interventions including, in addition to detoxification, 'enhanced' drug treatment services with a moderate intensity programme of 12–16 weeks and 'intensive' treatment lasting for at least 6 months which will be appropriate for prisoners serving longer sentences. In addition, during 2000, the Home Office commissioned research under the Drugs Strategy on the rates and causes of drug-related mortality among recently released prisoners.

Sources of epidemiological information in the UK

The following sections outline different epidemiological approaches to assessing the extent of substance misuse with illustrative examples from the UK to demonstrate how trends and patterns can be identified as well as the limitations and difficulties associated with the different approaches. The decision about what information to collect and the method of collecting it will depend on the purpose for which the information is needed and the scale and level of the enquiry. For example, information may be required to assess the prevalence and nature of substance misuse, to plan appropriate treatment services, educational programmes or preventive strategies or to assess and evaluate the effect of programmes that have already been implemented. Similarly, information may be needed for national and international purposes or locally, within much smaller communities.

Drug seizures

Locally, information about illicit drugs can be obtained from figures about drug seizures and purchases made on the black market for investigation purposes. These data give some idea of the availability and purity of individual drugs. In the UK, the Home Office publishes data on seizures of all controlled drugs, thereby providing information on a wide range of substances, as well as information on drug offences. While changes in seizures and offenders do not necessarily imply changes in the prevalence of the misuse of controlled drugs, they may reflect changed demand for these substances. It is acknowledged, however, that other factors such as changes in the direction and effectiveness of enforcement effort, and changes in recording and reporting procedures may be significant.

In 1998, the number of drug seizures increased by 8%, compared with an increase of 14% in the previous year. As in earlier years, the majority of seizures were of cannabis (Fig. 2.1). The total number of seizures decreased in 1999, particularly for amphetamines (Table 2.1) although the quantity of amphetamine seized increased significantly. The number of heroin seizures increased during the early 1980s from 985 in 1982 to nearly 3200 in 1985. Since then, and particularly since 1994, heroin seizures have soared to 15 108 in 1999, up by 21% since 1997. In terms of the quantity, 2342 kg of heroin was seized in 1999, a 74% increase over 1998 and the largest annual quantity seized during the decade.[36]

The total number of cocaine seizures (including crack cocaine) rose to 8055 in 1999, a new peak, and it is of particular interest that the number of crack-cocaine seizures has increased dramatically over the past few years, from 140 in 1989, to the present level of 2436 in 1999. In view of this increase in the number of seizures, it is not surprising that the quantity of cocaine seized is also at record levels. The average purity of seized cocaine also appears to be rising.

Among the wealth of information available on drug seizures, the following points are of particular interest.

1. In all but two police force areas, heroin was the most frequently seized class A drug. Seizures of MDMA (Ecstasy) fell by 7% in 1998. Nevertheless, 2 095 000 doses were seized, compared with about 44 000 in 1990, but still well below the

Table 2.1. Heroin, cocaine and amphetamine seizures 1989–99

	1989	1990	1991	1992	1993	1994	1995	1996	1997	1998	1999
Number of seizures each year											
Heroin	2728	2593	2640	2968	3677	4480	6468	9830	12 474	15 188	15 108
Cocaine	1905	1489	1401	1487	1799	1672	2210	2765	3691	5207	5619
Crack	140	316	583	878	1155	1320	1444	1332	1745	2488	2436
Amphetamines	3322	4629	6821	10 570	11 719	12 970	15 443	18 261	18 575	18 629	13 194
Quantity seized (nearest whole kg)											
Heroin	351	603	493	547	656	744	1395	1070	2235	1348	2342
Cocaine[a]	499	611	1078	2248	717	2262	672	1219	2350	2962	2957
Amphetamines	108	304	421	569	975	1305	819	2625	3296	1810	2017

[a]Excluding crack.
Source: Home Office.

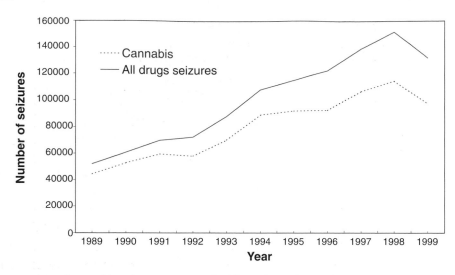

Fig. 2.1   Number of cannabis seizures compared with total number of drug seizures, UK 1989–99. (Source: Home Office.)

peak in 1996 of 5795000 doses, when some very large individual seizures were made. The number of seizures involving LSD in 1998 was 609, a drop of 240 (28%) on the previous year and the lowest figure since 1988. The availability, or popularity, of LSD appears subject to considerable fluctuations. Methadone seizures have increased significantly since 1992, when quantities were negligible, to 1550 in 1998, representing 82.5 kg.

    2. In 1992 there were 3000 seizures involving class C drugs, mainly benzodiazepines, milder stimulants, less potent analgesics and anabolic steroids. Of these, 2840 were for benzodiazepines, including 870 for temazepam. From 1 September 1996, anabolic steroids became controlled under the Misuse of Drugs Act 1971 (Modification) Order 1996 and the Misuse of Drugs (Amendment) Regulations 1996. There were 171 seizures of this drug in 1998, an 11% increase on the previous year.

Persons dealt with for drug offences

The number of persons dealt with for drug offences is yet another indicator of the prevalence of illicit drug misuse, although the figures need careful analysis and interpretation. In summary, the number of drug offenders has continued to rise, and the total number reported to the Home Office in 1998 was 153 156, 13% more than in 1997. This number has increased year on year since 1988, but fell in 1999. Unlawful possession remains the most common offence (Fig. 2.2). The majority of offenders are found in possession of cannabis but there has been a steep rise in offences related to heroin and cocaine (Fig. 2.3).[36]

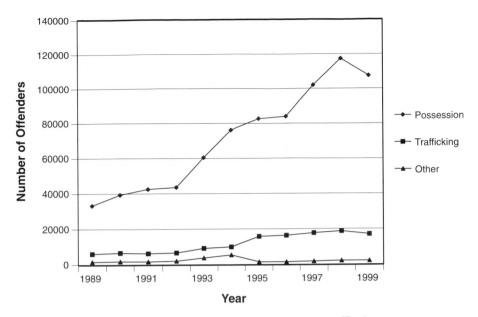

Fig. 2.2   Drug offenders by type of offence, UK 1989–99. (Source: Home Office.)

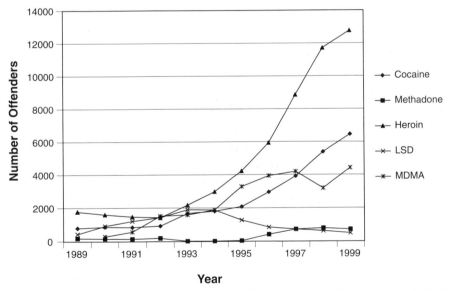

Fig. 2.3   Drug offenders by type of drug, excluding cannabis, UK 1989–99. (Source: Home Office.)

Drug-related crime

A topic of continuing interest and concern is the causal relationship between crime and substance misuse – how much crime is due to substance misusers offending merely to support their drug habit? 'Drug-related' crime includes acquisitive crime (e.g. theft, shop lifting, fraud and burglary), drug-dealing and prostitution. The relationship is important because such facts are often used, simplistically, as a reason to decriminalize illicit drug use. The complexity of this issue is demonstrated by the finding that most crack cocaine addicts have long-standing criminal records before using the drug; however, those who do not often turn to acquisitive crime to fund their drug misuse.[37]

One interesting approach is to test the urine of all arrestees – not just drug offenders – for the presence of drugs. One such study carried out in 1997 found that 61% had recently taken at least one illegal substance and, 2 years later, this figure had increased to 69%.[38,39] Nearly half of those testing positive in 1997 believed that their drug use was associated with their criminal behaviour, particularly the need to steal for money to buy drugs. Relatively high proportions of arrestees had used cocaine or opiates (18% and 10% respectively). Property offenders were more likely to be drug-takers than offenders against the person, alcohol/drug offenders or disorderly offenders, and a comparatively high proportion of property offenders in 1997 tested positive for opiates (23%) or cocaine (14%) compared with other offender groups. Almost half the shoplifters tested positive for opiates and 3 in 10 for cocaine.

Prescription audit

Another way of investigating patterns of drug use is to assess drug distribution by means of prescriptions.[40] This can provide information on individual drugs or drug classes prescribed either for the total population or for selected populations. It also, of course, allows trends and patterns of prescribing practices to be studied.

Thus it can be seen from Table 2.2 and Fig. 2.4 that the total number of prescriptions issued by GPs increased steadily over the period 1991–2000 and that the number of prescriptions for drugs that act on the nervous system, after dipping in the mid-1980s, has been increasing since 1991. Within the overall total, there has been a gradual, albeit fluctuating, decline in the number of prescriptions for hypnotics while the number of prescriptions for anxiolytics has remained steady. Perhaps the most striking feature however is the steady increase, over the last 10 years, in the number of prescriptions for opioid analgesics; in 2000, for example, there were 6.8 million prescriptions for these drugs, compared with 3 million in 1991. These drugs are a frequent substance of misuse, and rising prescription figures, such as those shown in Table 2.2, can act as an early warning system if abuse is becoming widespread. The increased prescription of antidepressants over this time period may be a reflection of the introduction of a large number of new drugs, such as the Selective Serotonin Re-uptake Inhibitors (SSRIs) which have fewer and more tolerable side effects than earlier drugs.

Of course it is possible to analyse prescription data in more detail – even by

Table 2.2. Total number of prescriptions and number of prescriptions of preparations acting on the nervous system, by selected therapeutic subgroups, England 1991–2000

	Millions of prescriptions										Percentage change 1991–2000
	1991	1992	1993	1994	1995	1996	1997	1998	1999	2000	
All classes	406.5	425.1	445.4	456.1	473.3	484.9	500.2	513.2	529.8	551.8	35.7%
Central nervous system	74.7	77.1	80.3	81.8	86.0	89.3	92.8	96.8	100.4	103.6	38.7%
Hypnotics	12.0	11.4	11.0	10.8	10.6	10.6	10.6	10.6	10.6	10.6	−11.7%
Anxiolytics	5.5	5.3	5.1	5.1	5.1	5.2	5.4	5.5	5.6	5.8	5.5%
Barbiturates	0.2	0.2	0.1	0.1	0.1	0.1	0.1	0.1	0.1	0.1	−50.0%
Antipsychotics	3.5	3.8	4.0	4.3	4.5	4.8	5.1	5.4	5.6	5.9	68.6%
SSRI antidepressants	0.5	1.2	1.9	2.7	3.8	5.1	6.6	7.6	8.9	10.4	1980.0%
Other antidepressants	8.4	8.7	8.9	9.1	9.4	9.8	10.3	10.8	11.2	11.6	38.1%
Stimulants and centrally acting appetite suppressants	0.5	0.4	0.4	0.3	0.3	0.3	0.3	0.2	0.3	0.3	−40.0%
Opioid analgesics	3.0	3.2	3.3	3.7	4.1	4.6	5.1	5.7	6.2	6.8	126.7%
Antiepileptics	4.8	5.0	5.1	5.3	5.5	5.7	5.8	6.1	6.4	6.7	39.6%
Drugs used in substance dependence	0.4	0.6	0.7	0.7	0.8	0.9	0.1	1.1	1.2	1.5	275.0%

Data is based on all prescriptions dispensed by community pharmacists and appliance contractors, dispensing doctors and personal administration.

SSRI, selective serotonin reuptake inhibitor.

Source: Department of Health, Statistics Division 1E, Prescription Cost Analysis System.

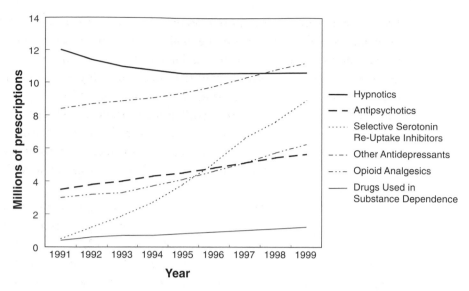

Fig. 2.4   Number of prescriptions for certain therapeutic subgroups acting on the nervous system, UK 1991–99. (Source: Department of Health.)

individual drugs. This shows for example that within the large number of prescriptions for benzodiazepines, there have been more prescriptions for shorter-acting drugs such as temazepam and lorazepam, which have become popular because, when taken as hypnotics, they have less 'hang-over' effect and, when taken through the day as anxiolytics, there is much less drug accumulation in the body. However, it now appears that dependence on these drugs is more severe and that withdrawal is correspondingly more difficult from these shorter-acting drugs.

Although the information obtained from prescription audit is fascinating, great care needs to be taken in its interpretation, because the method has obvious limitations. For example, a proportion of people who receive prescriptions do not get them dispensed (and are therefore not included in an audit of retail pharmacists) and a proportion of people who have their prescriptions dispensed do not take (all of) their drugs. In other words, it must not be forgotten that the sampling unit is a prescription and not a patient. Furthermore, changes in prescribing may be misrepresented; for example, changing from the practice of giving long-term prescriptions for large amounts of a drug to giving short-term prescriptions for small amounts would appear in the statistics as an increase in the total number of prescriptions, even if the amount prescribed is the same or less.

Index of Addicts

Historically, the main source of epidemiological information about addiction in the UK was the Home Office Index of Addicts, but this was closed in 1997. Before

1968, it was primarily based on a system of inspecting the books of dispensing pharmacists and reports from the police. Voluntary notification by medical practitioners also contributed to this knowledge base. From 1968 to May 1997, however, doctors had a statutory duty to notify the Home Office of any patient whom they considered to be dependent on certain controlled drugs (cocaine and, from 1973, a number of opiate drugs). The index of addicts was derived from these notifications and annual statistics were published giving the total number of notified addicts at the end of each year, their sex and age, the number of new (i.e. notified for the first time) and re-notified addicts, the drugs reported to be used at notification and so on.

However, as many addicts obtain drugs illicitly and are intent on concealment from any authority, the official statistics could only represent a proportion, and probably a changing proportion, of the total number who were actually addicted. Furthermore, at any time there were many people misusing the same drugs who were not (yet) addicted to them. A further disadvantage of the Index was that notification was not required for a large number of controlled drugs, such as amphetamines and barbiturates, which were and are misused and can cause dependence, and, of course, doctors did not always fulfil their statutory obligation to notify. Thus, although the primary function of the Index – to reduce the possibility of an individual receiving certain drugs from more than one doctor simultaneously – was largely achieved, the data it provided were of limited value, because those who were notified were probably only a small proportion of regular users. Nevertheless, even this quality of data was generally considered useful for picking up trends and for illustrating general patterns within a restricted group of drug users.

Number of addicts

The Home Office Index was closed on 30 April 1997 and this account can therefore only extend to that date. Up to and including 1996, it showed a steady, almost relentless increase in the number of notified addicts since 1987, with an increase of 17% between 1995 and 1996. Thus the total number of addicts notified to the Home Office increased from 14 785 at the end of 1989 to 27 976 by the end of 1993 and 43 372 by the end of 1996, a total increase of 193%. Within this huge increase, in 1996 there were 18 281 new notifications, the highest number of new addicts ever recorded in a single year, and 24% more than in the previous year (Fig. 2.5). Altogether, new notifications accounted for 42% of the total.[41]

It has been suggested that some of this increase may have been the result of efforts to attract more addicts into treatment because of fear of AIDS. There may also have been a greater awareness of notification procedures and obligations as a result of the establishment of Regional Substance Misuse Databases (see below) by

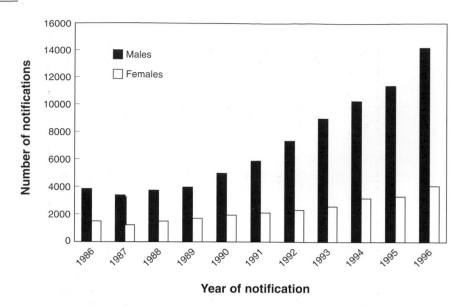

Fig. 2.5   New drug addicts notified to the Home Office, UK 1986–96. (Source: Home Office.)

Health Authorities and also because doctors were sent reminders about the requirement to re-notify addicts in their care.

Age and sex (Table 2.3, Fig. 2.6)

The age of new addicts remained relatively stable from 1986 to 1996, with an average age of 26–27 years. However, the number in the under-21 years age group increased after 1989 and very sharply, by 35%, between 1995 and 1996. In 1996, 74% of new addicts were under the age of 30 years and 20% were less than 21 years old. The average age of all addicts (not just new addicts) has fallen steadily since 1992, after having gradually risen since the mid-1980s.

Although the number of new female addicts increased over the years, they formed a smaller proportion of the total than previously. In 1996, for example, 22% of new addicts were female, compared with 28% in 1990. It can be seen from Table 2.3 and Fig. 2.5 that the majority of new addicts are men aged between 21 and 34 years of age.

Drugs of addiction (Table 2.4, Figs. 2.7, 2.8)

The common drugs to which addiction was reported in the Index were, in order of frequency, heroin, methadone, cocaine, morphine and dipipanone. A fifth of notified addicts were reported to be polydrug addicts.

Heroin was the most common drug of addiction for new addicts in the 1980s, with the proportion increasing from 72% in 1980 to 93% in 1985, perhaps

Table 2.3. Age and sex of new addicts, UK 1986–96

	1986	1987	1988	1989	1990	1991	1992	1993	1994	1995	1996
Age group in years											
Under 21	1261	975	1063	982	1178	1225	1698	2051	2453	2962	3984
21–24	1460	1386	1464	1598	1949	2194	2760	3202	3734	4120	5046
25–29	1262	1063	1324	1576	1946	2293	2701	3141	3645	3835	4695
30–34	705	618	696	767	964	1128	1253	1639	1896	1991	2487
35–49	374	373	478	561	732	943	1080	1218	1390	1459	1731
Over 50	41	33	35	44	39	67	81	89	104	122	133
Not recorded	222	145	152	111	115	157	90	221	247	246	205
Total	5325	4593	5212	5639	6923	8007	9663	11 561	13 469	14 735	18 281
Percentage new addicts under 21 years	25	22	21	18	17	16	18	18	18	20	22
Average age of new addicts	25.8	26.1	26.3	26.8	26.9	27.3	26.9	26.9	26.4	26.2	25.9
Males	3837	3372	3723	3952	4991	5899	7342	8981	10 293	11 422	14 205
Females	1488	1221	1489	1687	1932	2108	2321	2580	3176	3313	4076
Total	5325	4593	5212	5639	6923	8007	9663	11 561	13 469	14 735	18 281

Source: Home Office.

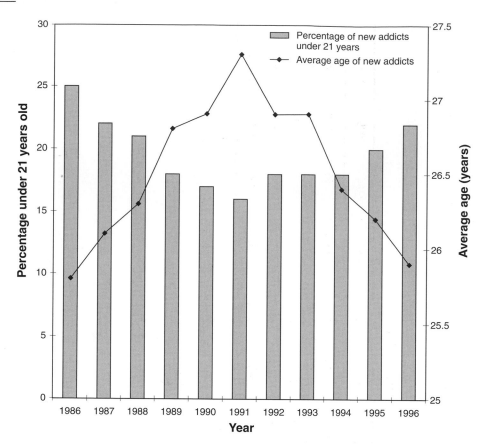

Fig. 2.6   Average age of newly notified addicts and percentage under 21 years of age, UK 1986–96.

reflecting ease of availability at that time. In 1996, some 15 271 new heroin addicts were notified, an increase of 32% on new notifications in 1995. A record number (4724) of people were reported as newly dependent on methadone in 1996. This was an increase of 6% on the previous year – a slower rate of increase than in previous years. About 13 900 re-notified addicts were reported to be dependent on methadone in 1996, 7% more than in 1995. These increases probably reflect the fact that more new addicts are being treated with methadone.

The number of new cocaine addicts fell in 1996 to 1714, reversing the upward trend of previous years. Nevertheless, despite very large seizures of cocaine, its misuse has, so far, not created a significant demand for medical treatment.

The number notified as addicted to dipipanone fell slightly in 1996, from 215 to 194, continuing the downward trend of recent years. The total is now substantially less than in the early 1980s, suggesting that the stricter controls placed on its prescription have been successful in controlling availability.

Among re-notified addicts, heroin and methadone remained the most common

Table 2.4. New drug addicts and type of drug to which addiction reported, UK 1986–96

	1986	1987	1988	1989	1990	1991	1992	1993	1994	1995	1996
Cocaine	520	431	462	527	633	882	1131	1375	1636	1809	1714
Methadone	659	627	576	682	1469	2180	2493	3362	3990	4468	4724
Heroin	4855	4082	4630	4883	5819	6328	7658	9063	10 607	11 620	15 271
Other	616	523	471	495	585	479	449	379	338	255	264
Total[a]	5325	4593	5212	5639	6923	8007	9663	11 561	13 469	14 735	18 281

[a]An addict may be reported as addicted to more than one drug.

Source: Home Office.

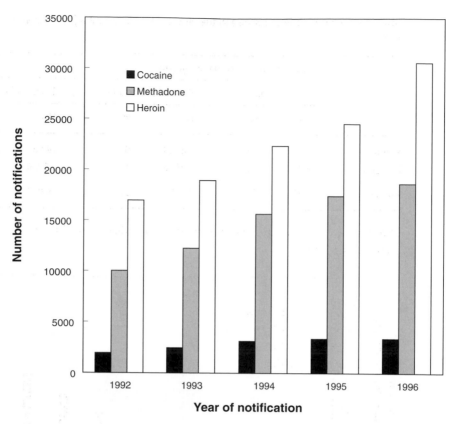

Fig. 2.7   Notification to the Home Office by drug of notification, UK 1992–96.

drugs of addiction in 1996, with 15 302 addicted to heroin and 13 893 addicted to methadone, 85% more than in 1992. As with new addicts, the increase in the proportion addicted to methadone is substantial: 55% in 1993. Altogether, notifiable drugs were prescribed to 9386 new addicts and 18 940 re-notified addicts at their first notification in 1996, with 99% being prescribed methadone, either alone or in combination with another drug.

Injecting status

Because of concern about the spread of HIV/AIDS, drug abusers' injecting status is of the greatest importance (Table 2.5). In 1996, just over half (51%) of all addicts whose injecting status was known were injecting their drugs and a higher proportion of re-notified addicts were injecting than new addicts. Despite the stability in the proportion of injectors, the number of addicts injecting increased to 19 011 in 1996. Of these, 2000 were aged under 21 years and must have started injecting after information about HIV/AIDS became widely available.

Table 2.5. All drug addicts notified to the Home Office by latest injecting status and sex, UK 1996

| | Number and percentage injecting[a] | | | | | |
| | New addicts | | Re-notified addicts | | Total addicts | |
	No.	%	No.	%	No.	%
Males	6259	48	8728	55	14 987	52
Females	1616	44	2408	47	4024	46
All persons	7875	47	11 136	53	19 011	51

[a]Percentages based on number of addicts for whom injecting status is known.
Source: Home Office.

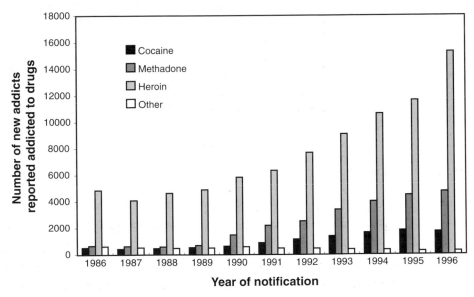

Fig. 2.8   New addicts and drugs of addiction, UK 1986–96.

Regional Drug Misuse Databases (RDMDs)

Until the mid-1990s, the only national figures available relating to the nature and extent of drug use were contained within the Home Office's Index of Addicts. The inadequacies of this system as an epidemiological tool have been outlined above and it has been recognized that more comprehensive information on a wider range of substance misuse was essential for effective service development and policy making at both local and national levels. In 1989 the Department of Health therefore required all Regional Health Authorities to establish databases to monitor trends in drug abuse and the use of drug abuse services, and nationally collated information (October 1992 to September 1999) is now available (for England). Separate databases were established for other countries in the UK. However, this system also has its drawbacks: although supposedly anonymized, data were originally required to be attributable; i.e. the drug user must be identified by initials, date of birth and postcode to enable data matching and the removal of duplicate client episodes. Apart from the ethical concerns raised by this practice (privacy, civil liberties), it is highly probable that some drug users and/or reporting drug agencies refused to provide attributable data, thereby compromising the epidemiological accuracy of the RDMDs. Because of these issues, the requirement for attributable data has now been dropped. A further limit to the comprehensiveness of the RDMDs arises because the Department of Health does not include data from certain agencies such as telephone helplines and prisons, and also excludes data where the primary substance of abuse is alcohol. Finally, it is worth noting that this method of recording information is a mixture of incident-reporting and case-reporting, with a potential lack of clarity in its results.

The South-West Thames Substance Use Database at the Centre for Addiction Studies (St George's Medical School) includes information on educational background, employment and other demographic variables as well as the subject's alcohol use. In addition to being more comprehensive than other databases, it maintains full confidentiality because all data is nonattributable; at the same time procedures are in place to prevent duplicate reporting. A similar, Europe-wide database has been developed by the Centre and this is used by the European Collaborating Centres on Addiction Studies (Appendices 2 and 3).

The databases collect information on all forms of drug misuse (not just notifiable drugs) and from a wide variety of sources. For example, of the reports made to the Drug Misuse Databases (DMDs) for the 6 months ending 31 March 2000, 47% have come from statutory Community Drug Teams, with non-statutory, nonresidential agencies accounting for 31%, GPs for 5% and outpatient DDTUs for 6%. In many respects, although they cover a much wider range of drugs, RDMD figures broadly confirm the picture produced by analysis of the Home Office Index, that most drug users presenting to services are men in their twenties and early thirties. In total, 74% of individuals reported to the RDMDs were using opiate drugs as their main drug (heroin 63% and methadone 9%) and 59% of those using heroin were known to be injecting it.[42]

Tables 2.6 and 2.7 illustrate the type of information that can be gathered about the sex and age of substance misusers, their injecting status and the substances of misuse.

Table 2.6. Age and gender of users starting agency episodes in 6 months ending 30 September 2000, UK

Age group (years)	Male	Female	All persons
< 15	255	114	369
15–19	3319	1664	4983
20–24	7229	2847	10 076
25–29	7380	2540	9920
30–34	5583	1768	7351
35–39	2930	990	3920
40–44	1276	404	1680
45–49	617	205	822
50–54	259	105	364
55–59	73	38	111
60–64	16	15	31
> 64	14	17	31
All ages	28 951	10 707	39 658

Mortality studies

Mortality studies by definition focus on the most serious forms of drug abuse – those from which the patient has died. Causes of death are numerous, they include overdose (suicidal, accidental or homicidal), side effects of drugs, complications of nonsterile self-injection and functional impairment that increases the risk of serious accident. Because there are so many possible causes of death and because many are not exclusively due to drug abuse, those that are, may be very difficult to identify among a large number of similar deaths that have nothing to do with drugs.[17,43,44]

However, the problem of mortality due to drug abuse can be tackled in many different ways:

- Analysis of a series of forensically examined cases;
- Analysis of national cause of death statistics;
- Cause of death surveys;
- Epidemiological studies on the mortality of drug consumers;
- Police records (drug-related deaths, road traffic deaths involving drug misuse, other criminal offences involving drug- or alcohol-related fatalities);
- Hospital records.

Clear differences exist in the indications, objectives, expense and amount of information obtained by these different methods. In most industrialized countries, cause of death statistics are the main source of data about drug overdose deaths and are often used for international comparisons. They are valuable

Table 2.7. All drugs of misuse by category and whether injecting the drugs, for users starting agency episodes in 6 months ending 30 September 2000, UK

Type of drug	Percentage of users of each drug as percentage of total number of users	Percentage injecting where injecting status was known	Number of users
Heroin	70	58	27 736
Methadone	20	7	7747
Other opiates	9	8	3405
Barbiturates	0	4	35
Benzodiazepines	21	2	8299
Amphetamines	8	36	3206
Cocaine	18	12	7224
Hallucinogens	1	3	379
Cannabis	27	—	10 861
Solvents	1	—	305
Alcohol	12	—	4730
Antidepressants	2	—	672
Other drugs	8	10	3281
Drug free/ no drug coded	0	—	15

Note: The percentages sum to more than 100% because individuals use drugs from more than one category.
Source: Department of Health.

because they are representative but they are always out of date because of delay in publication. In addition, as they are not substance specific, they cannot provide any evidence of new trends of drug abuse. This can be remedied to a certain degree by forensic toxicological analysis which can give an early indication of any increase in the number of deaths due to a specific drug. In England and Wales, for example, coroners' courts have proved to be a useful source of information about addict deaths. Since the coroner must be informed of any death arising from the use of drugs, whether occurring during treatment or as a result of mishap, abuse or addiction, a survey of coroners' courts' records provides accurate information on the number of addicts who die in a given period and whose death is in any way related to drug-taking.[45]

The following exemplify some of the approaches to studying drug-related mortality utilized in the UK.

Table 2.8. Deaths with underlying cause described as drug dependence or nondependent abuse of drugs, by type of drug, UK, 1985–95

	1985	1986	1987	1988	1989	1990	1991	1992	1993	1994	1995
Morphine type[a]	62	70	65	64	77	91	97	155	65	144	203
Methadone									74	114	116
Cocaine	0	2	1	2	2	3	0	0	3	6	3
Cannabis	1	2	0	0	1	0	0	0	0	1	0
Hallucinogens	0	0	1	0	0	0	1	2	0	0	0
Amphetamine type[b]	3	2	1	0	2	2	5	7	4	4	13
MDMA (Ecstasy)									2	10	6
Barbiturate type	7	14	10	7	15	7	16	6	13	35	43
Volatile substances	54	46	76	89	84	112	87	68	46	39	43
Morphine with other	4	7	12	10	14	15	18	29	21	17	30
Combinations excluding morphine	2	0	1	2	3	1	4	3	1	4	4
Unspecified drug dependence	22	21	24	19	27	24	31	26	45	48	53
Antidepressants	0	3	8	4	3	4	2	4	2	2	3
Other; mixed, unspecified, nondependent	35	28	29	24	17	35	46	45	46	65	85
Total	190	195	228	221	245	294	307	345	322	489	602

[a]Excludes methadone from 1993.
[b]Excludes MDMA from 1993.
Source: Home Office.

Home Office Index

In the UK, the Home Office Index used to be a further source of information about addicts' deaths because a separate list was kept of those addicts removed from the current index by reason of death. By definition, the information referred only to addicts known to the Home Office in the first place and, as already noted, this list was by no means complete anyway. However, the Home Office statistics also included national statistics of deaths where the underlying cause was drug dependence or nondependent use of drugs, or the use of controlled drugs (Table 2.8, Figs. 2.9, 2.10).[41]

In 1995, the last year for which the Home Office prepared the official UK mortality statistics, there were 1810 drug-related deaths nation-wide, according to this Home Office definition. Of these, about 600 (Table 2.8) were attributed to drug dependence (ICD9 304) or nondependent misuse of drugs (other than alcohol or tobacco but including volatile substances: ICD9 305). Four hundred and seventy deaths were recorded as resulting from accidental poisoning

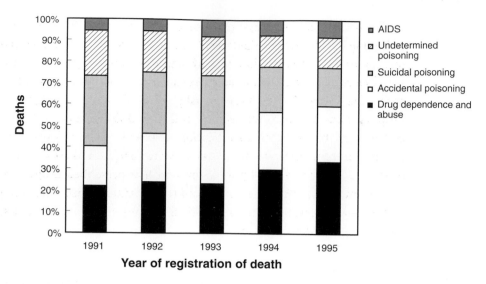

Fig. 2.9   Causes of death of addicts known to the Home Office, UK 1991–95.

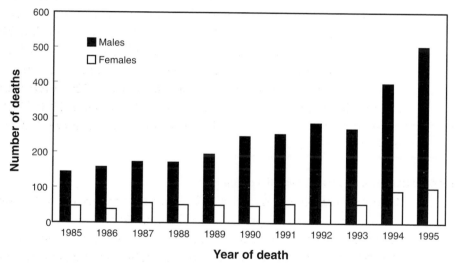

Fig 2.10   Deaths of addicts known to the Home Office by sex, UK 1985–95.

(E850-E866) by controlled drugs and 260 involved controlled drugs where it was undetermined whether the drugs had been taken purposefully or accidentally. In addition, some 350 people committed suicide with controlled drugs.

Of the 602 deaths in 1995 resulting from drug dependence or the nondependent misuse of drugs, about 53% used morphine-type drugs (including 19% involving methadone) and about 7% used volatile substances. Fifteen per cent of those who died were under 20 and about four fifths were of people under the age of 35.

The main Class A drugs (Misuse of Drugs Act 1971) used in accidental poisoning deaths were methadone (154), morphine (97) and heroin (60). Benzo-diazepines were involved in one sixth and dextropropoxyphene in one tenth of such deaths. About a third of suicides caused by poisoning involved at least one controlled drug. These were usually class C drugs, particularly dextro-propoxyphene and benzodiazepines, and class B drugs, mainly dihydrocodeine, codeine and barbiturates. Investigation of suicide using information from the Home Office Index showed that, over a 25-year period, addicts were at higher risk of suicide than the general population and that prescribed drugs, notably anti-depressants and methadone, influenced this heightened risk. The average annual suicide rates among newly notified addicts for the period were 69 (males) and 44.8 (females) per 100,000 person years.[46]

National Statistics

Figures published by National Statistics for England and Wales and by the General Register Offices for the rest of the UK, are another source of mortality data, classified using the Ninth Revision of the International Classification of Diseases (ICD-9). Using the National Statistics 'standard' approach, which is fairly similar to the Home Office definition except for the omission of AIDS deaths, there were 2922 deaths in England and Wales in 1998.[47] AIDS is of course a serious threat to substance misusers who inject their drugs and, of over 17 200 AIDS cases reported in the UK between January 1982 and June 2000, some 1380 (8%) probably acquired the virus through injecting drugs and, of these, nearly 1000 had died by the end of June 2000.

National database for misuse of volatile solvents

A national database on deaths associated with the misuse of volatile substances is based at St George's Hospital Medical School. The most recent reports show that deaths decreased slightly from 79 in 1996 to 70 in 1998, about half the rate in 1990.[48] These reductions reflect a decline in deaths from aerosols and glues, so that the majority of solvent-related deaths are now due to gas fuels and butane gas lighter refills. Altogether, volatile substances account for about 2% of all deaths of those aged 15–19 in the UK; they are much more common in males than females, and in the North of England, Northern Ireland and Scotland. It can easily be appreciated that this sort of information on emerging trends is particularly helpful in planning preventive strategies.

National Programme for Substance Abuse Deaths

The National Statistics total of drug-related deaths in 1997 and 1998 can be compared with a relatively new surveillance system, the National Programme of

Substance Abuse Deaths (np-SAD), which was established in 1997. This programme collects data direct from coroners and applies local expertise in mortality, addictions and epidemiology to extract a comprehensive picture of drug-related deaths in England and Wales. Rather than simply counting deaths where the coroners' verdict is 'drug dependence', or 'nondependent abuse of drugs', the np-SAD also investigates the causes of death, drugs present at post-mortem, drugs prescribed and whether the deceased was an addict or had a history of drug abuse. In its latest report, np-SAD recorded 1296 drug-related deaths in 2000, a decrease of 8% over the previous year[49] (Appendix 5).

Surveys

Surveys are widely used epidemiological tools to measure knowledge, attitude and behaviour in different populations. Where they are used in an assessment of substance misuse, they can be applied to whole populations or restricted to specific groups often identified by age. In the UK for example there are regular surveys of people's experience of crime, one component of which explores self-reported drug misuse. The most recent published report covers the 1998 survey in England and Wales[50] and offers a measure of prevalence of drug misuse among the general population. Young people aged 16–29 reported the highest level of drug misuse, with 49% saying that they had taken a prohibited drug at some time. However, only 25% had taken drugs within the last year and only 16% within the last month. Cannabis was the most widely consumed prohibited drug, with a significant increase between 1996 and 1998 in its use by young men. Other surveys include those undertaken by the Health Education Authority Survey which focuses on assessing the level of knowledge of risks associated with drug misuse; surveys of schoolchildren, surveys of adolescents and surveys of youth lifestyles. Out of the wealth of information gained by such surveys, the following points indicate the sort of areas that can be explored in this way and the information that can be obtained.

Recent drug users were more likely to have started smoking earlier and were twice as likely to describe themselves as fairly regular smokers. Recent drug users drank alcohol regularly and were more likely to imbibe than those who had ever used drugs (94% compared with 74%).[51]

Of 930 Scottish schoolchildren aged 11 and 12 years, 105 (11.4%) reported having used illegal drugs; there was a higher rate for boys (13.7%) than girls (8.8%). Of those who had used drugs, 79.4% reported having used cannabis but other drugs were extensively used too. Current use rates were much lower and cannabis again dominated the picture. Use of drugs by a family member was found to be an important factor influencing drug use by these young people.[52] By the age of 13 years, over 90% of children could recognize the commonly used drugs; 60%

of 14-year-olds and 80% of 16-year-olds had encountered or been offered drugs. In Northumbria the rate of drug-taking increased from 34% at the age of 13 years to 51% a year later. The corresponding figures for West Yorkshire were 21% and 34% – illustrating the differences that can occur just within one country. Volatile substances and 'popping' were features of drug-trying in early adolescence; LSD and amphetamine were tried in mid-adolescence and ecstasy after the age of 16 years.[53]

The 1998/99 Youth Lifestyles Survey looks at offending behaviour including unreported, unrecorded and undetected crime among people aged 12–30 years, interviewed in the British Crime Survey and those living at addresses next door.[54] About one third (32%) of males aged 12–30 years reported ever having used drugs compared with 22% of females, but there were big differences between different age groups. Only 3% of 12- to 13-year-olds had used an illegal drug, compared with a peak of 54% among 21-year-olds. The level of offending amongst drug users aged 12–17 years was 15 times higher than for nondrug users. Amongst 18- to 30-year-olds, male drug users were twice as likely to offend than nonusers whereas the ratio was three to one for females in this age group. Serious or persistent offenders were more likely to use opiates or cocaine.

Accident and emergency (A & E) departments

As psychoactive drugs such as hypnotics, anxiolytics and antidepressants have been prescribed more widely, the morbidity associated with their use has become apparent. Undoubtedly, the most important morbidity in terms of sheer number is that of drug overdose. Such is its frequency that the margin of safety between the therapeutic dose of a psychoactive drug and the dose required for serious overdose or death is at times a property with commercial significance.

The majority of cases of drug overdoses are seen in hospital A & E departments which are, therefore, excellent places to study this particular morbidity, to monitor the whole range of drug problems and, by including all who attend with a drug-related problem, to identify trends in drug abuse in the general population. These departments offer several advantages for undertaking this kind of epidemiological research. Perhaps most important of all is the fact that although administration and organization may vary, some sort of emergency facility exists in all health care systems so that there is a ready-made, cost-effective set-up available, world-wide, ready to monitor drug-related problems. Another advantage of A & E departments is that they are 'neutral' ground for those with drug-related problems. For those who have taken a drug overdose, for example, the underlying psychosocial reasons are ignored, at least temporarily, while the acute consequences of the overdose are treated by a medical team. It is probable that patients seen in this 'neutral', comparatively nonjudgmental situation are more representative than those in more highly selective situations such as specialist drug treatment units, prisons or remand homes. The value of A & E departments as a neutral ground is enhanced by an awareness of medical confidentiality which facilitates the gathering of accurate data on sensitive issues. Nevertheless, it must be noted that studies in these departments, while providing valuable information about drug-taking in society as a whole, say little about individual patterns.

If A & E departments are to be utilized on a large scale for this type of research, the monitoring procedure must be planned very carefully. All studies must be prospective in nature because notes taken during an emergency situation are rarely sufficiently detailed for comprehensive data to be gleaned from them retrospectively. However, any prospective study must be aware of the busy conditions prevailing in A & E departments and the questionnaire, designed to elicit maximum information, should also be brief and simple so that the staff of the department, whose main responsibility is to the patient and not to research, can complete it easily.

An important decision to be made when planning the investigation is whether to study incidents or individuals. When individual patients are identified, valuable information is obtained about the comparatively small group of individuals who attend A & E departments repeatedly. They are important partly because they generate a lot of work and also because the health care response they initiate is clearly inappropriate to their needs, suggesting that an alternative response should be sought. However, having information that positively identifies patients poses difficult problems of confidentiality while that information is being processed.

The largest survey of A & E departments, both geographically and in terms of duration, is that being carried out in the USA by the Drug Abuse Warning Network (DAWN).[55] This receives reports from hospital emergency rooms, medical examiners (i.e. coroners) and crisis intervention centres, which provide some indications of drug-abuse trends in large urban populations. A specially trained reporter recruited from the staff of each hospital and located in the A & E department is responsible for identifying patients with a drug-related problem and for completing the DAWN questionnaire. This focuses on two main issues: the drug(s) used and the drug user. As more than one drug may be used in a particular incident, more drug 'mentions' are recorded than drug-related incidents; no identifying information about the patients is collected.

In contrast, a survey carried out in 1982 in A & E departments in London specifically identified patients with drug-related problems by recording their name, date of birth and address so that they could be traced if they presented to hospital on more than one occasion during the period of the survey.[56] Information was also elicited about the drug(s) of abuse and self-poisoning, the underlying reason for the drug overdose, the source of supply of drugs, their method of administration and any history of drug overdoses taken in the 12 months prior to the survey.

The potential of using A&E departments to monitor substance misuse has been acknowledged in the National Plan, which has as one of its research objectives for 2000–01, 'to put forward proposals to examine the feasibility of collecting data on drug-related attendances at Casualty Departments'.[57] Because the picture is constantly changing it is essential for epidemiological research to be regular and, in some situations, continuous. In A & E departments, for example, ongoing research could form a sensible early warning system to identify new drugs of abuse so that responses could be swift and appropriate. Ideally such research should be taken in several centres, even internationally, but then great care must be taken about the data that is recorded. Soft data, such as the dependence status of the patient or the motivation of an overdose, is difficult to categorize even with careful operational definitions so that there is always a large 'unknown' group. In contrast, hard data on age, sex and drug(s) taken is easy to elicit and record. However, even with hard data a uniform system of tabulating results must be decided on in advance if valid comparisons are to be made. For example, uniform age and drug classification systems are essential if research done in one department is ever to speak to that done in another.

Other epidemiological approaches

There are many other potential sources of information about drug abuse. Individually, they often deal with highly selective groups of the population and provide unrepresentative information. Together, however, they contribute to a more complete picture about the trends in drug use and drug abuse.

Possible sources of information are:

Drug-dependence treatment, services, rehabilitation centres and voluntary agencies. Various types of surveys in these places can provide information about the characteristics of clients, treatment and outcome.

Toxicology laboratories. Now that reliable methods have been developed for the qualitative and quantitative measurement of drugs in body tissues and fluids, toxicological analysis is playing an increasingly important role in providing firm data about drug use. Where this is done, it is a good, cost-effective method of gathering data on drug-related health problems.

Hospital discharge diagnoses

Drug-related disease. One way of finding out about drug-related problems is to monitor public health data on the frequency of reports of various types of pathology such as HIV/AIDS, viral hepatitis, fetal damage, etc., on the assumption

Table 2.9. New AIDS cases notified to the end of June 2001, identifying the number who acquired it through injecting drug use, UK

Year	New AIDS cases notified	
	Total	Injecting drug users
1985 or earlier	408	3
1986	474	7
1987	681	16
1988	908	28
1989	1082	64
1990	1244	82
1991	1387	88
1992	1578	84
1993	1785	153
1994	1851	139
1995	1764	151
1996	1425	118
1997	1064	77
1998	767	44
1999	715	27
2000	718	34
2001	142	6
Total	17 993	1121

There were also 311 AIDS cases notified involving sex between men who had also injected drugs. These cases are *not* included in the 'injecting drug users' column above.
Source: Department of Health.

that these problems are sufficiently closely linked to drug consumption to be reasonable indicators (Table 2.9). The advantage of this method is its simplicity and low cost, and if data is gathered promptly and routinely it should provide early information about the extent of drug abuse. However, the simplicity and economy are offset by the lack of the specificity of a particular morbidity for psychoactive drug abuse. To give an extreme example, it would be hopeless to try and monitor drug abuse by reports of skin rashes – many drugs can cause rashes as can a variety of infections and allergic conditions.[58] It follows that the disease or disturbance must be relatively specific for the drug in question and that the majority of cases must be due to that drug.

Another difficulty is that monitoring of public health data depends on the identification of cases in different centres with an epidemiological picture being built up by multicentre reporting of fairly low frequencies. Case definition and case recognition will probably vary from centre to centre and may vary in time with changing medical awareness. Other factors also combine to make morbidity an unreliable indicator of drug abuse: the proportion of casualties presenting to medical agencies may vary at different times and at different centres and the percentage of those who take drugs and sustain a particular complication may also vary from time to time. Hepatitis, for example, used to be a reliable indicator of heroin dependence, but for a variety of reasons, now seems a much less certain marker.

Because of difficulties such as these, attempts to design indirect indices of drug misuse similar to those designed for alcohol are unlikely to succeed, although specific morbidities can be useful in providing an early warning of new drugs being misused, of geographical spread to new areas and of involvement of new population groups. For example, public health laboratory services in the UK publish a quarterly bulletin giving information on HIV/AIDS.[59] The most recent issue has identified 6% of AIDS cases (1121/17993) being accounted for by heterosexual injecting drug users and a further 2% (311 cases) by homosexual injecting drug abusers. About 10% (3608/42125) of HIV cases were contracted by heterosexual drug abusers and a further 2% (629 cases) by homosexual injectors.

International information on drug abuse

The problems of drug abuse that have preoccupied the UK during the last 30 years have not been confined to this country. There is a world-wide concern about all aspects of drug abuse, although specific drug problems may be of greater importance in some areas than in others.

The European Monitoring Centre on Drugs and Drug Addiction (EMCDDA) was set up in 1993 to provide the European Union and its Member States with 'objective, reliable and comparable information at European level concerning drugs and drug addiction and their consequences'. It is based in Lisbon and became fully operational in 1995. The EMCDDA's main tasks include (a) collecting and analysing existing data; (b) improving data-comparison methods; (c) disseminating data and information; and (d) cooperating with European Union institutions, international partners and with non-European Union countries.[60] The information processed by the Centre focuses on the following areas:

• Demand and reduction of demand for drugs;
• National and European Community strategies and policies;
• International cooperation and the geopolitics of supply;
• Control of the trade in narcotic drugs, psychotropic substances and precursors;

- Implications of the drugs phenomenon for producer, consumer and transit countries.

In much of Europe, the changes in the patterns of drug abuse have been very similar to those in the UK during the same period.[61] Cannabis, for example, became popular in the 1960s in much of Western Europe as did LSD (Appendix 1(c)), although to a much smaller extent. Elsewhere, especially in Sweden, amphetamines were the preferred drugs and their intravenous use has become common and remains a problem today. The influx of illicit heroin into Europe first from South-East Asia, and later from South-West Asia, caused serious problems of opiate dependence in many countries. In Poland, however, the problem was with home-grown heroin, prepared from the straw of opium poppies which were grown quite legally to provide the poppy seeds found in so many Polish dishes.

Other notable trends in drug abuse have been the rapid spread of cocaine and solvent abuse and changes in the pattern of barbiturate abuse. The latter drugs, once the cause of serious problems in several countries, have become less important as they are now prescribed less and heroin has become so easily available. More recently, as in the UK, benzodiazepines have largely taken their place as drugs of abuse often used in combination with other drugs, particularly alcohol.

International audit [62–69]

One way of finding out about patterns of drug use is to investigate the supply situation by obtaining information about the production of drugs and their importation and exportation. In practice, reliable data can only be obtained about licit sources of supply, but a global overview of the situation is maintained by the International Narcotics Control Board (Chapter 12), which collects statistics on drug production and consumption from almost all countries and collates this with information about illicit drug activity internationally. Analysis of this data provides information on the development of new trends in drug consumption and can give early warning of rapidly increasing use that might suggest abuse.

The World Customs Organization (WCO) and the International Criminal Police Organization (Interpol) also have invaluable information on drug trafficking and seizures.

Demand and supply of opiates for medical and scientific purposes

While focusing on the abuse of drugs, it should not be forgotten that many have legitimate and important medical uses. Not least among these are the opiates, which are widely used for the treatment of severe pain, particularly in cancer patients. Despite the increasing use of morphine for this purpose, expansion and diversification of the licit opioid market has been somewhat slow during the last

25 years and has not kept up with the increased requirements expected of a growing population. However, the global consumption of opiates was relatively stable in the five year period between 1995 and 1999, at an annual average of 241.5 tons in morphine equivalent. Thus global licit opioid consumption was 240 tons in morphine equivalent in 1999. Of this, codeine is the most widely used natural opioid used as a cough suppressant and an analgesic with an average annual consumption of around 170 tons in recent years (173.4 tons in 2000), representing about 75% of total licit opiate consumption. Between 1978 and 1998, global codeine consumption increased at an annual rate of only 1–2%. As far as morphine itself is concerned, global consumption for medical purposes was relatively low and stable for many years up to 1984 when it amounted to about 2.2 tons. Since then, it has risen almost 10-fold (20.2 tons in 2000). Global consumption of dihydrocodeine, having stabilized at approximately 30 tons per annum in morphine-equivalent for the last 6 consecutive years, declined in 2000 to 26.5 tons. However, consumption of oxycodone has followed an upward trend, with a gradual increase during the period 1980–95 followed by a sharper increase from a level of 3 tons per annum to 12.8 tons in 1999 and 18.5 tons in 2000. Other semisynthetic or synthetic opioids with significant or increasing consumption levels are buprenorphine, hydrocodone, hydromorphone and fentanyl.[62]

However, these global figures for opiate consumption conceal significant inequity of access to analgesics because morphine and its derivatives are not equally available in all countries in the world. For example, the average per capita consumption of morphine in 1998 in the 10 countries with the highest morphine consumption levels, was 31 g per 1000 inhabitants; in the 10 countries with the next highest consumption levels, the corresponding figure was 16 g per 1000 inhabitants; in the next 60 countries (whose total national morphine consumption exceeded 1 kg), average per capita consumption was only 2 g per 1000 inhabitants. In the remaining 120 countries there was little or no opioid consumption for licit medical purposes.

Total licit global production fluctuates from year to year, according to climatic, social and political conditions. However, global production of opiate raw materials increased steadily from 1996 to 1999 in terms of both the area harvested and the quantity produced. The area harvested fell sharply in 2000 but the total quantity of morphine-equivalent that was produced remained fairly steady (384.3 tons). In 2000, India was the major producer (146.2 tons morphine-equivalent), closely followed by Australia (112.0 tons). Other producer countries are: France (40 tons), Turkey (35.8 tons), Spain (34.8 tons), other countries (15.5 tons). The production of opiate raw materials declined in 2001 and it is predicted that it will reduce further in 2002.

It is important that a balance between production and licit requirements is maintained because this controls the amount of this highly prized drug that is available for diversion to the black market. In fact, the amount of such diversion is small in comparison with the volume of illicit transactions, indicating that international control measures are largely effective for this group of substances. In 1999 and 2000, production exceeded demand by about 160 tons; this permits the maintenance of reserve stock so that opioid analgesic supplies can be maintained even if the crop suffers a major failure.[63]

Medical requirements and availability of psychotropic substances

Just as for opioid drugs, the national supply of psychotropic substances should correspond as closely as possible to medical need. National drug requirements may be assessed in a number of ways, including morbidity rates and regular surveys of consumption, although both methods have their limitations.[58] Comparison of consumption data between countries and regions appears to be a useful indicator and throws up some interesting differences. For example average per capita consumption of benzodiazepines is much higher in Europe than in any other region. Specifically, in 1997–99, consumption of benzodiazepine-type sedative hypnotics in Europe was four times higher than in America, six times higher than in Asia and 25 times higher than in Africa. Similarly, benzodiazepine-type anxiolytic consumption in Europe was one and half times that in America, three times that in Asia and seven times that in Africa. However the consumption of amphetamines and anorectic drugs is about 10 times higher in the USA than in any country in Europe. Again, these intercontinental differences hide significant differences between countries in the same continent. It is worth noting that excessive drug consumption that is medically unjustified and which occurs predominantly in industrialized countries, together with street / parallel / unregulated markets, that occur predominantly in developing countries, have a number of general and country-specific causes and driving forces, of which the most important are their commercial, sociocultural and educational environments. For example newly gained wealth or affluence appears to be associated with quickly growing drug consumption in countries and territories experiencing rapid economic growth, e.g. Malaysia, Singapore, Thailand.[64,65]

The diversion of psychotropic substances

The control of psychotropic drugs under the international conventions has been less successful, resulting in large diversions of these drugs into the illicit market. This has frequently involved drugs such as stimulants, sedative hypnotics and tranquillizers, mainly in developing countries, and suggests that current control mechanisms are inadequate. Moreover, for several years, some parties to the 1971 Convention on Psychotropic Substances (see Chapter 12), have failed to bring

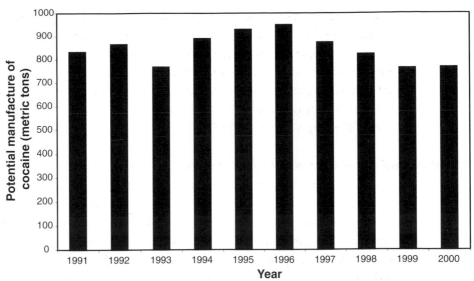

Fig. 2.11   Potential global manufacture of cocaine, 1991–2000. (Source: United Nations Drug Control Programme (UNDCP).)

some of these drugs under the control of national legislation, enabling traffickers to exploit these gaps. Despite these setbacks, the world-wide reduction in stocks of methaqualone in line with declining medical requirements is an example of how the system can work well, and there has been a similar reduction in stocks of the stimulant fenetylline.

Production (Figs. 2.11–2.13)

Global production of illicit drugs can be considered both in terms of the tons of drugs produced and the areas under cultivation. Firstly it is interesting to note that the global area devoted to opium poppy cultivation is at its lowest level since 1988 and was 17% lower in 1999 than in 1990, while the area under coca cultivation has reduced by 14% over the same period. This suggests that efforts at crop eradication and crop substitution are bearing fruit, although this is partly offset by higher yields per acre. The global production of opium has declined from more than 5700 tons in 1999 to an estimated 4700 tons in 2000. This trend is due mainly to a decrease in production in Afghanistan, which accounted for about 69% of global production in 2000 compared with 31% in 1985, 41% in 1990, and 79% in 1999. Opium production in Myanmar accounted for 23% of global production in 2000 while other countries in Asia continued to account for less than 5%, and Latin America for about 3%. Thus, although a record harvest of opium in Afghanistan in 1999 had an impact on global production in 1999, the rate of increase in the 1990s was lower than during the preceding decade.

In 1999 potential heroin production was more than 570 tons and the total

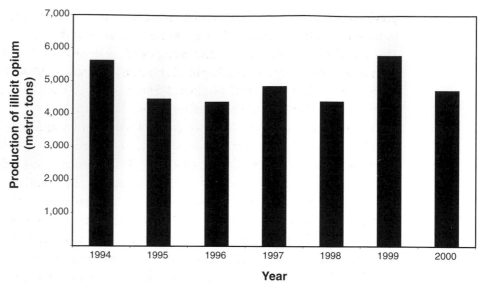

Fig. 2.12   Global production of illicit opium, 1994–2000. (Source: UNDCP, 2001.)

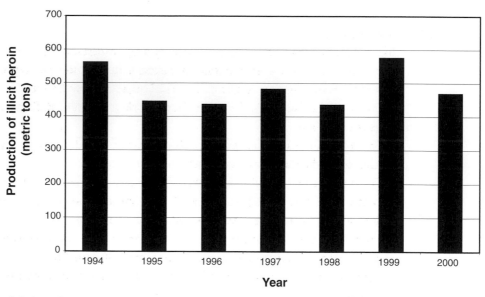

Fig. 2.13   Global production of illicit heroin, 1994–2000. (Source: UNDCP, 2001.)

amount of opiates seized amounted to 85 tons (in heroin equivalent), an interception rate of 15%. Thus the potential availability of heroin to the world market in 1999 was about 500 tons in comparison with 360 tons in 1998 and 400 tons in 2000.

Global illicit coca production was more or less stable in 2000 compared with previous years. Globally, the potential annual manufacture of cocaine is assessed to have fluctuated between 800 and 900 tons per annum throughout the 1990s. This stabilization is the result of decreasing trends in Peru and Bolivia which have been offset by an increase in Colombia. It is estimated that, in 2000, about 75% of cocaine available in the world originated from Colombia, with Peru and Bolivia accounting for 21% and 4% respectively.

Globally, it appears that the production of illicit opium and coca is concentrated in fewer countries than previously and, when viewed as a whole, the total areas under production are remarkably small. Unfortunately, this only serves to emphasize how so small an area can maintain global supplies – and how easily this could be moved, if conditions change in the current areas of production.

In contrast to the opium poppy and the coca bush, cannabis is grown widely all across the world with significant amounts growing wild, particularly in the Commonwealth of Independent States, in the Russian Federation and in Kazakhstan. It is also grown indoors under conditions of intense (hydroponic) cultivation, in many industrialized countries. This has led to tetrahydrocannabinol (THC) concentrations in cannabis increasing from 10% to 30% during the 1990s.

Trafficking (Figs. 2.14–2.20)

The extent of drug trafficking is assessed by drug seizures, which can be measured in terms of their number, the amount seized and the countries reporting them. Using such information, major drug trafficking routes can be identified:

- From Afghanistan, via Pakistan, Iran, Turkey and the Balkans to Western Europe: opiates;
- From the Andean countries of South America to the USA, either directly or via Mexico or the Caribbean: cocaine;
- From Mexico to the USA: cannabis. Global cannabis seizures increased significantly in 1999, reaching almost 4000 tons, an increase of 36% over 1998 and 46% above the average level recorded during the 1990s;
- From Morocco to Spain and other European countries: cannabis resin. Global seizures of cannabis resin amounted to almost 900 tons in 1999 and the main consumer market continued to be Western Europe which accounted for 77% of global volume.

Western Europe remains the primary source of amphetamine and Ecstasy-type substances although, in recent years, Eastern Europe has emerged as an additional manufacturing zone for amphetamine. However, stimulant seizure statistics reflected a decrease for the first time in 1999. The production of Ecstasy-type substances remains more or less concentrated in Western Europe and from there it is trafficked world-wide. The second region where amphetamine is produced, trafficked and consumed in large quantities is East and South-East Asia. Western

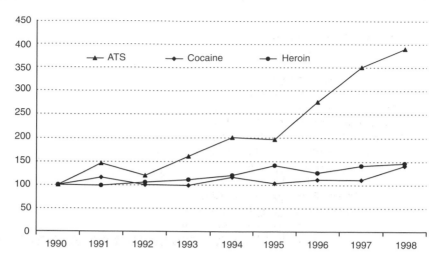

Fig. 2.14   Trends in global seizures of amphetamine-type stimulants (ATS), cocaine and heroin, 1990–98 (index: 1990=100). (Source: UNDCP, 2000.)

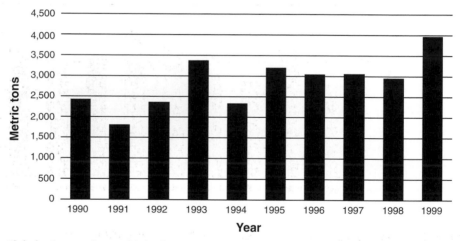

Fig. 2.15   Global seizures of cannabis herb, 1990–99. (Source: UNDCP, 2001.)

Europe and East and South-East Asia have each accounted for approximately 40% of global stimulant seizure volume in recent years and North America for about 20%. However, in 1999 a very large seizure (16 tons) occurred in China.

It is worth noting that, in recent years, there has been a proliferation and diffusion of trafficking and a divergence from these now well-established routes. In particular, various African countries are increasingly linked into the process.

Consumption (Figs. 2.21–2.23)

Estimates of drug abuse in different countries are based on the frequency with which they report drug problems in international monitoring surveys. Drugs

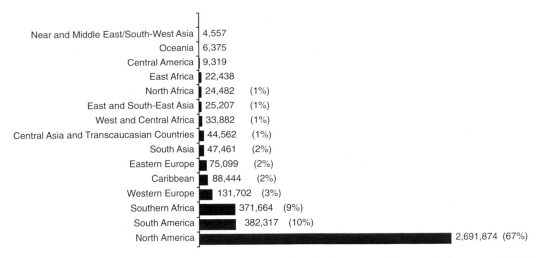

Fig. 2.16   Percentage by region of seizures of cannabis herb in 1999 (kilograms). (Source: UNDCP, 2001.)

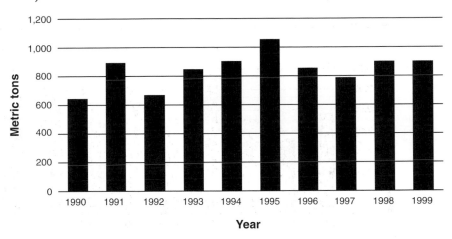

Fig. 2.17   Global seizures of cannabis resin, 1990–99. (Source: UNDCP, 2001.)

come to light as problems because of demand for treatment, emergency room attendances, their use in overdose, drug-related morbidity etc. – as described earlier in this chapter.

Global drug problems

A brief description of drug problems in other parts of the world is helpful in putting the UK's problems into an international perspective. Knowledge of these problems is gained from information about illicit drug production, trafficking and consumption and although individual pieces of information may be of limited value, together they can build up a useful picture.

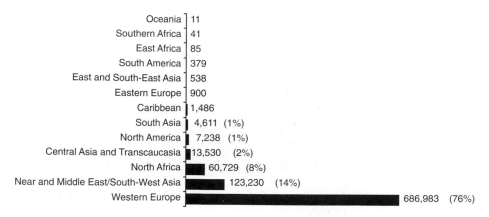

Fig. 2.18   Percentage by region of seizures of cannabis resin in 1999 (kilograms). (Source: UNDCP, 2001.)

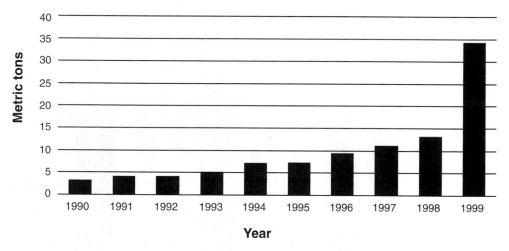

Fig. 2.19   Global seizures of amphetamine-type stimulants (excluding Ecstasy), 1990–99. (Source: UNDCP, 2001.)

Africa

Cannabis is the main problem drug in treatment demand in Africa and there is illicit cultivation in 22 countries in the continent. Indeed, Morocco is the world's largest producer of hashish (cannabis resin) while Nigeria and South Africa are major sources of marijuana. Both forms of cannabis are produced for domestic consumption and for smuggling – primarily to Europe. According to Interpol, 22% of the cannabis herb seizures made worldwide in 2001 were effected in Africa with Morocco as the source of 60–70% of cannabis seized in Europe.

There is a long history of the abuse of psychotropic drugs, particularly stimulants, and particularly in West Africa and this remains a problem, with the bulk of drugs being smuggled in from Europe. Methaqualone is mainly abused in south-

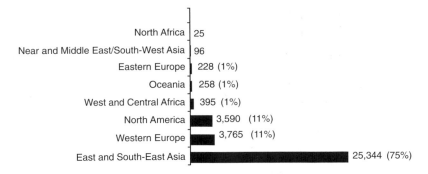

North Africa | 25
Near and Middle East/South-West Asia | 96
Eastern Europe | 228 (1%)
Oceania | 258 (1%)
West and Central Africa | 395 (1%)
North America | 3,590 (11%)
Western Europe | 3,765 (11%)
East and South-East Asia | 25,344 (75%)

Fig. 2.20   Percentage by region of seizures of synthetic-type stimulants (excluding Ecstasy) in 1999 (kilograms). (Source: UNDCP, 2001.)

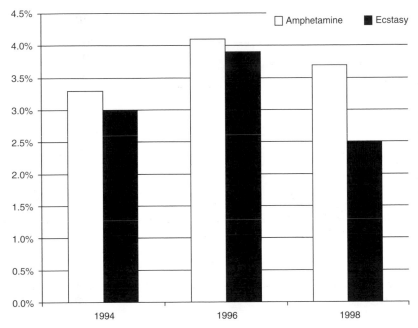

Fig. 2.21   Use of stimulants in Spain. (Source: Observatorío Español Sobre Dragos, *Informé 3*, Madrid, 2001.)

ern and East Africa and to some extent in West Africa. It is estimated that up to 80% of the methaqualone illicitly manufactured world-wide may be abused in South Africa.

However, the abuse of opiates and cocaine is increasing in Africa and, in Egypt for example, where hashish has long been the main problem drug, opiates became prominent in the 1990s, accounting for 45% of all cases in treatment, followed by benzodiazepines (32%). While opiate abuse is beginning to show up on the eastern coast of Africa, down to South Africa, cocaine abuse is more common in

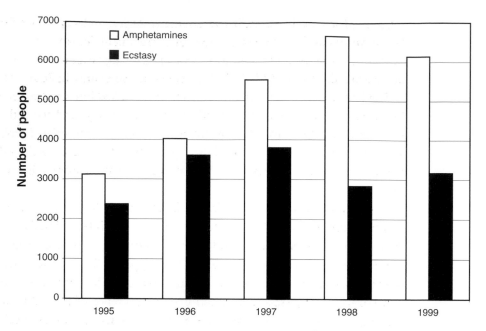

Fig. 2.22   Use of stimulants in Germany (combined result of new and old provinces weighted by size of population), annual prevalence (age 18–59 years), 1995–99. (Source: UNDCP, 2000.)

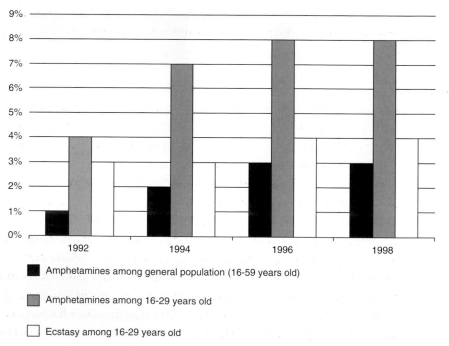

Fig. 2.23   Use of stimulants in the UK (annual prevalence), 1992–98. (Source: Home Office, *Drug Misuse Declared in 1998: British Crime Survey*, 1999.)

western Africa, again extending to southern Africa. Indeed, in the Republic of South Africa cocaine accounts for 15% of all treatment demand compared to only 3% for opiate abuse and the abuse of crack is growing faster than the abuse of any other drug; the abuse of MDMA (Ecstasy) is also spreading in South Africa.

The countries of West Africa are increasingly linked into the trafficking routes for cocaine (and heroin) from South America to Europe and the spillover from these markets is undoubtedly influencing the nature of drug-related problems that are now being reported. In addition, in Nigeria, the use of 'Zakami' (*Datura metel*), a plant that grows wild in some parts of the country, is an emerging problem.

In the Horn of Africa, khat (*Catha edulis*) poses a different problem. Its trade and consumption are not prohibited or controlled by international treaties, and it is grown in Ethiopia, Kenya and Yemen. Although most is consumed locally, freeze-dried and vacuum-packed leaves are shipped to Europe and some countries have introduced national control measures to prevent its importation. Within the Horn of Africa, large scale consumption of khat is reflected in treatment demand.

Drug abuse appears to be increasing in most countries in Africa; specifically, the age of initiation to drug abuse is falling and the number of women and children abusing drugs is growing. Although the rate of injecting drug abuse is still relatively low, this practice is particularly worrying because the prevalence of HIV/AIDs is high in most parts of the continent. In South Africa for example, there has been a 40% increase in the number of injecting heroin abusers over the last 3 years.

South America

Despite significant reductions in the extent of illicit coca bush cultivation in Bolivia and Peru in recent years, the overall capacity of the region to manufacture cocaine does not seem to have been significantly reduced. Indeed, the illicit production, manufacture, traffic and abuse of cocaine is the cause of serious economic and social problems in several South American countries with Colombia, Peru and Bolivia accounting for 98% of global coca leaf cultivation. However, within these three countries there has been a marked shift in production and Colombia, which used to be the smallest producer, is now the largest. The reasons underlying this change are interesting because they demonstrate how several different events interlink. In Peru, which used to be the main source of coca leaves and coca paste for conversion to cocaine hydrochloride in Colombia, government action to curtail illicit cultivation was aided by a fungus infection that destroyed most of the crop. At the same time, air transport of coca paste between these two countries was successfully interrupted, leaving the cocaine laboratories in Colombia without easy access to their source material. However, the ongoing civil war in

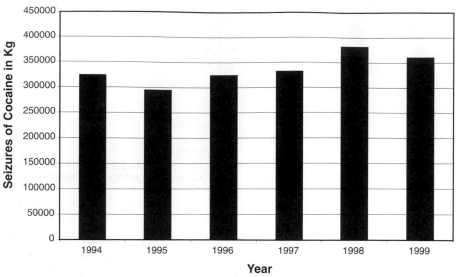

Fig. 2.24   Global seizures of cocaine. (Source: UNDCP.)

Colombia and the consequent political instability facilitated the expansion of domestic cultivation on a large scale and, although the Colombian government has a comprehensive plan including extensive eradication programmes (Plan Colombia), it has not been possible to reduce significantly production of cocaine hydrochloride. Furthermore, rather than exporting all of their coca leaves and paste to Colombia, some is now utilized within Peru and Bolivia for the domestic production of cocaine hydrochloride – although this is on a very small scale in comparison with Colombia, which accounts for 90% of all cocaine hydrochloride seizures in the Andean region (Appendix 1(a)). Seizures of cocaine and its derivatives in Colombia amounted to 64 tons in 1999 and this increased by more than 100% in 2000, with seizures of coca leaf also increasing by almost 200%. In 2000, according to Interpol, the countries in the Andean subregion produced an estimated 700–900 tons of cocaine (Figs. 2.24, 2.25).

With this level of local production, it is not surprising that cocaine-type substances (cocaine hydrochloride, crack cocaine and related products) are the main problem drugs in South America, responsible for 61% of treatment demand and accounting for most drug-related violence and crime. Nevertheless, drug problems in South America are not confined to cocaine. Cannabis is cultivated in most countries, mostly for domestic consumption and, in addition, illicit poppy cultivation has been introduced because the associated profits are higher than those from growing cocaine. Indeed, Colombian heroin production, although small in global terms, is important regionally and has substituted for South-East Asian heroin in the lucrative US market; in the late 1990s, 65% of heroin seized in

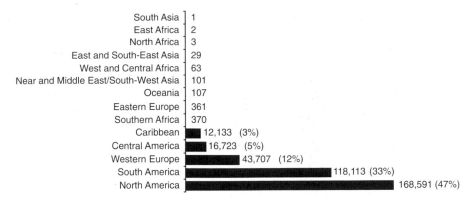

Fig. 2.25   Percentage by region of seizures of cocaine in 1999 (kilograms). (Source: UNDCP, 2001.)

the USA originated in Colombia. Although heroin seizures have significantly increased in recent years in Colombia, the abuse of heroin in most countries in South America continues to be negligible. Argentina and Chile have the highest prevalence of cocaine abuse in the region and it is estimated that in Rio de Janeiro approximately 3000 street children are involved in drug trafficking.

Solvent abuse poses major problems in many South American countries, particularly among the large population of street children in the urban slums. The abuse of tranquillizers is widespread in Peru and Bolivia but there is very little statistical data from other countries. Seizures of MDMA (Ecstasy) have become more common and this substance has become fashionable among the youth of several countries in the region.

Central America and the Caribbean

The strategic location of the Caribbean region has led to its being an important transit area for cannabis and cocaine being imported into North America and, to a lesser extent, into Europe. Indeed, transit traffic in cocaine constitutes the greatest drug problem in the region and this has led to domestic drug problems too, with an associated increase in drug-related deaths. It is estimated that nearly half of the cocaine that arrives in the USA each year (approximately 375 tons) comes through Central America and the Mexican land corridor. However, drug traffickers have diversified their activities from cannabis and cocaine to psychotropics (mainly MDMA) and heroin. There is a long history of cannabis cultivation in the region and this continues today; most is intended for local use leading to high levels of problem drug use, although some is smuggled into the USA and Canada.

North America

Cannabis is the most commonly abused drug in North America, with significant amounts being smuggled in from South and Central America. It is estimated that there were over 19 million cannabis users in the USA alone in 1997, and cannabis accounts for 23% of demand for treatment. This reflects the high concentration of THC in cannabis that is grown hydroponically in the USA and Canada which leads to higher morbidity rates, and also the fact that some cannabis users have treatment orders as a result of court cases. The use of cannabis increased only slightly in 1999 which was considered not to be significant by the US Household Survey. Both annual and monthly prevalence rates in the USA are significantly below the levels reported a decade earlier and, as there has not been a significant increase in Canada and Mexico, cannabis use in North America as a whole can be considered stable. However, the use of cannabis in combination with stimulants is increasing in both the USA and Canada, including the practice of smoking 'blunts' (cannabis packed in cigar wrappers) which are dipped in phencyclidine (PCP).

Although cannabis remains important in terms of the numbers using it, cocaine is the main problem drug in North America, accounting for more than 40% of treatment cases. Several multi-ton seizures of cocaine were made in the Pacific in 2001, including one that amounted to 13 tons – the largest maritime seizure ever made. Against this background, it is perhaps not surprising that the estimated number of cocaine users in the USA alone in 1997 exceeded 4 million, including more than 1 million crack cocaine users. Despite these large numbers, the overall level of cocaine abuse in the USA remained unchanged between 1998 and 1999, with an annual prevalence rate of 1.7% of the population aged 12 years and above, and a monthly prevalence rate of 0.8%. All of the indicators show a decline in cocaine use in the USA with the rate of cocaine abuse among adolescents declining by 14% during the same period. The serious nature of cocaine-related problems is reflected in the demand for treatment that it generates, although there are signs that the latter is also decreasing. Thus in 1997, 222 000 people were treated for cocaine abuse (29% of all demand for treatment) compared with 267 000 people (40%) in 1992. Most demand for treatment was related to crack cocaine.

In Mexico, the abuse of cannabis, cocaine and heroin is increasing although it has remained at a level that is considerably lower than in Canada and the USA.

In comparison with cannabis and cocaine, relatively small numbers abuse opiates in North America. For example, in 1997, there were an estimated 597 000 abusers in the USA; nevertheless they generated more than 25% of all demands for treatment. Overall, heroin abuse has declined – due, it is claimed, to the effect of educating people about the harmful consequences of drug abuse.

In addition to methamphetamine abuse, which is widespread in western Canada and the USA, MDMA of Western European origin is increasingly being abused by young people in North America. It has spread beyond the 'rave' scene to other settings and other age groups such as schoolchildren as young as 12 years old. There has also been an increase in abuse of other 'club' drugs such as ketamine and

GHB (gamma hydroxy-butyric acid) which have just come under international control. In addition, there is evidence of increasing abuse of methylphenidate by adolescents, who steal or purchase tablets from children being treated for attention deficit hyperactivity disorder (ADHD). Potentially, this is a huge source of stimulant drugs for abuse because of the massive increase during the 1990s in the diagnosis and pharmacological treatment of ADHD in the USA, which now accounts for 90% of global manufacture and consumption of this drug (> 13 tons per year). Altogether, in the USA in 1999, nine million persons over the age of 12 years had abused prescription drugs, including opioids, depressants and stimulants and widely prescribed oxycodone and amphetamine-type stimulants are finding their way to illicit markets.

East and South-East Asia

South-East Asia continues to be a major producer of illicit opium, with poppy cultivation taking place mainly in Myanmar. Indeed, in 2001, following the ban on opium cultivation in Afghanistan, Myanmar accounted for most of the world's illicit poppy cultivation. Although the Lao People's Democratic Republic is another large producer, the area under opium poppy cultivation has been successfully reduced in China and in the northern provinces of Viet Nam. There have also been major changes in the trafficking patterns in this part of the world. Traditionally, the so-called Golden Triangle was the major outlet for heroin from South-East Asia, with Thailand accounting for almost 60% of all seizures in the late 1980s. A decade later, this had fallen to only 5%, but seizures in the People's Republic of China increased from 4% to 77% over the same period. Most of these seizures were of heroin that had originated in Myanmar and were intended for the North American market, via Hong Kong and Taiwan, although more is now used within China itself. Interestingly, a poor opium harvest in 1999 led to a sharp downturn in seizures in the region. The abuse of opiates remains a serious problem, in particular in China, the Lao People's Republic, Myanmar and Viet Nam and there continues to be a relationship between trafficking in heroin and the prevalence of heroin abuse.

Interestingly, HIV of the same viral subtype is found to have spread along the length of the trafficking route; this is closely linked to the spread of drug abuse by injection. At the same time many new drug abusers are increasingly choosing to ingest substances such as MDMA (Ecstasy) in tablet form or to inhale the fumes of methamphetamine. The wide availability of and increasing illicit demand for amphetamine-type stimulants has been confirmed by the number of seizures, which has increased sharply in the region since the end of the 1990s. A new development is the increasing abuse of ketamine in dance clubs in some cities in South-East Asia.

Stimulant abuse is common in several countries in East Asia, most notably Japan, the Republic of Korea and the Philippines, where methamphetamine is the main problem drug, accounting for more than 90% of treatment demand. In Thailand too, where opiates have long been the main problem drug, the number of methamphetamine users is now thought to exceed the number of heroin users. Recently there have been sharp increases in the number of MDMA abusers in some countries in the region. Most of the MDMA has been manufactured in European countries but some laboratories in the border area between Myanmar and Thailand may already be manufacturing relatively inexpensive MDMA for local abuse (Appendix 1(d)).

South Asia

The opium poppy is cultivated legally in India, and small quantities are diverted into illicit channels. At one time, far greater problems were posed in this region by transit traffic in heroin from South-West and South-East Asia. However, this appears to have been reversed and, over the last decade, seizures of heroin and morphine in India fell by over 60%. Nevertheless it is estimated that there are about 3 million people abusing opiates in India, representing a prevalence rate of 0.5%. Heroin abuse has been accompanied by increased evidence of HIV infection. Heroin abuse is also a serious problem in Nepal and Sri Lanka, and has been reported in urban slums in Bangladesh. Buprenorphine is abused in a number of countries in the region and, in Bangladesh, its abuse by injection largely accounts for the increasing number of individuals who abuse drugs by injection.

There is large-scale cannabis cultivation in parts of Sri Lanka, while Nepal remains an important source of cannabis resin for countries in Europe as well as India.

Cocaine abuse remains very limited in South Asia although the number of seizures has increased in recent years, particularly in India.

Growing abuse of psychotropic substances has been reported by every country in the region and, on average, about 10% of all drug abuse in India involves prescription drugs. Although there has been a decline in the illicit manufacture of methaqualone in India, the seizure of tablets of Indian origin has been reported in South Africa; methaqualone abuse has also started to spread in those African countries that serve as transit points. There has been a significant increase in the flow of ephedrine into Myanmar from India and flow of methamphetamine through the traditional heroin route from Myanmar to India – an indication that the abuse of amphetamine type stimulants may become a problem in India.

West Asia

Afghanistan and neighbouring parts of Pakistan appear to be the main sources of large quantities of cannabis resin that is smuggled into Europe along various

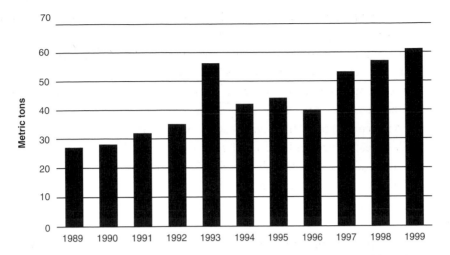

Fig. 2.26   Global seizures of heroin and morphine, 1989–99. (Source: UNDCP, 2000.)

trafficking routes. There is also considerable illicit traffic in cannabis in CIS member states, with cannabis growing wild over extensive areas in Kazakhstan and in the Russian Federation. The illicit cultivation of cannabis in the Bekaa valley in Lebanon, which had been eradicated in the early 1990s, was resumed in 2001.

As well as being involved in the production of cannabis, Afghanistan accounted for 79% of global opium production in 1999. The combination of drought and the implementation of successful programmes reduced its production by 28% in 2000 to about 3300 tons, with a significant impact on the world market. However, it is estimated that Afghanistan holds stockpiles equivalent to 2–3 years' supply. A decree in July 2000 totally banned the cultivation of the opium poppy in Afghanistan, which led to a major reduction in new supply. Production by Afghanistan in 2001 is estimated to have been in the region of 200 tons, which is comparable to the amount of opium produced in the mid-1980s. However, opium poppy cultivation increased again at the end of 2001. At the time of writing, there is uncertainty about the future contribution of Afghanistan to the global illicit market.

For many years Afghanistan has been the main source of opium and heroin for its neighbouring countries (Iran, Pakistan, India, Central Asia) as well as for Eastern and Western Europe. The trafficking routes have proliferated steadily – via Iran, Turkey, Pakistan, Central Asian republics – and more than half of the world seizures in 1997–98 were made in South-West Asia, with Iran accounting for 9% of seizures in 1987–88 and 42% in 1997–98. In 1999 Iran accounted for 80% of the total amount of opium seized in the world and 90% of the total morphine seized. For the first time it seized more heroin than any other country in West Asia (Figs. 2.26, 2.27). These increases reflect a number of different factors: increased production of opium in Afghanistan, the increasing use of Iran as a trafficking route and

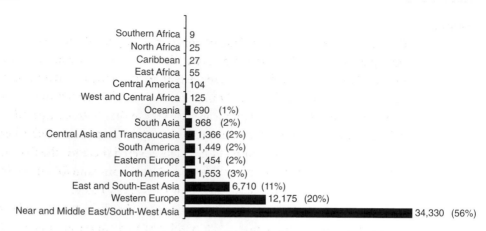

Fig. 2.27   Percentage by region of seizures of heroin and morphine in 1999 (kilograms). (Source: UNDCP, 2001.)

the increased efforts of the Iranian authorities to stop trafficking. The effects of the increased production of heroin locally (Appendix 1(a)) are only too clear in Pakistan, where opium abuse used to be the most common form of substance abuse; this was superseded by heroin abuse by inhalation ('chasing the dragon'), which in turn, since the late 1990s, has been overtaken by the injection of heroin as the preferred route of administration. The ban on opium cultivation in Afghanistan has had a significant impact on the illicit market for opium, leading to a relative shortage of opium and opium residue in Iran and Pakistan. Although the purity of heroin decreased, the proportion of heroin abusers continued to increase since heroin was more available than opium.

The abuse of benzodiazepines, often in conjunction with opium and heroin, is widespread in Afghanistan and Pakistan. The flow of illicit drugs, in particular heroin from Afghanistan, in the countries of Central Asia increased in 2001 where there are indications of a serious increase in the number of drug abusers and a rapid increase in drug abuse by injection. In Uzbekistan, for example, the number of injecting drug abusers doubled between 1998 and 2001 and, in Tadjikistan, Turkmenistan and other Central Asian Republics, there has been a rapid increase in the number of people abusing opiates.

Although the extent of cocaine abuse and trafficking in West Asia remains insignificant, numerous seizures of small quantities of cocaine have been made in countries in the eastern Mediterranean area, in Lebanon, Israel and Turkey. The abuse of stimulants, including amphetamine, metcathinone and fenetylline (Captagon) is endemic in parts of West Asia and in 2000 there were significant seizures of MDMA in Israel and Turkey and CIS member states.

Europe

Cannabis remains the main drug of abuse in Europe, with huge quantities being smuggled in from Africa and West Asia. There is also a more local 'indoor' source in the Netherlands and, to a lesser extent in the UK, Germany, Scandinavian countries and Eastern Europe. This is associated with varieties of cannabis with a very high THC content, ranging from 10–30% in the 1990s compared with 5–7% before then. Albania has continued to be a major source of cannabis herb and, in 2001, illicit opium poppy cultivation was discovered there for the first time. It has been estimated that there are more than 22 million cannabis users in Europe, representing 3.5% of the population aged 15 years or more.

The cultivation of poppy for culinary purposes has been traditional in countries such as Poland and some of the CIS republics; a recent development is the use of poppy straw to prepare an abusable extract of opium ('Kompot' or 'liquid heroin'). This practice has long been endemic in Poland but is now spreading to other countries. However, Afghanistan is the major source of illicit heroin in Europe, accounting for 70–90% of the market there. The turmoil in the former Yugoslavia and the opening of borders of former socialist countries has led to considerable diversification in trafficking routes.

France uses buprenorphine for long-term opioid maintenance treatment on a wider scale than most other countries and has about 55 000 injecting drug users on buprenorphine maintenance on the basis of a belief in its lower abuse liability and low diversion potential. All physicians are allowed to prescribe buprenorphine for maintenance therapy. However, recent studies show that a significant proportion self-inject and more stringent regulation has been recommended. Some other European countries have now also started to use buprenorphine for the treatment of opioid dependence. However, whereas in France this is within a 'low threshold' policy, Germany has adopted a 'high threshold' policy.

A newer problem is the increasing traffic in and abuse of cocaine in Europe, most of it originating in Colombia. The main entry points are in Spain and the Netherlands, which together accounted for 63% of all European cocaine seizures in 1997–98. However, increasingly, other cities in Portugal, the UK, Germany, Italy, Belgium, France and Switzerland are being used as well as seaports in the Nordic and Baltic countries – demonstrating yet again the continuing diversification of trafficking routes. This illegal market has, until now, been less well organized than in North America, but there is some evidence emerging of the growing involvement of criminal groups from Colombia, Russia and Italy. Despite this growth, cocaine seizures in Europe still account for less than 11% of the global total (Fig. 2.28).

Other important drug problems in Europe include the illicit manufacture of amphetamines (Appendix 1(b)) and of hallucinogenic amphetamines (e.g.

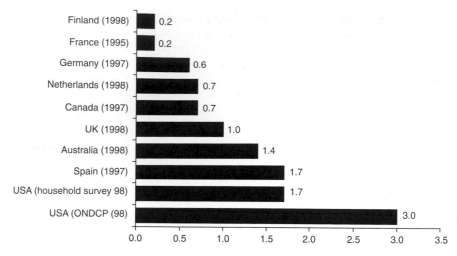

Fig. 2.28   Cocaine abuse in North America, Australia and Europe, annual prevalence (percentage of youth and adult population). (Source: UNDCP, 2000.)

Ecstasy), which are traditionally used by young adults in nightclubs and all-night parties. A worrying trend of the late 1990s is the extent to which the production of Ecstasy is spreading outside Europe, to Israel, South America, South Africa and Australia and also the extent to which European Ecstasy is trafficked outside Europe with huge increases reported from several regions. Seizures of MDMA and similar synthetic drugs increased during 2000 throughout Western Europe, with a large number of seizures in France, Germany and the UK. In France, for example, the number of seizures doubled during 2000. However seizure statistics for 2000 show a decline in amphetamine seizures for the second successive year.

Finally, it should be noted that the long-standing drug problems in Europe have been compounded by the political changes there. Factors such as the relaxation of border controls, both in and between Western and Eastern Europe; growing international trade with CIS countries, which frequently lack appropriate drug control mechanisms and where drug-associated crime is increasing at a formidable rate; the war in former Yugoslavia and the consequent political instability; all make the traffic in illicit drugs much easier to conduct than formerly.

Oceania

Although substance misuse does not constitute a major problem in many parts of this region, Pacific islands are increasingly being used as transit points. Cannabis is cultivated in Australia and New Zealand but in addition to this some is smuggled in from Papua New Guinea and from South-East Asia. Heroin comes in from Asia while cocaine originates in South America. Illicit trafficking in and abuse of heroin continue to be serious problems in Australia. Seizure data indicate that it remains

Table 2.10. Estimated global number of drug abusers (annual prevalence) in the late 1990s

	Illicit drugs of which:	Cannabis	Amphetamine-type stimulants[a]	Cocaine	Opiates of which:	Heroin
Global (million people)	180	144.1	28.7	14	13.5	9.2
As percentage of global population	3.0	2.4	0.5	0.2	0.2	0.15
As percentage of global population age 15 years and above	4.2	3.4	0.7	0.3	0.3	0.22

[a]Amphetamines (methamphetamine and amphetamine) and substances of the ecstasy group.
As drug users frequently take more than one substance, the total is not identical with the sum of the individual drug categories.
Source: UNDCP, DELTA.

widely available, that its price has fallen and its purity remains high. With the exception of Australia, the availability of and demand for cocaine are low in this region. In 2000 the total amount of cocaine seized in Australia reached a record high level, more than twice the total amount seized in 1999. Stimulants such as amphetamine are manufactured illicitly, mostly for markets in Australia and New Zealand, while hallucinogenic amphetamine abuse is becoming more common, mostly under the control of gangs of motorcyclists. The demand for MDMA has been increasing in New Zealand.

Summary

The global picture of drug abuse seems to have two major components which used to be quite distinct, but which have now merged. There is the traditional form of drug abuse using crude plant material which contains only a low concentration of active drug. This type of abuse by adults of opium, coca and cannabis has been going on for centuries and continues today in the areas where the plant is grown. In addition, there is the abuse of highly potent, synthetic or semisynthetic substances mostly by young people in industrialized countries who often abuse several different types of drugs. It is this latter type of drug abuse that has been spreading rapidly world-wide and that has been given back to the countries where the traditional use of the drug originated. Thus Thailand and Pakistan now have a major problem with heroin abuse and Bolivia with cocaine abuse.

It is now apparent that the distinctions that used to be made between producer/ supplier and consumer countries no longer have any meaning. Consumer countries are simultaneously suppliers of other drugs, while those that supply the world

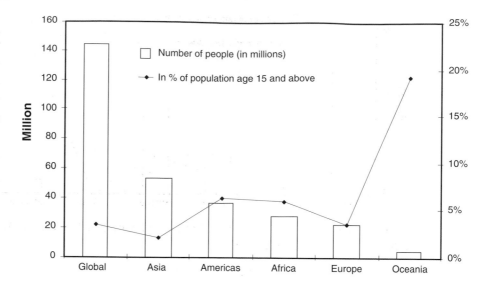

Fig. 2.29   Estimated number of cannabis abusers (annual prevalence) in the late 1990s. (Source: ODCCP, *World Drug Report 2000.*)

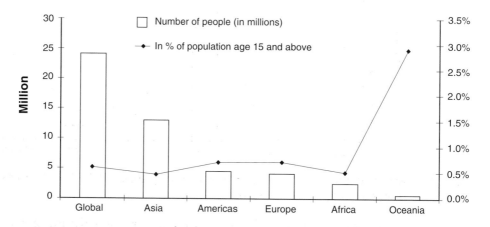

Fig. 2.30   Estimated number of amphetamine abusers (annual prevalence) in the late 1990s. (Source: ODCCP, *World Drug Report 2000.*)

markets themselves import drugs. The notion of transit countries is also some-what out of date as they are often involved in both supply and consumption too. Underlying this 'globalization' of the drug abuse problem is the internationaliz-ation of, and cooperation between, the powerful drug cartels. They are skilled at identifying the weak links in the international drug control measures – countries that are not parties to the international drug control treaties (see Chapter 11) and those that have not fully implemented their provisions. They take advantage of

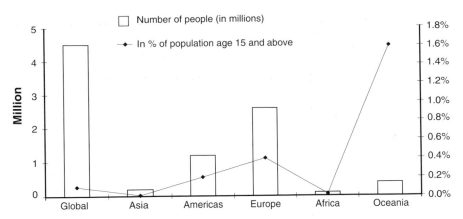

Fig. 2.31   Estimated number of Ecstasy abusers (annual prevalence) in the late 1990s. (Source: ODCCP, *World Drug Report 2000.*)

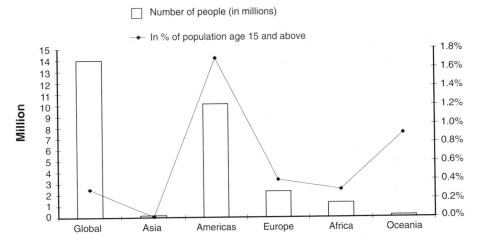

Fig. 2.32   Estimated number of cocaine abusers (annual prevalence) in the late 1990s. (Source: ODCCP, *World Drug Report 2000.*)

countries that, because of political unrest, terrorist activities or civil war, are unable to ensure governmental control over some parts of their territories and to maintain adequate law enforcement, customs and pharmaceutical control.

Certainly as drug abuse spreads throughout the world, the target population is definitely the young. At first it was predominantly young males that became involved – often students – and drug use often became associated with protest movements. It soon spread, however, to involve those from deprived social backgrounds as well, and to involve nearly as many females as males.

When these broad trends in the patterns of drug abuse are considered against a background of global demographic trends, it is possible to make some guesses about what will happen to drug abuse in the future. It seems likely, for example, in

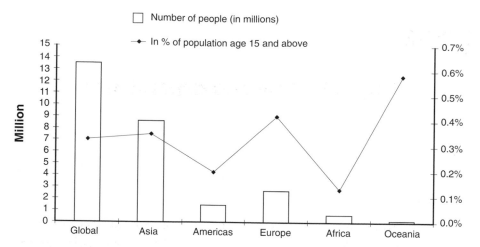

Fig. 2.33   Estimated number of opiate abusers (annual prevalence) in the late 1990s. (Source: ODCCP, *World Drug Report 2000.*)

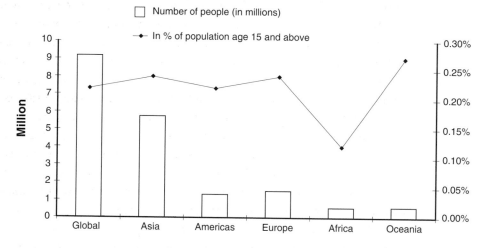

Fig. 2.34   Estimated number of heroin abusers (annual prevalence) in the late 1990s. (Source: ODCCP, *World Drug Report 2000.*)

industrialized countries, with a falling birth rate and an aging population, that there will be an increase in drug abuse by the elderly, which is most likely to involve prescribed drugs. In contrast, in many poor countries with an exploding birth rate, there will be a massive increase in the juvenile and young adult population just at the time when illicit drug abuse is becoming entrenched. Never has there been a greater need for effective, preventive action.[62–69]

Drugs of abuse and dependence

Opioids

The parent drug of this class is opium, obtained from the opium poppy *Papaver somniferum*, which grows in large areas of South-East Asia and the Middle East (Turkey, Iran, Afghanistan, Pakistan, Myanmar, Thailand, etc.), as well as in other parts of the world (e.g. Poland). After the poppies have bloomed, the unripe seed capsules are incised with a knife and the milky exudate that oozes out is allowed to dry. It becomes a brown, gummy mass which is scraped by hand from the seed capsule. This, dried further and then powdered, is crude opium which may be smoked in special pipes, chewed, or inserted as small pellets into cigarettes. 'Prepared' opium is a boiled-down aqueous solution of raw opium, prepared for opium smokers by repeated boiling and filtration to extract all possible opium and to remove all impurities. The final boiling leaves a thick, sticky paste.

Crude opium contains a number of chemical compounds called alkaloids which possess the same or similar properties as opium. The major alkaloids obtained from opium include morphine (10% by weight) and codeine. Traditionally, the term 'opiates' was used to describe these naturally occurring substances and the semisynthetic drugs that are derived from them (e.g. diamorphine/heroin) while 'opioids' described totally synthetic drugs (e.g. dextromoramide, methadone, pethidine) with similar properties. More recently, with the discovery of so-called opioid receptors that bind all of these drugs, the term 'opioid' has come to be used as the collective description of the naturally occurring alkaloids, semisynthetic derivatives and totally synthetic drugs. However, in general usage 'opiates' and 'opioids' are often used interchangeably.

Effects

The outstanding property of opioid drugs is their ability to relieve pain. It was this that inspired Thomas Sydenham in 1680 to say 'Among the remedies which it has pleased Almighty God to relieve his sufferings, none is so universal and so efficacious as opium', and it is this property that continues to set opioids among the most useful therapeutic agents available today.

The analgesic action of opioids is probably due not only to their direct action at one or more sites within the nervous system,[1] but also to the way in which they make pain seem more tolerable. This in turn is related to the euphoriant effect of opioids – their ability to induce a state of mental detachment and of extreme well-being. However, in some individuals, some opioids induce not euphoria, but the opposite mental state of dysphoria.[2,3]

Opioids also have a sedative effect on the nervous system causing inability to concentrate, drowsiness and sleep. In addition they depress the respiratory centre, the part of the brain that controls breathing, so that respiration becomes progressively slower and more shallow. Higher doses cause respiratory arrest (breathing stops), unconsciousness and death. Opioids also control cough by suppression of the cough reflex.[1]

A stimulant effect on specific areas of the brain may cause nausea and vomiting and also a very characteristic sign of opioid administration, the constricted, or 'pin-point' pupil of the eye (miosis). The action of opioids on the muscles of the intestines causes constipation, accounting for their use in antidiarrhoeal preparations.

Tolerance

Tolerance develops to many, but not all, of the effects of opioids so that increasing doses have to be taken to obtain the desired effect (of analgesia or euphoria, for example). Ultimately a regular user may be consuming a daily dose of opioid many times greater than that which would kill an opioid-naive individual. If drug administration is interrupted in a regular user, by a period of imprisonment, for example, tolerance is lost and if the old dose is suddenly resumed, it leads to intoxication which may be fatal. Cross-tolerance occurs between different opioids; this means that theoretically it does not matter which opioid an addict takes. If he or she cannot obtain the preferred opioid (usually heroin), a more easily available one may be substituted.

Finally, it should be noted that tolerance does not usually develop to miosis (pupil constriction) so that regular opioid users retain the characteristic, pin-point pupils.

Physical dependence

Physical dependence on opioids develops if drug administration is regular and continuous, but becomes apparent only if regular administration of the drug ceases. While opioids are being taken there is no objective evidence of the existence or the severity of physical dependence. If drug administration is interrupted, or if other drugs that oppose the action of opioid (opioid antagonists) are given, the symptoms and signs of the abstinence syndrome develop (Table 3.1). Its severity is an indication of the degree of physical dependence that had developed.

Table 3.1. Opiate abstinence syndrome: symptoms and signs

Grade 0
Drug craving
Anxiety
Drug-seeking behaviour

Grade 1
Yawning
Sweating
Running eyes and nose
Restless sleep

Grade 2
Dilated pupils
Gooseflesh ('cold turkey')
Muscle twitching
Hot and cold flushes; shivering
Aching bones and muscles
Loss of appetite
Irritability

Grade 3
Insomnia
Low-grade fever
Increased pulse rate
Increased respiratory rate
Increased blood pressure
Restlessness
Abdominal cramps
Nausea and vomiting
Diarrhoea
Weakness
Weight loss

The severity of physical dependence depends on the particular opioid being taken, the dose and the duration of chronic administration. As tolerance to opioids develops, the daily dose is increased, and the severity of dependence increases too. However, it reaches a maximum or 'ceiling' for each drug, beyond which further increases of dose have little effect on the degree of physical dependence as measured by the severity of the abstinence syndrome. Each opioid has its own capacity to induce physical dependence; drugs such as codeine and dextropropoxyphene, even in very high dosage, do not cause physical dependence to match that caused by morphine or heroin.

Opioid abstinence syndrome

The signs and symptoms of opioid abstinence may be graded (Table 3.1) to indicate the different stages and the severity of the abstinence syndrome. This grading is clinically convenient, if somewhat arbitrary, as the symptoms and signs of any particular grade may not all be present simultaneously.

The severity and timing of the abstinence syndrome, its onset, peak and duration of symptoms, all depend on a variety of factors, including which opioid was being taken, its dose and for how long it had previously been taken. Generally, an opioid with a short duration of action, such as heroin, has an abstinence syndrome of earlier onset, shorter duration and greater intensity than a longer-acting drug such as methadone. Similarly, the larger the dose of opioid, the more intense the symptoms and signs of withdrawal. The personality of the addict, his or her expectations and the ability to tolerate the discomfort of withdrawal are also important.

The opioid abstinence syndrome, although extremely unpleasant, is rarely life endangering in an otherwise healthy person. It is, however, very distressing for the individual concerned who can think of nothing except an overwhelming and urgent need for opioids. Consciousness is unimpaired so that the addict is painfully aware of what is happening and feels generally so wretched that he or she may say anything, whether true or not, in an attempt to receive earlier attendance from a doctor and quicker relief of symptoms.

The abstinence syndrome can be immediately relieved by the administration of any opioid; not necessarily the one that has been taken previously. Other sedative drugs may provide partial symptomatic relief, but will not reverse the symptoms and signs of the abstinence syndrome in the way that opioids do.

Psychological dependence

Psychological dependence on opioids is severe and accounts for the desire and craving for drugs that eventually disrupt the addict's life, which may become wholly devoted to obtaining more drugs. Unfortunately, psychological dependence does not end when drug withdrawal has been achieved. It persists long after the pain and discomfort of the abstinence syndrome have abated and accounts for the high relapse rate of opioid addiction.

Opioid receptors

Although opiates, in one form or another, have been used by humans for centuries, it is only during the last 25 years or so that considerable progress has been made in understanding their mechanism of action. The first step was the discovery within the brain of opioid receptors.[4] These are specialized sites on the cell membranes, with a very specific shape to which opioids bind. Drugs which fit the receptor and activate it are called agonists. Other drugs, which bind to the receptor but do not activate it, thereby preventing other opioids from binding to it, are called antagonists. There appear to be three major categories of opioid receptors, designated mu (μ), kappa (κ) and delta (δ), with subtypes of each category.[5] Each type of receptor is activated only by opioids conforming to its particular shape and therefore has different sensitivities to different opioids and develops selective tolerance to different opioids. They are distributed differently throughout the central and peripheral nervous systems, with the μ and δ receptors concentrated in areas involved in the transmission and perception of pain and the control of respiration.

That most important property of opioids – the ability to induce analgesia – appears to be mediated by the supraspinal activation of μ receptors and by the activation of κ receptors in the spinal cord. Other opioid effects related to μ receptor stimulation include euphoria, miosis, respiratory depression and reduced gastrointestinal motility. In contrast, stimulation of κ receptors is often associated with dysphoria. The effects of δ stimulation have not yet been fully established but all three types of receptor are found on presynaptic nerve terminals and have an inhibitory effect on transmission across synapses, by reducing the release of neurotransmitters.[6]

Opioid receptors have now been identified not only in humans but in all vertebrates examined so far, as well as in some invertebrates. An obvious implication is the existence of naturally occurring (endogenous) opioid(s) in these animals,[7,8] as it seems very unlikely that a receptor which is so widely distributed in the Animal Kingdom should have as its only ligand a substance of plant origin. To date, three distinct 'families' of endogenous opioid peptides have been identified:

1 The enkephalins (Met- and Leu-enkephalin) which are composed of five amino acids each, identical except for the fifth amino acid;
2 Beta-endorphin with 31 amino acids;
3 Dynorphin with 17 amino acids.

They are coded by separate genes, occur in different anatomical cell groups in the brain and may have distinct biological functions. All three known classes of opioid peptides are found in one or more sites that are known to be part of the body's intrinsic system for pain modulation under physiological conditions, and it appears that endogenous opioids activate the δ receptors which modify transmission in pain pathways.[1]

What then of dependence on opioids? Do changes occur in this system of opioid transmitters and receptors to account for certain individuals becoming (or remaining) opioid abusers? So far, progress in this field has been limited, although interesting: tolerance develops to endogenous opioids in vitro and in vivo and cross-tolerance develops between morphine and endogenous opioids. An abstinence syndrome can be precipitated by the opioid antagonist, naloxone, in rats dependent on endogenous opioids and, even more interesting, human beta-endorphin, administered intravenously to opioid-dependent individuals produces a marked improvement in the abstinence syndrome. Its beneficial effect on diarrhoea, vomiting, tremor and restlessness lasts for several days, suggesting that endogenous opioids may well be deficient in the abstinence syndrome, their production perhaps having been suppressed by the administration of opioid drugs. Assays of endogenous opioids in dependent individuals have, however, produced inconclusive results. This might be because the assays were done on opioid peptides in blood, and it is unlikely that blood levels reflect levels in the central nervous system. Furthermore, blood levels may be less important than rates of biosynthesis and turnover.

Studies on opioid receptors have similarly been unhelpful as neither the number of receptors nor their properties (ability to bind opioids) seem to be altered in the dependent state. However, it appears that chronic (agonist) action at μ or κ receptors can cause tolerance and physical dependence within the neural systems which are affected by these receptors. Thus withdrawal of the agonist drug – that is, one which binds to and activates the receptor – after a long period of administration, or its displacement by a drug with antagonist properties, precipitates a withdrawal syndrome which is quite specific for the receptor type. μ receptor physical dependence, for example, produces severe withdrawal manifestations with intense drug-seeking behaviour. There appears to be little cross-tolerance between the different receptors so that a drug with κ agonist properties cannot suppress the withdrawal syndrome caused by a μ agonist withdrawal.[9]

Different opioid drugs

There have been many attempts to separate, by means of chemical modification, the desirable analgesic action of opioids from their dependence-producing property. Many new drugs have been synthesized either by changing the chemical structure of naturally occurring opioids, or by synthesizing completely new drugs. These are often introduced with extravagant claims that they do not cause dependence. As their use becomes more widespread, however, their dependence-producing potential usually becomes more obvious, and so far all of the clinically useful opioid analgesics share similar structural characteristics and possess a general similarity of action. Any differences between them tend to be differences of degree rather than of nature.

In particular, it has been found that morphine and all the closely related morphine-like opioid drugs have a high affinity for the μ receptor (which was, in fact, named μ for the drug morphine). They have less affinity for κ and δ. Thus all of these drugs can be described as μ agonist opioids, or as prototype μ agonists.

Their low affinity for κ receptors probably accounts for the fact that they rarely cause hallucinations or dysphoria.

Morphine

Morphine is a naturally occurring opioid alkaloid. It was first isolated in 1803 and was named after Morpheus, the Greek god of sleep and dreams, because of its sedative, sleep-inducing properties. Although it can be taken orally, the development of the hypodermic syringe facilitated its widespread clinical use. It is still frequently used in the management of severe pain, but suffers from the drawback that it often causes nausea and vomiting. Perhaps for this reason it is not particularly popular as an illicit drug of abuse or dependence.

Papaveretum (omnopon)

Papaveretum is a mixture of morphine and other opium alkaloids. It is often used for preoperative medication, but is rarely abused, and then usually by members of the medical profession.

Diamorphine (heroin)

Diamorphine was first marketed as the 'heroic' (or powerful) cure for morphinism. It was claimed to be nonaddictive, but this soon proved to be untrue. Illicit production occurs in large quantities in fairly primitive 'laboratories' close to the source of opium. This requires the chemical acetic anhydride and international controls on the availability of this substance is one way of controlling illicit heroin production. Once manufactured, heroin, in the form of a white powder, is much easier to transport and smuggle than opium and is now available in most places in the world, its source varying according to local and international politics (Appendix 1).

Heroin is a more potent analgesic than morphine, and is used medicinally in a dose of 5–10 mg 4 hourly. It is less likely to cause nausea or constipation and has a much greater euphoric effect. Perhaps for these reasons it is the drug of choice of most opioid-dependent individuals. It may be taken orally or administered by intramuscular, intravenous (mainlining) or subcutaneous (skin-popping) injection. A popular way of taking it is called 'chasing the dragon', in which the heroin is heated on a piece of foil and the resultant fumes are inhaled. This method, although just as likely to cause dependence, is safer than injecting, which is associated with a number of serious complications. Because 'chasing the dragon' is easier and safer than injecting, it may encourage those who would not have dared to inject, to experiment with heroin and subsequently become addicted. In time, as the individual's habit becomes larger and therefore more expensive to maintain, or if heroin is in short supply (and again more expensive), it is more likely to be taken by intravenous injection. This delivers all the available drug right into the bloodstream providing the addict with the best 'kick' ('high', 'rush') possible for that dose of heroin.

Methadone (physeptone)

Methadone is a synthetic opioid analgesic with a long duration of action (about 24 hours) so that once daily administration to an opioid-dependent individual is sufficient to prevent the onset of the abstinence syndrome. For this reason it is the opioid most frequently prescribed in the treatment of opioid dependence. Although also available in tablet or injectable form, it is usually prescribed as methadone mixture which is unsuitable for injection and has little black market value. Most addicts receive between 30 and 80 mg methadone daily. Despite cross-tolerance between the different opioids, opioid-dependent individuals claim to be able to tell the difference between heroin (their drug of choice) and methadone, which does not give them the euphoric 'high' that they seek. In addition, methadone often causes increased sweating, a side effect which does not seem to occur with other opioids and for which there is no physiological explanation.

Although methadone is a potent analgesic it is rarely prescribed for this purpose.

L-alpha acetylmethadol (LAAM)

LAAM is a derivative of methadone and was initially developed as an analgesic. Although it has been available since 1993, it has only recently been licensed in the UK for the treatment of opioid dependence. It is very long-acting and can prevent opioid withdrawal symptoms for more than 72 hours. Hence, as an alternative to methadone, it requires only three times weekly administration. However, the onset of action is much slower than with methadone and the time taken to reach maintenance levels is correspondingly longer (8–20 days, compared with 5–8 days for methadone). It is reputed to have less euphoriant effect and, because it is metabolized more slowly, it produces a long, even plateau in blood levels. The danger of overdose is increased due to cumulative toxicity if illicit opioids are used and the treatment of opioid-dependent individuals with LAAM should always be under the supervision of a specialist.[10]

Pethidine (Pethilorfan, Pamergan; meperidine, Demerol in USA)

Pethidine is a synthetic opioid widely used clinically as an analgesic in childbirth and postoperatively. It is a frequent drug of abuse for opioid-dependent individuals in the medical or related professions.

Dipipanone (with cyclizine as Diconal); dextromoramide (Palfium)

These are two synthetic opioid drugs which, during the late 1970s and early 1980s, were very popular with opioid-dependent individuals in the UK.[11] They were often prescribed by independent doctors whom the addicts consulted because the drug dependence treatment units (DDTUs) were (and are) unwilling to prescribe the injectable opioids which the addicts sought. Although intended for oral use, Diconal tablets were often crushed, dispersed in water and injected, resulting in the expected complications of self-injection. Tablets surplus to requirement were sold on the black market. Because of the increasing frequency of dependence on dipipanone, it was brought under the same control as heroin and cocaine, so that only doctors with a licence from the Home Office may now prescribe dipipanone to addicts. More recently, because illicit heroin is widely available on the black market, dextromoramide and dipipanone have become less attractive to addicts.

Dextropropoxyphene (Doloxene)

Dextropropoxyphene is a mild opioid analgesic derived from methadone, but with less addictive and analgesic potential. Although available in capsule form, it is much more popularly combined with paracetamol as Distalgesic. Abuse of Distalgesic is not uncommon and overdose is particularly serious, because of the combination of hepatotoxicity due to paracetamol and respiratory depression due to dextropropoxyphene.

Codeine

Codeine is another alkaloid found in crude opium. It is a much less effective analgesic than morphine and is therefore used for the relief of mild to moderate pain only; it is often combined with aspirin or paracetamol. Its constipating effect is utilized in the treatment of diarrhoea and it is also used as a cough suppressant. It must not be forgotten, however, that codeine and its derivatives (pholcodine, dihydrocodeine) are opioids with a liability for abuse and dependence, albeit less than that of morphine or heroin. As some of these preparations (e.g. codeine phosphate and pholcodine syrups and linctuses) are available without prescription, 'over the counter', opioid addicts can buy them easily. They sometimes use them to supplement supplies from other sources or to prevent the onset of the opioid abstinence syndrome.

Opioid antagonists and agonist-antagonists

During the search for effective opioid analgesics free from the dependence liability of morphine and heroin, new drugs have been identified which are devoid of analgesic properties, and which oppose or antagonize the respiratory depressant effects of opioids. These drugs (e.g. naloxone, naltrexone) are known as opioid antagonists.

It is now understood that their properties arise because they bind to opioid receptors but do not activate them. For example, naloxone is a μ receptor antagonist which also binds to a lesser degree to κ and δ receptors. It antagonizes the effect of morphine and related drugs by displacing them from their receptor sites. However, binding to receptors and activating them is not an 'all or none' phenomenon. Some drugs, described as partial agonists, may bind to a receptor but not activate it fully. In so doing they may displace a full agonist, thus reducing or 'antagonizing' its effects. Thus partial agonists are commonly described as agonist-antagonists and, unlike the full agonists, their effects do not increase in proportion to the dose administered, but appear to have a 'ceiling'. It is also important to appreciate that as well as having different affinities for the different receptor sites, a particular drug may be a full agonist at one receptor and an antagonist or partial agonist at another.

Because classical opioid dependence appears to be so firmly linked to μ receptor activity, it seems likely that a partial μ agonist might have less abuse and dependence liability than the prototype μ agonists. Much recent research has therefore concentrated on the mode of action of different drugs at the different receptor sites and a number of agonist-antagonist opioids are now available. However, the abuse liability of a particular drug is more than the mathematical sum of its activity at several receptor sites. Other factors, such as its solubility, the ease with which it enters the nervous system and the firmness with which it binds to the receptor site may all be important. Unfortunately, there is no single animal species which can provide a completely reliable model for predicting the abuse and dependence liability of opioid drugs and these problems usually become apparent only when the drug has become widely available for use by humans outside the laboratory setting.

Pentazocine (Fortral)

Pentazocine is a partial μ agonist with agonist activity at κ receptors too. It may precipitate withdrawal symptoms in opioid-dependent individuals. When administered by injection it is a more potent analgesic than codeine or dihydrocodeine, but it sometimes causes hallucinations and thought disturbance, presumably because of κ receptor activation. High doses may also cause respiratory depression, raised blood pressure and tachycardia.

Some of the psychotomimetic effects of pentazocine are not blocked by naloxone, suggesting that it also affects other receptor sites within the brain. Two such receptors are the phencyclidine receptor site and a receptor which also binds to dopaminergic drugs. This interaction of pentazocine with both opioid and nonopioid receptors perhaps accounts for the range of side effects associated with its use.

Although the dependence liability of pentazocine is less than that of morphine or heroin, cases of abuse and dependence have been reported and in certain places abuse became widespread. In some places in the USA, for example, pentazocine abusers used to add crushed tablets of the antihistamine tripelennamine, which is known to enhance the reinforcing and analgesic effects of pentazocine, to crushed tablets of pentazocine and inject this mixture, known as 'Ts' and 'blues', subcutaneously or intravenously. The effect was said to be indistinguishable from the 'rush' or 'high' caused by heroin and lasted 5–10 minutes; this practice has become less common. Repeated injection of this mixture may cause convulsions. However, the non-μ actions of pentazocine at other receptors, which cause progressive increases in dysphoria and other undesirable subjective effects, tend to limit its abuse potential.

Self-injection with pentazocine causes characteristic fibrotic changes in the skin and muscle.

Buprenorphine (Temgesic, Subutex)

Buprenorphine is a partial μ receptor agonist with a long duration of action because of tight receptor binding. It is an effective analgesic which is administered sublingually (under the tongue) or by injection. Oral administration is unsatisfactory because the drug is metabolized very rapidly by the liver.

An unusual property of buprenorphine is that, after chronic administration, the onset of the abstinence syndrome is delayed. There are few, if any, signs of withdrawal during the first 48 hours and only mild signs from the 3rd to the 10th day. In one study, more marked withdrawal effects were reported on the 14th day. Heroin addicts dependent on a small dose of opioid can be transferred on to buprenorphine, which can be withdrawn fairly easily because of the delayed onset of the abstinence syndrome. While they are taking buprenorphine, the subjective effects of self-administered heroin are reduced, presumably because buprenorphine is acting as an antagonist on the μ receptors.[12,13] Thus theoretically the rewarding properties of heroin are impaired and the likelihood of future administration should be reduced. However, if buprenorphine is given to individuals dependent on large doses of opioids, its antagonist properties precipitate the onset of withdrawal symptoms. Despite early optimism, the abuse potential of buprenorphine is causing concern. Opioid addicts are clearly able to identify buprenorphine as an opioid when it is administered in sufficient quantity (0.8–2.0 mg) and there are reports of abuse and dependence from several countries. Tablets intended for sublingual administration are being crushed and injected by addicts.

It is interesting that naloxone in doses of up to 4 mg does not precipitate the buprenorphine withdrawal syndrome, although higher doses can reverse the effects of buprenorphine and should theoretically precipitate withdrawal in dependent individuals.

Buprenorphine has recently been licensed in the UK for the treatment of opioid addiction but has been used more extensively in France over the last few years as substitution therapy for opioid addiction. The doses are very much higher than for analgesia, an average dose for an opioid addict being in the range of 8–12 mg daily.[14]

Butorphanol

Butorphanol is an agonist-antagonist opioid with affinity to μ and κ receptors. Like other μ agonists it has analgesic and respiratory depressant properties and like other κ agonists it can cause psychotomimetic symptoms. It can precipitate symptoms of withdrawal when administered to morphine-dependent individuals. Although butorphanol has positive reinforcing properties in animals, there have been only occasional reports of dependence upon it. This is probably because, like pentazocine, it tends to produce undesirable subjective effects, rather than the sought-after euphoria induced by morphine and other prototype μ agonists.

Nalbuphine (Nubain)

Like pentazocine, nalbuphine is a partial μ agonist with a high affinity for κ receptors but it is less likely than pentazocine to cause dysphoric symptoms. It can reverse the respiratory depression caused by full μ agonists and precipitates the withdrawal syndrome if given to individuals dependent on these drugs. Experienced morphine users usually recognize nalbuphine as morphine-like, and after a period of chronic administration of nalbuphine, naloxone precipitates a mild withdrawal syndrome. So far, however, there have been very few cases of abuse.

The drugs mentioned in this section do not form a comprehensive list of opioid analgesics. They were selected because they are common, or fairly common, drugs of abuse or dependence, or because they are used to treat opioid dependence. Other opioids are available and may more rarely be the subject of abuse; dependence upon them is similar to that described in this section.

Sedative hypnotics

Sedative hypnotic drugs can be conveniently classified into two groups:
1 The barbiturates, which dominated this area of therapeutics for half a century;
2 The more modern nonbarbiturates which were developed because of all the disadvantages and dangers of the earlier drugs.

Since the 1960s the benzodiazepine nonbarbiturates have been of overwhelming importance in terms of the number of prescriptions issued and the number of individuals receiving these drugs. However, both barbiturate and nonbarbiturate sedative hypnotic drugs have many similar pharmacological properties.

Effects

Sedative hypnotic drugs have a depressant effect on the brain. In small doses they relieve anxiety, inducing a sense of relaxation. In a slightly larger dose they cause drowsiness and sleep, shortening the time until its onset and prolonging its duration. Even when taken in small, hypnotic doses, these drugs have a 'hang-over' effect the following day, often leaving the patient feeling 'drugged' and drowsy. Slowing of performance occurs, measurable under laboratory conditions and manifesting itself in daily life by an inability to concentrate, to make quick decisions or to carry out tasks as quickly and efficiently as usual. Driving a car or operating machinery after taking them the night before may therefore be hazardous.

In excessive doses, such as those taken in deliberate self-poisoning, sedative hypnotic drugs cause a prolonged deep coma with respiratory depression (slow, shallow breathing) and low blood pressure. Death, due to respiratory failure, may occur quite suddenly and unexpectedly with barbiturates, although an overdose of a benzodiazepine alone is unlikely to be fatal.

Tolerance

Tolerance develops rapidly to some of the effects of sedative hypnotics drugs. After taking them for a few days or weeks, the patient is again taking longer to go to sleep and the duration of sleep returns to normal. To achieve the original and desired improvement in sleep the dose has to be increased. After a while the habitual user may show little sign of sedation and may be sleeping for only an hour or two more than usual on a night-time dose that would be profoundly sedating for anyone not used to taking these drugs.

Tolerance also develops to the anxiolytic effect of these drugs, so that they rapidly become ineffective if prescribed in a normal, therapeutic dosage. It is dangerous to increase the dose, however, because this increases the risk and the severity of physical dependence.

Physical dependence

Physical dependence on sedative hypnotics drugs is characterized by the manifestations of the abstinence syndrome, and by a state of chronic intoxication which develops in those who habitually take very large doses.

It is difficult to be precise about the dose or the duration of consumption of these drugs necessary to cause physical dependence, because it varies according to the criteria of dependence that are adopted. For example, withdrawal of therapeutic doses of benzodiazepines given for only a few weeks may lead to anxiety, depression, tremor and somatic symptoms. Because these are often similar to the symptoms of the original illness, it used to be thought that they were evidence that treatment should be continued for longer. Now, however, it is appreciated that they are genuine symptoms of withdrawal (rebound) and that during this stage, anxiety may increase to an intensity above that in the predrug period. This type of rebound phenomenon is particularly marked in patients stopping medium-acting benzodiazepines, such as lorazepam, and the importance of prescribing these drugs for short periods only (2–4 weeks) is stressed. Another form of rebound anxiety occurs, particularly with shorter-acting compounds, when there may be interdose anxiety associated with falling blood levels as the time for the next dose approaches.

Similarly, withdrawal of the normal hypnotic dose of sedative hypnotics drugs may precipitate nightmares, broken sleep with vivid dreams and increased REM (rapid eye movements) which may persist for several weeks. This is known as rebound insomnia and its appearance following the abrupt withdrawal of benzodiazepine hypnotics suggests that even modest doses can cause mild physical dependence. Higher doses (say diazepam 60 mg daily) taken over a period of 1–2 months would be sufficient to cause noticeable physical dependence with many of the signs listed below, although there is considerable individual variability of response and some people may be vulnerable to severe consequences of withdrawal, having taken a much smaller dose.

Sedative hypnotics abstinence syndrome

The symptoms and signs of sedative hypnotic withdrawal develop progressively. They include weakness, anxiety, tremor, dizziness, insomnia, impaired concentration, loss of appetite, nausea and vomiting, dysphoria, headaches, incoordination, heightened sensory perception, lethargy, depersonalization, tiredness, blurred vision, facial burning sensation, hot and cold feelings with sweating and muscle aching. All of these symptoms may be experienced when patients are withdrawn from long-term treatment (3 months) with a benzodiazepine administered in normal dosage.[15–17] Perceptual symptoms vary considerably from patient to patient and can be very distressing. It should be emphasized that these symptoms are genuine manifestations of withdrawal and are not a resurgence of the original condition for which the sedatives were originally prescribed; thus patients who were prescribed benzodiazepines for nonpsychiatric reasons may experience perceptual symptoms, anxiety and insomnia when their medication is stopped. The abstinence syndrome usually begins within 2 days of drug withdrawal although it may be delayed for over a week; it may occur despite dose tapering, but usually subsides over a period of a few weeks.

If larger doses of sedative hypnotics have been taken, withdrawal will lead to an increased pulse rate (more than 100/min) with a further increase (of more than 15/min) on standing. Standing is also associated with a fall in blood pressure. There is muscle twitching and tremor, increased reflexes and dilated pupils. These unpleasant, but not particularly dangerous symptoms may, however, be followed by *grand mal* convulsions (fits) which may progress to life-threatening status epilepticus, in which the patient has fits continuously. A psychotic state, resembling alcoholic delirium tremens in which the patient is very agitated and confused and suffers auditory and visual hallucinations may also occur.

Although the sedative hypnotic withdrawal syndrome is the same in its broad outline regardless of which class of drug is responsible, there are differences between different drugs. Fits and delirium are more common after barbiturate withdrawal, while milder symptoms such as anorexia, agitation and insomnia are more common after benzodiazepine withdrawal.[18]

Chronic intoxication

Because there is an upper limit to tolerance to sedative hypnotic drugs and because dependent individuals often increase their daily consumption beyond this point, chronic intoxication is a common feature of their condition. This resembles intoxication with alcohol and is characterized by difficulty in thinking, slow and slurred speech, poor comprehension and memory, and emotional lability. Irritability and moroseness are common. It is interesting that abusers seem less aware of their mood changes and behavioural impairment when taking high doses of benzodiazepines than with high doses of barbiturates.

Chronic intoxication with barbiturates, which is now less common than formerly, is accompanied by neurological symptoms and signs: nystagmus (jerky, involuntary movements of the eyes), double vision, squint, difficulty in visual accommodation, unsteadiness and falling. With larger doses the increasing sedation leads to the subject falling, sleep and eventually respiratory depression and death. In fact, one of the main risks of chronic barbiturate use and the consequent development of tolerance is that the gap between the intoxicating dose and the fatal dose is dangerously reduced.

Psychological dependence

Psychological dependence on sedative hypnotic drugs is manifested by craving for the drug and by drug-seeking behaviour. Animals will perform an action repeatedly to obtain these drugs, thereby demonstrating their reinforcing properties. However, sedative hypnotics are less powerful reinforcers of behaviour than are opioids or cocaine, and undoubtedly cause less severe psychological dependence.

Although psychological dependence on barbiturates has long been recognized, it was thought at first that benzodiazepines were free from this disadvantage. However, the considerable difficulty experienced by many benzodiazepine users in managing without their drugs, even when they were withdrawn gradually to prevent the onset of physical symptoms, has contradicted early beliefs and hopes. It is now recognized that benzodiazepines can and do cause psychological dependence and that this is closely related to the dose that is taken and the duration of administration.[19] For this reason the indications for prescribing them are now defined very strictly, and it is recommended that they should be prescribed in the smallest effective dose for a period that does not usually exceed 4 weeks.

Different sedative hypnotic drugs

Barbiturates

Barbiturate drugs are all derived from a single chemical substance, barbituric acid. The first to be synthesized was barbitone (Veronal) which was introduced into clinical practice in 1903 when it was welcomed as the solution to one of man's oldest and most intractable problems – insomnia.

Over the years many different barbiturates have been synthesized. Some very short-acting barbiturates are administered intravenously for the induction of general anaesthesia (e.g. thiopentone, methohexitone). Other, long-acting compounds such as phenobarbitone and methylphenobarbitone are used to treat epilepsy. Neither of these two types of barbiturates have been involved in problems of abuse and dependence and concern has centred on barbiturates of medium duration of action which used to be prescribed for the treatment of anxiety or insomnia. These include amylobarbitone, butobarbitone, pentobarbitone and quinalbarbitone. The similarities between all of these drugs are more striking than their differences.

Nonbarbiturate, nonbenzodiazepine sedative hypnotics

Because of the disadvantages and dangers of barbiturates and particularly their dependence liability and their serious effects when taken in overdose, many attempts were made to synthesize safer sedative hypnotics. These include drugs such as meprobamate (Equanil), glutethimide (Doriden), dichloralphenazone (Welldorm) and methaqualone which, when they were introduced, were hailed, like the barbiturates before them, as an answer to the prayer for a safe hypnotic. Clinical experience, however, revealed that their effects on the nervous system are similar to those of barbiturates, that tolerance develops together with physical and psychological dependence. When taken in overdose all of these drugs show features of poisoning similar to those of barbiturate overdose although some, such as glutethimide, which is no longer marketed in the UK, are particularly dangerous. Methaqualone used to be available in combination with an antihistamine (Mandrax) and became a very common drug of abuse. None of these drugs is important therapeutically now.

Benzodiazepines

Because the above drugs were no more satisfactory than barbiturates, the search continued for safer and better alternatives. The benzodiazepines were introduced into clinical practice in the 1960s and an enormous number have now been synthesized. Like barbiturates they possess powerful antiepileptic properties, although they are rarely used in the long-term treatment of epilepsy because their effectiveness wanes within a few months. However, a benzodiazepine (diazepam or clonazepam) is the drug of choice for the emergency treatment of the life-threatening condition of major status epilepticus. In addition, benzodiazepines have muscle relaxant properties permitting their use for the relief of muscle spasm or spasticity. They differ from earlier sedative hypnotics drugs in being much safer when taken in overdose. Indeed, very large doses of benzodiazepines rarely cause sufficient respiratory depression to kill the patient unless another drug or alcohol has been taken simultaneously. Their safety in overdose is a very important property in societies where deliberate self-poisoning with psychoactive drugs has become very common.

The main advantage of benzodiazepines over older drugs in this class is their ability, in low doses, to relieve anxiety without causing undue sedation. This was undoubtedly the basis for their early popularity, when their potential for producing dependence was not appreciated, and a vast range of benzodiazepines were synthesized. Their similarities are more striking than their differences, which mostly depend on their duration of action. The early benzodiazepines (e.g. diazepam, chlordiazepoxide) are long-acting drugs, mainly because they are converted in the body to active metabolites such as desmethyldiazepam which itself has a half-life of 72 hours or more. These drugs have the disadvantage that they often cause a prolonged hangover, leaving the patient feeling 'drugged' for some time. For this reason, shorter-acting benzodiazepines (e.g. lorazepam, oxazepam) were developed, which bypass desmethyldiazepam in their metabolic pathways and which are more suitable as daytime anxiolytics and as hypnotics with minimal hangover.[19] However, these short-acting drugs cause rapid rises and falls in blood levels so that withdrawal phenomena are more common and patients may crave the next tablet to relieve their distressing symptoms. Dependence on them often seems more severe and more difficult to treat than dependence on benzodiazepines with a longer duration of action,[20] although there is insufficient scientific evidence that a particular benzodiazepine is any better or worse than any other, in terms of therapeutic effectiveness or dependence liability.[21]

Flunitrazepam (Rohypnol)

Flunitrazepam has recently emerged as a drug of abuse that is giving rise to particular concern. It is a potent sedative hypnotic which gives an increased feeling of power and self-esteem, leading to a belief that everything is possible. It may be associated with loss of episodic memory and impulsive violence, particularly when taken with alcohol. It is often used as a cheap way of becoming intoxicated.[22]

Flunitrazepam has gained notoriety as the 'date rape drug', with men accused of slipping it into the alcoholic drink of unsuspecting women victims and then sexually abusing them. The drug is colourless, odourless and tasteless and leads to drowsiness, impaired motor skills and, importantly, anterograde amnesia. This makes it difficult to obtain accurate information about the alleged sexual abuse. It is therefore recommended that if a woman who appears intoxicated complains of sexual abuse, a urine specimen should be analysed for flunitrazepam.[23,24]

Cross-tolerance

It is not surprising that cross-tolerance develops between different barbiturates and that any barbiturate can be taken to prevent or treat the abstinence syndrome caused by withdrawal of another. It is perhaps less expected that a considerable degree of cross-tolerance also exists with other central nervous system depressants such as alcohol, benzodiazepines and other nonbarbiturate hypnotics including chlormethiazole. The existence of this cross-tolerance emphasizes the intrinsic similarities of all of these drugs, whatever their differences in terms of chemical structure, etc.[19,25]

The discovery of separate benzodiazepine receptors in human brain tissues may go some way towards explaining the differences that do exist. These receptors are associated with the receptor sites for the neuroinhibitor γ-aminobutyric acid (GABA) and benzodiazepines appear to act by promoting the depressant effect of GABA on the brain, thus inducing sedation and sleep. It is interesting that the benzodiazepine receptor is just one component of a large, macromolecular structure which has binding sites not only for benzodiazepines but also for barbiturates and GABA and that all three receptor sites appear to influence channels in the cell membrane for chloride ions. In particular, benzodiazepines increase the frequency of GABA-induced opening of the chloride channels and, in the absence of GABA, they are ineffective. Both benzodiazepines and sedative barbiturates increase GABA binding – an observation that may underpin some of their clinical similarities.

The effects of benzodiazepines in relieving anxiety and in blocking seizure activity is correlated with their affinity for receptor sites and, in the light of knowledge gained from the study of opioid receptor sites, it is not surprising that benzodiazepine antagonists have been identified, such as flumazenil, that compete with agonist drugs by occupying the receptor sites and blocking their action. Partial agonists have also been identified, that occupy the receptors but have only a limited action, as well as inverse agonists, which have opposite effects on the receptors to those induced by benzodiazepines and can cause seizures and anxiety.[26]

There are two subtypes of benzodiazepine receptor (BZD_1 and BZD_2, or omega$_1$ and omega$_2$) which are widely but differentially distributed throughout the central nervous system, with high densities in the cerebral cortex, the limbic system and the cerebellum. In addition 'peripheral-type' receptors have been identified both in nonneural tissue as well as the central nervous system.

Stimulant drugs

Amphetamine

Amphetamine is the general name given to a class of synthetic drugs that are similar in effect to a substance produced by the body called adrenalin. Adrenalin acts as a transmitter in part of the nervous system known as the sympathetic nervous system, which prepares the body for 'fight or flight', releasing sugars stored in the liver and increasing heart and respiration rates. Amphetamines, because they mimic many of the effects of adrenalin, are known as sympathomimetic amines. They appear to act by releasing the neurotransmitters noradrenalin and dopamine, by inhibiting their reuptake and perhaps also by a direct agonist action on the receptor sites for these two chemicals. There is extensive illicit manufacture of amphetamine and methamphetamine (Appendix 1).

The least potent of the amphetamines is amphetamine sulphate, which was marketed in 1932 as a nasal decongestant in the form of an inhaler (Benzedrine). It was soon realized that one of the side effects of Benzedrine was sleeplessness and it was thus that the stimulant effect of amphetamine was revealed.

Amphetamine sulphate is in fact a mixture of two forms of amphetamine, chemically indistinguishable and differing only in the direction in which they rotate plane polarized light. Dextrorotatory amphetamine (D-amphetamine) is approximately twice as powerful a central stimulant as the racemic compound which contains both forms of amphetamine, and three to four times as potent as laevorotatory amphetamine (L-amphetamine).[27]

Effects

Amphetamine is a powerful central stimulant producing an elevated mood and making the user feel energetic, alert and self-confident.[28] Task performance that has been impaired by boredom or fatigue is improved, accounting for the popularity of amphetamine among students working for examinations. Feelings of hunger and fatigue are reduced and there is increased talkativeness, restlessness and sometimes agitation. Some individuals may, however, become anxious and irritable.[29] Because it is a sympathomimetic drug, amphetamine causes increased heart rate and blood pressure, palpitations, dilated pupils, dry mouth and sweating; L-amphetamine has a greater effect on the cardiovascular system than D-amphetamine.

Acute intoxication with amphetamine is characterized by dizziness, sweating, chest pain, palpitations, hypertension and cardiac arrhythmias. Body temperature may be raised and convulsions often occur.

Tolerance

Tolerance develops to some but not all of the effects of amphetamine. Those taking it for its euphoric, mood-elevating effect find that they have to escalate the dose progressively to maintain this effect and may take 250–1000 mg daily. However, because they have also become tolerant to its cardiovascular effects they do not suffer from adverse side effects. Because tolerance also develops to the appetite-suppressant effect of amphetamine, it is not effective in the treatment of obesity. It is, however, useful in the treatment of narcolepsy, a rare condition in which the sufferer keeps falling asleep suddenly and inappropriately; tolerance does not develop to the awakening effect of amphetamine and narcolepsy remains one of the few therapeutic indications for amphetamine (10–60 mg daily). Amphetamine and its derivatives have a paradoxical effect on hyperkinetic children, reducing their antisocial behaviour and increasing their attention span. As tolerance does not develop to these effects, amphetamine is sometimes used in the management of this condition,[27] although the effect of long-term treatment is not clear.

In addition to the development of tolerance, amphetamine can also produce sensitization, which is sometimes called 'reverse tolerance'. It has been observed in animals, when single daily doses of the drug that do not, at first, cause hyperactivity or stereotyped behaviour, can start to induce this behaviour if injections continue over a period of several weeks. This effect is believed to be mediated by the release of dopamine in the striatum (part of the mid-brain) and it has been suggested that this is the basis of the stereotyped behaviour that is sometimes observed in amphetamine and cocaine addicts.

Cross-tolerance develops between different amphetamines, but not between amphetamine and cocaine, despite their many similarities.

Physical dependence

Although chronic amphetamine users may escalate their dose until they are taking large quantities, the existence of physical dependence is disputed. After long-term use, or after a binge of drug-taking lasting a few days, abrupt withdrawal is commonly followed by feelings of fatigue, depression and hunger, and a need for sleep (the 'crash'). Although these may be the manifestations of a withdrawal syndrome it has been suggested that they are the normal reaction to the lack of sleep and food that occurs with chronic amphetamine use.[30] Depression at this time may be so severe that suicide is a real risk.

Psychological dependence

Psychological dependence on amphetamine undoubtedly develops and chronic users experience intense craving and exhibit drug-seeking behaviour. This craving may last, with varying intensity, for several weeks, responding to emotions and to drug-related stimuli. Laboratory experiments on animals confirm that amphetamine has powerful reinforcing properties.

Adverse effects

The most serious consequence of amphetamine abuse is a psychotic illness, which may be difficult to distinguish from schizophrenia. It is characterized by paranoid delusions and by auditory and visual hallucinations. It usually develops if amphetamine has been taken for a long time and the dose has been escalated. It is particularly common if methylamphetamine is injected, but can occur with oral use and may even develop after a single, oral dose of amphetamine. The symptoms usually remit within 1 week of drug withdrawal.

Another complication of chronic amphetamine abuse is automatic, stereotyped behaviour in which some action such as tidying a handbag, fiddling with a radio or touching/picking at the skin on the face or extremities may continue for hours at a time. Scratching or picking at the skin is often associated with tactile hallucinations and with delusions of being infested with parasitic insects.

Amphetamine-type stimulants

Since the introduction of amphetamine into medical practice many other drugs have been synthesized for their stimulant or appetite-suppressant effects. Methyl-amphetamine, an injectable amphetamine, was available in the 1960s, but was withdrawn from retail pharmacies when there was a veritable epidemic of intravenous methylamphetamine abuse, with many cases of psychosis. Benzphetamine was used for the treatment of obesity because of its appetite-suppressant properties, but problems of dependence soon became apparent. Since then a range of drugs have been produced. Most are chemically similar to amphetamine, have rapidly become drugs of abuse and have been brought under strict control. They include methylphenidate (Ritalin), phenmetrazine (Preludin), diethylpropion (Apisate), phentermine (Duramin) and mazindol (Teronac). Slight modifications of chemical structure have produced drugs such as fenfluramine and chlorphentermine with less stimulant properties, but their role in the long-term management of obesity remains questionable.

Methylphenidate

Methylphenidate warrants special mention because of the recent upsurge in its prescription. This is reflected by the increase in its global (licit) manufacture from 2.8 tonnes in 1990 to 15.3 tonnes in 1997. This is predominantly due to increased consumption in the USA, which accounts for about 85% of total world production, but the same pattern is occurring in other countries too. For example, manufacture and importation for consumption has increased in Spain (484%), UK (277%), New Zealand (107%) and The Netherlands (64%).[31]

This growth is because methylphenidate is increasingly being prescribed in the treatment of attention-deficit disorder (ADD) and its variant, attention-deficit hyperactivity disorder (ADHD). These are now the most commonly diagnosed childhood behaviour disorders occurring most frequently in boys, aged 6–14 years and characterized by inattention, impulsivity and sometimes hyperactivity. There is evidence that methylphenidate is effective at reducing these symptoms in the short term, while children continue to take medication. However, because of the difficulty of separating this condition from unacceptable/undesirable behaviour due to underlying social problems, there is growing concern that methylphenidate is now being used as a pharmacological solution to complex and difficult underlying relationship and parenting problems. These concerns are heightened by inexplicable differences between different physicians in their rates of prescribing. For example, in some schools up to 20% of children may be receiving methylphenidate, while in others none do. This is particularly worrying when the long-term effects of psychotropic drugs on children are not known. In addition, with such a large pool of legitimate methylphenidate available, it is not surprising that some finds its way into the illicit market, with some adolescents purchasing or stealing tablets from those who have them on prescription. Methylphenidate tablets may then be crushed and snorted.[32]

In response to growing concern in the UK – both about the increased prescription rate and about equity of access to treatment – guidance on the use of methylphenidate for ADHD has been issued by the National Institute for Clinical Excellence. This states that treatment should only be initiated by child and adolescent paediatricians or psychiatrists with expertise in ADHD, and that, ideally, it should be part of a wider, comprehensive treatment programme involving advice and support to parents and teachers. Children receiving treatment should be monitored regularly, and the need for continued therapy should be carefully assessed under specialist supervision.[33] It is to be hoped that these measures will ensure that methylphenidate prescription is restricted to genuine cases of ADHD and that leakage to the illicit market is minimized.

Pemoline

Pemoline is an amphetamine-like drug which decreases appetite and has central stimulant effects. Its therapeutic usefulness is rated as low and in large doses it may produce hyperactivity, dyskinesia, seizures, insomnia and hallucinations.

The euphoric effects induced by pemoline are significantly less than those of amphetamine and its reinforcing properties appear very limited. In addition, it is not soluble in water so that there is less likelihood of it being injected. It is perhaps not surprising therefore that there have been few case reports of dependence on pemoline, although large quantities are diverted illicitly, mainly to countries in West Africa. Abuse has been reported from several countries and pemoline has been suspected in some cases of drug abuse by athletes and in the doping of racehorses.

Cocaine

Cocaine is an alkaloid prepared from the leaves of the coca bush *Erythroxylum coca*, which grows in the mountainous regions of Central and South America (Colombia, Bolivia, Peru). Traditionally, the leaves were (and are) chewed by the natives – apparently without ill effect – to alleviate fatigue, hunger and cold. They were used by the Incas in religious ceremonies as well as socially and for medicinal purposes.

Cocaine itself was first isolated in the 1880s and its oral consumption became widespread throughout the USA and Europe as it was included in tonics, patent medicines, soft drinks and even wine.[34] Its pharmacological properties were investigated by Sigmund Freud who noted its local anaesthetic and psychic effects. He initially recommended it as a cure for morphine addiction, but later became aware of its dependence liability.

The process of extracting cocaine is carried out in illegal factories often situated in the jungle close to where the coca shrubs are grown. Cocaine hydrochloride of a high degree of purity is obtained. It is a white powder, easy to transport and smuggle and is often diluted ('cut') with adulterants such as sugar, amphetamine or local anaesthetics (Appendix 1).

Routes of administration

Cocaine may be administered by almost any route. Intravenous use has long been popular with 'serious' drug users because the drug reaches the brain rapidly and subjective effects, including an intense rush or high, are reported within 1 or 2 minutes. They also abate rapidly, over the next 30 minutes or so.

A common way of taking cocaine is by sniffing (snorting) it. A line of cocaine hydrochloride (20–30 mg) is laid out and inhaled through a straw and the drug is absorbed through the vascular mucous membranes lining the nose. Because cocaine causes vasoconstriction (narrowing of the blood vessels), drug absorption is slowed and there is no rush. However, a period of pleasurable stimulation and euphoria occurs, lasting for 20–40 minutes. Sniffing is simpler than injecting and carries no risk of infective complications, but repeated intranasal use of cocaine damages the nasal mucous membrane causing chronic inflammation (rhinitis) and sometimes a perforated nasal septum.

Smoking cocaine has recently become popular. This practice originated in South America in the 1970s when coca paste, a crude derivative of coca leaves, was mixed with tobacco or marijuana and smoked.[35] Cocaine hydrochloride is unsuitable for smoking because it decomposes at high temperatures. However, when the cocaine alkaloid is freed from its hydrochloride base by a chemical reaction involving ether, it has a melting point of 98 °C and is volatile at temperatures above 90 °C. It therefore vaporizes very easily when heated, and the drug is rapidly and efficiently absorbed from the lungs.

Another form of cocaine freebase is crack, which is prepared by a simple process of 'cooking' cocaine with baking powder and water. The baking powder precipitates out any impurities or adulterants, leaving pure, crystalline cocaine which is cracked into chips which are marketed in small phials. Because each phial contains only a very small quantity of cocaine it is comparatively cheap, so that cocaine, once available only to the wealthy, has become accessible to many more people.

Purified cocaine base is usually smoked in a glass water pipe, or it may be sprinkled on a tobacco or marijuana cigarette. It produces a sudden, intense high, (the 'rush' or 'flash') comparable to that produced by intravenous injection, because the cocaine is absorbed very rapidly by the large surface area of the lungs and reaches the brain within seconds. The euphoria abates equally quickly, leaving the user feeling restless and irritable and craving for another dose. The cocaine user often appears unable to titrate or adjust the dosage and the frequency of administration and the quantity inhaled escalates rapidly. Inhalations may be repeated as often as every 5 minutes during binges that may last from hours to days. Smoking continues until supplies are finished or the user falls asleep exhausted.

Effects

Cocaine is a powerful central nervous system stimulant producing increased energy, wakefulness, activity and confidence and facilitating social interchange. Most important of all it is a powerful euphoriant, giving the user a great feeling of well-being.

This euphoriant property is utilized when cocaine is included in elixirs (e.g. 'Brompton Cocktail') used for the treatment of pain in terminally ill patients. These elixirs also contain heroin or morphine, and cocaine counteracts what might otherwise be an undesirable degree of sedation.

The physical effects of cocaine include a raised pulse rate, blood pressure and temperature, and dilated pupils. In addition to its local anaesthetic properties, cocaine also causes local vasoconstriction (narrowing of blood vessels) so that it was once widely used in ear, nose and throat surgery because it reduced haemorrhage. Now, however, it has been replaced by less toxic synthetic local anaesthetics.[36] It is still used in eye drops for ophthalmic surgery.

Very large doses, taken by those who are not used to it, cause hypertension, cardiac arrhythmias and convulsions. Death may occur due to cardiac or respiratory arrest. There have also been reports of intracerebral haemorrhage in young adults following stimulant abuse and this often seemed to be related to an underlying vascular malformation which does not withstand the hypertensive surge following stimulant administration. Mortality and morbidity from this cause is greater than in those who have not used illegal drugs and may be due to the intensity and duration of vasospasm being worsened by the use of cocaine, together with an underlying poor state of health.[37]

Tolerance

It used to be believed that tolerance to cocaine did not occur and that large doses were taken only in a search for greater euphoria, rather than because small doses were no longer effective. These observations were based on cocaine users who snorted cocaine hydrochloride intermittently, in what was described as 'usual' recreational doses, which were probably insufficient to induce tolerance.

Now that pure cocaine freebase is available, a very different picture is emerging. Some users may take huge doses – 30 g in 24 hours has been reported – that would undoubtedly be toxic to a cocaine-naive individual, but which the regular user can take without serious complication because of the development of tolerance to the hyperthermic, convulsant and cardiovascular effects of cocaine. It is less clear whether tolerance develops to the euphorigenic properties of cocaine; if it does, this would contribute to dose escalation. However, as the dose and frequency of consumption increase, dysphoric effects of cocaine, such as irritability, suspiciousness and restlessness occur, suggesting that there is a ceiling to tolerance of cocaine's psychic effects.

Tolerance does not seem to develop to the reinforcing effect of cocaine.

Physical dependence

A variety of symptoms have been described following cocaine withdrawal by users who habitually consume very large doses. The symptoms include lethargy, depression, apathy, social withdrawal, tremor, muscle pain and disturbances of eating and sleeping (as well as EEG (electroencephalograph) changes). When severe, they form a syndrome known as the 'crash', which begins 15–30 minutes after a 'binge' and which may last for a few hours or up to a few days, accompanied by dysphoria and high levels of craving.[38,39] There may also be excessive sleepiness, paranoid ideas, agitation and suicidal thoughts. When this acute phase subsides, there is a longer period, lasting for several weeks, when anxiety, craving and dysphoria may recur and when the risk of relapse is high. Only later, in the 'extinction' phase, which lasts for 3–12 months, do symptoms subside completely but, even then, exposure to particular cues may stimulate craving again.[40,41] Despite long-standing opinion to the contrary, it is difficult to believe that the crash could be anything but the cocaine abstinence syndrome, although it does not cause the major physiological disruption associated with the more familiar abstinence syndromes of opioids, alcohol or sedative hypnotics.

Psychological dependence

Cocaine causes severe psychological dependence with craving and drug-seeking behaviour so intense that the normal pattern of life is disrupted and everything becomes subservient to the need to obtain cocaine. In the early stages, a weekend user, accustomed to having a good time if he or she takes cocaine, finds that nothing is quite as enjoyable without it, and eventually that he or she is incapable of enjoying anything if cocaine is not taken. Consumption extends gradually through the week and it is then often taken specifically to relieve stress, because of the learned experience of 'feeling better' after cocaine. Severe psychological dependence may develop quite rapidly, often without the user being aware that his or her drug use is problematic.

In animals, cocaine is a powerful primary reinforcer: laboratory animals exposed to cocaine will repeat an action more and more frequently in order to obtain more cocaine and, given free access to it, will take the drug to the exclusion of food so that they lose weight and die.[41,42] Until recently there was little evidence that cocaine has such compelling effects in humans and it was thought to be a 'safe' recreational drug, often glamorized as the drug of the 'rich and famous', for whom sniffing was the most usual route of administration. The advent of pure cocaine freebase has dramatically changed this view. Not only has it become apparent that cocaine can cause tolerance and physical dependence, but new patterns of consumption of cocaine have developed, with freebasers smoking cocaine almost continuously until either they or the supply of drug are exhausted – a behaviour pattern remarkably similar to that observed in laboratory animals. It has been suggested that this pattern of drug use is caused by the high concentrations of cocaine in the brain that are achieved by smoking cocaine freebase, and that last for only a few minutes before a rapid decline in concentration occurs. It is possible, for example, that it is the sharp contrast between the 'rush' and withdrawal that generates the drive to use more drug within a short period.

Mechanism of action

The mechanism of action of cocaine is complex and is not fully understood. However, it is now known that there are specific cocaine receptors in the central nervous system that bind cocaine molecules and which affect the brain's dopaminergic system by inhibiting the reuptake of dopamine from synapses. The consequent increase in dopamine at the synapse is thought to be associated with euphoria but, with long-term use, the excessive dopamine is metabolized, leading to reduced dopamine concentration. This in turn leads to changes in the post-synaptic receptors which are thought to be associated with craving.

Cocaine also acts on the noradrenergic and 5-hydroxytryptamine systems within the brain, inhibiting the reuptake of these neurotransmitters. The consequent increase in noradrenalin at synapses leads to the stimulatory effects of tachycardia, hypertension, sweating, tremor, mydriasis, etc.[38]

Cocaine toxicity/psychosis

As the dose and frequency of use of cocaine increase, adverse reactions may occur. These start with feelings of anxiety, restlessness and apprehension and progress to suspiciousness, hypervigilance and paranoid behaviour. Stimulation of the nervous system occurs causing muscle twitching, nausea and vomiting, increases in pulse and blood pressure, irregular respiration and sometimes convulsions. In cases of severe toxicity, this is followed by depression of the nervous system with circulatory and respiratory failure, loss of reflexes, unconsciousness and death.

Cocaine psychosis has also been described with persecutory delusions and repetitive (stereotyped) behaviour such as compulsively taking a watch or radio apart and reassembling it or repeatedly tidying or rearranging a set of objects. There may be auditory hallucinations and sometimes tactile hallucinations, classically described as a sensation of insects crawling under the skin ('cocaine bugs') and causing incessant picking at the skin, or scratching. These symptoms are indistinguishable from the toxic symptoms caused by other stimulants such as amphetamine, but last for a shorter time and may come to medical attention less often.[43–45]

Because of the adverse effects of cocaine when it is taken in high dosage, the cocaine user finds him or herself in a dilemma. The unpleasant symptoms of drug withdrawal and above all the intense craving for cocaine, making discontinuing it almost impossible, but continued consumption of large doses leads to the unpleasant symptoms outlined above. Other drugs, such as alcohol and other central nervous system depressants, may then be taken to counteract the unwanted effects of cocaine and the drug abuser may become (unwittingly) physically dependent on them too. Overdose and intoxication with these drugs is also common. It should also be noted that cocaine is often adulterated with synthetic local anaesthetics such as procaine or lignocaine which, when consumed in large doses, may cause convulsions.

Khat

Khat is a tree, *Catha edulis*, that grows at high altitude in East Africa, Yemen and Democratic Yemen, where the leaves and young shoots have been used for their stimulant effect for hundreds of years. Modern methods of transport have made it easy to export khat and to bring regular supplies of fresh leaves to markets in towns and cities in Democratic Yemen, Ethiopia, Somalia, Yemen, Kenya and Tanzania. Recent reports suggest that it is now exported widely in vacuum packs for the benefit of expatriate communities.

Nowadays khat is usually chewed, although in the past an infusion of the leaves was prepared (Arabian or Ethiopian tea). The khat leaves are plucked from the twig and are chewed; the juicy extract is swallowed and the leafy residue is kept as a wad in one side of the mouth. In Yemen it is usually taken in a group setting at special parties, drinks are served and tobacco is smoked either as cigarettes or in a water pipe.

One alkaloid, cathine, was identified in khat a century ago. More recently, other substances, including cathinone, have also been isolated. Although these constituent chemicals are controlled substances under international conventions, khat itself is not controlled.

Effects

Khat affects the digestive system, commonly causing anorexia and constipation. Stomatitis (inflammation of the mouth), gastritis and dyspepsia have also been reported.[46] In the cardiovascular system there is a temporary increase in pulse rate and blood pressure, palpitations and flushing of the face.

Khat is chewed because of its ability to produce cerebral stimulation. Because of this it was traditionally consumed by tribal people when travelling, and nowadays is taken by long-distance lorry drivers and by students preparing for examinations. It produces a general sense of well-being and when taken in a group setting (as it traditionally is) it elevates the mood of the group and promotes social interaction.[47] After a few hours, however, the mood of the group changes and some participants become restless and irritable. It may cause sleeplessness which in turn may lead to the abuse of alcohol or sedative hypnotic drugs. It has been reported that khat may (rarely) cause a toxic psychosis or schizophrenic reaction in predisposed individuals.[48]

Dependence

There is no evidence of a clear-cut abstinence syndrome and thus no evidence of physical dependence on khat. Psychological dependence does develop, and in cities in Somalia and Yemen it is estimated that a consumer may spend 25% of his daily earnings on khat, thus causing financial hardship to his family.[49,50]

Although the problems associated with the use of khat may seem minor in comparison with those of other drugs of abuse, khat should not be ignored. Until recently it had been used only locally where it was grown, and even now because the leaves must be fresh when they are chewed, their area of distribution has remained fairly localized. However, the active ingredient of khat, cathinone, has now been isolated and, in experiments on laboratory animals, has been shown to have primary reinforcing properties similar to those of cocaine.[51] If pure cathinone were to become available on the street, it is possible that it would cause severe psychological dependence and that it would be extensively abused. Already, in countries where khat is not cultivated and has to be imported, its use raises major socioeconomic issues and these, together with the medical complications of its use, have been considered by some countries serious enough to warrant the introduction of preventive measures (prohibition).[52]

There are clear similarities between the present state of khat abuse and the way in which cocaine abuse began. Already, khat is being cultivated for export. It would indeed be tragic if the rest of the world waited in ignorance while a new drug of dependence and abuse was systematically extracted, marketed and exported. The lessons learned from the history of cocaine should not be forgotten too quickly.

Hallucinogens

Lysergic acid diethylamide (LSD)

LSD was first synthesized in 1938 by Hofmann. It is derived from ergot, a fungus that grows on rye grains and is a white, crystalline powder soluble in water and effective in such minute quantities that doses are measured in micrograms. It is taken orally and its effects can be felt with a dose of only 25 μg although a more usual dose would be 100 μg.[53] It was originally sold on sugar cubes and on small, flat strips known as microdots, and is now available on squares of paper, rather like stamps (Appendix 1).

The physical effects of LSD consumption are apparent within a few minutes. They include nausea, headache, dilated pupils, raised pulse rate, a small and variable alteration of blood pressure and perhaps an increase in body temperature.

The mechanism of action of LSD and related drugs is not clear. They act at multiple sites in the central nervous system, with an agonistic action at presynaptic receptors for 5-hydroxytryptamine (5-HT, serotonin) in the mid-brain, where the firing rate of neurones was sharply reduced following small systemic doses of LSD.[54]

Effects

The psychological effects of LSD are very variable, depending on the expectations and mood of the subject and the setting in which the drug is taken. Their onset follows the somatic symptoms and they persist for several hours.

Characteristically there are changes in perception, especially in the more experienced user. These affect all senses, particularly vision, and may take many different forms: stationary objects appear to move and change shape; some things become minute while previously ignored details loom large and assume importance; colours become more intense. There is often a 'cross-over' of perceptions (synaesthesia) so that sounds are 'seen' or 'felt' and colours are 'heard'. Distortions of body image are common: a limb may appear to shrink, or become enormous and may seem completely separate from the rest of the body. The perception of time is often distorted too, with 'clock' time passing very slowly.

Although LSD and similar drugs are often described or classified as hallucinogens, these perceptual changes are often illusions (the altered perception of an existing object) rather than true hallucinations (perception in the absence of stimulus). The latter do occur sometimes, although auditory hallucinations arise less frequently than in naturally occurring psychoses.

In addition to these striking perceptual changes, LSD also affects thinking processes and mood, and induces feelings that are rarely, if ever, experienced at other times. The user may feel that he or she has achieved union with and a unique understanding of mankind, God and the universe, but often lacks the language to describe what has obviously been a profound experience. Sometimes the experiences are wonderful and exalting, although they may be overwhelmingly frightening. It is thus not surprising that the mood of the LSD user is labile, moving through anxiety, apprehension, gaiety and depression in a way that may be incomprehensible to an observer. The subject may be withdrawn and introspective, preoccupied with these experiences and, because LSD also affects thought processes, may show impaired concentration, distractibility and illogical thinking and be totally out of touch with others and unable to explain what is happening.

It should now be apparent why LSD and other similar drugs are often described as psychedelic or mind-expanding; it enables the user to experience a mental state which he or she would otherwise be unlikely to achieve. There is no evidence, however, that these apparently profound and, at the time, very meaningful experiences affect the personality or subsequent behaviour in a beneficial way. However, at one stage, LSD was used as an aid to psychotherapy, because it was believed that it would enable events of psychodynamic importance to be relived.

Specific receptors have not been identified for LSD but it seems likely that its effects are due to agonist activity on serotonin receptors. Serotonin, also known as 5-hydroxytryptamine (5HT), is a neurotransmitter, widely distributed throughout the central nervous system and elsewhere in the body, which acts by regulating ion channels in the cell membrane so that the concentration of potassium and calcium in the cell is changed. There are different types of 5HT receptors and LSD has greatest affinity for the 5-HT$_2$ receptor, where it acts as a partial agonist.[29]

Tolerance and dependence

Tolerance to the effects of LSD develops so rapidly that a second dose of the drug taken within 24 hours has less effect than the first, and after three or four daily doses, subsequent administration has little or no psychological effect. Because of this there is no incentive to take it regularly on a daily basis, psychological and physical dependence do not develop and withdrawal phenomena are not observed. Tolerance is lost equally rapidly and after 3 or 4 days of abstinence, full sensitivity to the effects of LSD is regained. Chronic users usually take LSD once or more a week, often in large doses. Tolerance to the cardiovascular effects of LSD is less pronounced.

Adverse effects

The most common adverse effect of LSD is a 'bad trip' – an unpleasant, often terrifying drug experience that leads to a temporary episode of overwhelming anxiety and panic which may last for up to 24 hours. A bad trip cannot be predicted or prevented and may happen to any user, even after a number of previously pleasurable experiences. Its occurrence is presumably related in some way to the mental state of the user and the setting in which drug consumption occurred.

Serious, even fatal, accidents may occur during a period of LSD intoxication. They may be due to the individual's belief in supernatural powers or in an ability to perform the impossible – such as flying, walking on water, etc. Such events receive much publicity but occur only rarely.

Spontaneous, involuntary recurrences of the drug-induced experience (flashbacks) are fairly common after LSD use and may be troublesome if they occur frequently. They may also be precipitated by the use of another drug such as cannabis.

It is not clear whether LSD can cause prolonged psychotic illness. When such an illness does occur after LSD use, it is generally believed that it would have occurred anyway and that its onset was merely precipitated by LSD. Nevertheless, given the psychotomimetic properties of LSD, it is possible that it plays a more causal role in vulnerable individuals.[55]

Other hallucinogenic drugs

There are several drugs whose psychological effects are similar to those of LSD and which are also described as hallucinogenic, psychedelic or psychotomimetic. Many are derived from plants which have been used for a long time in religious rituals. Indeed it has been suggested that there are hundreds of thousands of species of hallucinogenic plants in the world. Mescalin, for example, is obtained from the peyote cactus which is traditionally chewed by Indians in Mexico, while psilocin and psilocybin come from a particular ('magic') mushroom in Mexico; lysergic acid monoethylamide, which has mild hallucinogenic properties, is found in the seeds of the morning glory plant; and there are hallucinogens in plants such as nutmeg, mace and deadly nightshade. Cross-tolerance occurs between LSD, mescaline and psilocybin.

In addition to naturally occurring drugs, a whole range of synthetic compounds are available, including DMT (dimethyltryptamine), DMA (dimethoxy-amphetamine) and DOM (dimethoxymethylamphetamine) which are similar in their effects to LSD, but also have some amphetamine-like properties. DOM is also known as STP (standing for serenity, tranquillity and peace) and has a longer duration of action than LSD.

Other drugs, such as MDA (methylenedioxyamphetamine) and MMDA (methoxymethylenedioxyamphetamine) are probably LSD-like but have other properties as well.

The particular problems posed by these new drug analogues are discussed in the section on 'designer' drugs.

Phencyclidine (PCP)

PCP also produces changes in mood and perception, but is quite distinct from the psychedelic drugs described above. It is related to pethidine and induces a marked sensory blockade. First introduced as a veterinary anaesthetic, its property of causing patients to feel detached from bodily sensations and therefore unaware of pain, suggested a revolutionary approach to anaesthesia for humans.[56] However, this was soon abandoned because it so often made patients agitated and deluded. It became, however, a drug of abuse, particularly in the USA where it is known as 'angel dust'. It is relatively easy to synthesize illicitly and is often passed off as LSD. It is usually smoked or snorted.

Effects of PCP vary according to the dose consumed but as there is great individual variation of response, even small doses may cause profound effects in some people. The desired effect is a euphoric sensation of floating, usually accompanied by mild numbness of the extremities, but the cerebellar effects of PCP simultaneously cause staggering gait, slurred speech and nystagmus.[56] Slight increases in dose may precipitate severe muscular rigidity, hypertension and a noncommunicative state. The risk of convulsions and coma becomes greater if more than 20 mg is consumed.

The psychological effects of PCP are very unpredictable; there may be perceptual disturbances, hallucinations, elevation of mood, restlessness, anxiety or paranoia. Sometimes the patient is frankly psychotic and there may be aggressive and bizarre behaviour.[57] The acute effects of PCP last for 4–6 hours, followed by a long period of 'coming down'.

Tolerance and dependence

Tolerance to the effects of PCP develops in animals and humans. Most of those who abuse it probably take it about once a week, although some people have 'runs' of using it for 2 or 3 days at a time. Craving for the drug occurs in some people and the depression and disorientation that occurs after a run of drug use may represent a mild abstinence syndrome. The fact that monkeys will self-administer PCP (but not LSD) also suggests that it may have some dependence potential. However, it is rarely abused in Europe (as yet).

Cannabis

Cannabis is obtained from the Indian hemp plant *Cannabis sativa*, which is grown in many countries as a source of rope fibre. When the plant is fully grown, its flowers and upper leaves are covered with a sticky resin which contains psychoactive substances collectively known as cannabinoids. There are probably more than 50 of these, of which the most important is Δ-9-tetrahydrocannabinol (THC). The potency of a particular preparation of cannabis is related to its THC content, which in turn depends on the part of the plant that is gathered and the environmental conditions, particularly the climate, where it is grown. Certain varieties of *Cannabis sativa* are cultivated specifically for their resin in some tropical countries in the Caribbean, South America, South-East Asia, Indian Subcontinent, etc. Hydroponic cultivation of cannabis is now undertaken in some countries, where the climate is unsuitable for traditional methods and, combined with careful plant selection, leads to very high concentrations of THC (20–30%).

Preparations

Various preparations of cannabis are available, often known by different names in different countries.

1 *Bhang*: the dried leaves and flowering tops of uncultivated plants, which are infused and drunk;

2 *Marijuana*: the dried leaves and flowering tops of uncultivated plants, which are smoked;

3 *Ganja*: small upper leaves and flowering tops of cultivated female plants, which are smoked. It is about three times as potent as marijuana;

The THC content of these three herbals preparations is between 1% and 10%.

4 *Hashish/charas/cannabis resin*: the pure resin from the flowering tops and leaves of female plants. It is in the form of a sticky brown cake which is usually smoked. The THC content varies between 8% and 15%.

5 *Liquid cannabis/hashish oil*: this is obtained by subjecting cannabis resin to extraction with a nonaqueous solvent. After filtration and evaporation, a brown syrupy liquid is obtained into which tobacco is dipped before smoking. It may contain up to 60% THC.

An average marijuana cigarette in the UK usually contains 300–500 mg of herbal material with a THC content of perhaps 1–2%. Even if smoked by an experienced user, only 50% of the available THC is absorbed and so the estimated dose of THC from one cigarette is in the region of 2.5–5.0 mg. However, the dose may also vary because heat converts some inactive compounds into THC and can inactivate psychoactive cannabinoids.[58] With the introduction of varieties of cannabis with very high concentrations of THC, the THC content of individual cigarettes can now be much higher than previously.

Absorption and fate of THC

THC is absorbed very quickly across the large surface area of the lungs and plasma concentrations peak very quickly (10–30 minutes). THC binds tightly to blood proteins but, because it is so fat soluble, it is readily absorbed by organs such as the brain which have a high fat content and is released only slowly back into the bloodstream. It is metabolized (broken down), mostly in the liver, to 11-hydroxy THC, which is 20% more potent than THC itself, and to other products with unknown or relatively little psychoactive effect.[59] The effects of a single marijuana cigarette are apparent within minutes and last for 2–3 hours. When cannabis is consumed orally, the onset of action is slower than if it is smoked and a larger dose is required to obtain the same effects, which then last longer.[60]

Because of their fat solubility, THC and its metabolites remain for long periods of time in the fatty tissues of the body. Thus, 5 days after a single injection of THC, 20% remains stored and 20% of its metabolites remain in the blood; complete elimination of a single dose may take 30 days. Given this slow rate of clearance, it is likely that repeated administration may lead to accumulation of THC and its metabolites in the body.[61] An awareness of these pharmacokinetics is relevant to any discussion about the long-term effects of cannabis.

Effects

The physical effects commonly associated with cannabis use include dryness of the mouth, hunger, reddening of the eyes and reduced pressure in the intraocular fluid of the eyes. There may be increased blood pressure (together with postural hypotension) and a dose-related increase in heart rate. Chronic, high-dosage effects of cannabis are reported to include reduced testosterone level and sperm count, as well as reduced fertility in women and reduced fetal birth weight. Gynaecomastia may occur.

The psychological effects of smoking a marijuana cigarette are well known. The desired and sought after effects are of euphoria, self-confidence, relaxation and a general sense of well-being. There is often an altered perception of time, which may appear to be passing more slowly than usual, and the perception of hearing, taste, touch and smell may seem to the subject to be enhanced, although there is no objective evidence of this on formal testing. It may be difficult for the subject to concentrate and memory may be impaired. Sometimes these experiences are not pleasurable and the subject becomes anxious, agitated and suspicious, occasionally experiencing a severe panic reaction. Although there is no conclusive evidence, it is likely that the ability to drive a car safely is adversely affected by cannabis consumption.

The mental set of the subject and the setting in which cannabis is taken may both influence the drug-induced experience, although laboratory experiments have provided conclusive evidence that the psychological effects of cannabis are due to its THC content. In small doses, equivalent to smoking one marijuana cigarette, THC causes changes in mood (usually euphoria) and altered perception. With bigger doses (200–250 μg/kg; approximately 15 mg THC for an average, 70 kg man), there is marked distortion in visual and auditory perception, and hallucinations occur in most subjects together with sensations of depersonalization and derealization. Thinking becomes confused and disorganized and paranoid feelings are common. With even higher doses, a frank toxic psychosis develops.

It appears, therefore, that THC, the main constituent of cannabis, is a psychotomimetic drug; in other words it can produce a state similar to that of a psychotic illness and this effect depends on the dose that is administered. In the laboratory the reaction of the same individual to the same dose is reproducible on different occasions and some individuals are unusually sensitive to THC, experiencing psychosis even at low doses.

Two cannabinoid receptors have recently been identified in the brain, CB_1 and CB_2. CB_1 is the central receptor that binds 11-hydroxy THC, which inhibits the release of GABA into the synaptic cleft. There appear to be high levels of binding in the hippocampus, a part of the brain particularly associated with memory. This may account for some of the observed psychological effects of cannabis.[62]

Tolerance

The development of tolerance to the effects of cannabis has long been a controversial issue. In Western countries it is often claimed that cannabis does not cause tolerance, on the grounds that experienced users continue to obtain a 'high' from their first cigarette of the day. Indeed, the phenomenon of reverse tolerance has been described, when experienced users may report more subjective experiences than novices. These observations and opinions are contradicted by the experience of countries where heavy, regular consumption of cannabis is common. In these countries, very large doses may be consumed (hundreds of milligrams of THC) that would undoubtedly be toxic to a drug-naive individual, suggesting that tolerance to the effects of THC has indeed developed.

Laboratory experiments also confirm the existence of tolerance to cannabis-induced changes in mood, tachycardia (increased heart rate), decreased intraocular pressure and impairment of performance in psychomotor tests. Tolerance develops rapidly, within a few days of regular drug use, and decays rapidly when drug use ceases. It is generally much less obvious than tolerance to heroin or cocaine, and the irregular small doses of cannabis that are usually consumed in Western countries may not be sufficient to cause a noticeable degree of tolerance. Furthermore, there appears to be an upper limit to tolerance to cannabis, which may vary from individual to individual, and once this is reached further increases in dose may precipitate the onset of psychotic symptoms.

Dependence

Similar controversy surrounds the question of dependence on cannabis. Again, it is not surprising that dependence is reported most frequently in those countries where cannabis is consumed regularly and in large quantities. In this situation, cannabis withdrawal is followed by some discomfort and an abstinence syndrome, the hallmark of physical dependence, has been described. It is characterized by irritability, restlessness, decreased appetite, weight loss and insomnia. These clinical observations are supported by the observation under laboratory conditions of a withdrawal syndrome in volunteers who had taken high doses of THC for several weeks. This experiment confirmed that the syndrome is relatively mild, starting a few hours after the cessation of drug administration and lasting for 4–5 days.

The issue of whether tolerance develops to cannabis and its dependence liability is particularly important because of continuing discussions in many countries about its 'decriminalization'. The recent observation that monkeys self-administer THC is therefore of great interest.[63] In this experiment the monkeys gave themselves about 30 injections of THC during an hour-long session, self-administering a dose that was roughly equivalent to that obtained by a person smoking a marijuana joint. It was also noted that self-administration was blocked by a cannabinoid receptor blocker. This suggests that THC has primary reinforcing properties that are qualitatively similar to those of heroin and cocaine, both of which are drugs that animals will self-administer. However, there is no doubt that craving and drug-seeking behaviour, the hallmark of severe dependence, rarely occur among those who misuse cannabis.

Cannabis psychosis

World-wide, millions of people smoke marijuana and consume cannabis in different forms, and there have been many reports, from all over the world, of 'cannabis psychosis', a psychotic illness arising after the consumption of a large quantity of cannabis. It is characterized by the sudden onset of confusion, generally associated with delusions, hallucinations and emotional lability. Temporary amnesia, disorientation, depersonalization and paranoid symptoms are also common. This toxic mental state may persist for a few hours or a few days.[58,64,65] This syndrome is well recognized and frequently reported in countries, such as India, West Indies and in South-East Asia, where heavy consumption of cannabis is common,[66] but its existence is often questioned in the UK and other Western countries. Here, the THC content of the cannabis that is available is often low and even 'experienced' users usually smoke only a few cigarettes, perhaps two or three times a week, or even daily – a far cry from Jamaican heavy users whose consumption of THC is estimated to be 420 mg daily. As toxic psychosis is a dose-related effect of cannabis, it is only to be expected that there would be a smaller incidence of the syndrome in the UK, although it seems likely that there is a general lack of awareness of its existence and consequent underdiagnosis. Furthermore, it seems likely that many users are familiar with the effects of cannabis and are able to titrate their intake to avoid unpleasant effects. Mild intoxication is undoubtedly dealt with, without recourse to medical advice.[58]

It has also been suggested, although there is little firm evidence, that cannabis can cause a functional psychosis – a paranoid schizophrenia-like illness in a setting of clear consciousness. There are many alternative explanations for any apparent relationship between cannabis and psychosis: that the patient was psychotic anyway and cannabis use was incidental or merely aggravated the existing condition; that the patient was potentially psychotic and this was precipitated by cannabis, which cannot cause psychosis in a 'normal' individual; that the illness preceded and indirectly caused cannabis use. Although these and other explanations may be true, they do not preclude the existence of a cannabis-induced functional psychosis, and those who are experienced in the sequelae of prolonged and heavy cannabis abuse have observed subtle differences between true paranoid schizophrenia and the psychotic illness that sometimes develops in cannabis abusers.[67,68] For example, the latter are more likely to have hypomanic symptoms, but less likely to have 'schizophrenic-type' thought disorder. Their illness responds very swiftly to antipsychotic medication, but tends to relapse if cannabis use is resumed.

There is, however, no evidence that cannabis causes a chronic psychosis that persists after drug use is discontinued, although some patients may effectively 'maintain' themselves in a psychotic condition by continuing to consume large quantities of cannabis.[69]

Flashbacks

Flashbacks are spontaneous, involuntary recurrences of drug-induced experiences after the effects of the drug have worn off. They have been described following cannabis use, but the generally accepted wisdom is that they only occur if the patient has previously used other psychotomimetic drugs such as LSD[65] – although the flashback may then be of a cannabis-induced experience. In some cases flashbacks have occurred within hours of using cannabis; given the prolonged presence of THC in the body, these symptoms can hardly be said to be occurring in the absence of the drug.

Amotivational syndrome

Amotivational syndrome is a phrase coined to describe a condition of chronic apathy attributed to long-term, heavy cannabis use. It is characterized by the asocial, nondirectional behaviour of a 'drop-out' who appears to have none of the usual goals of life. There is controversy about whether the amotivational syndrome actually exists and, if it does, whether it is causally related to cannabis use or whether both conditions (cannabis use and amotivational syndrome) are manifestations of underlying psychopathology.

Chronic brain damage

It has also been suggested that prolonged use of cannabis eventually leads to brain damage or atrophy. Again, there is no conclusive evidence to support this hypothesis.

Volatile solvents

The inhalation or 'sniffing' of volatile solvents became a focus of attention in the UK during the 1970s and early 1980s, when it was closely related to the punk subculture. It was, however, like most forms of drug abuse not a new phenomenon but a 'variation on a theme' – an epidemic of a condition that previously had warranted only occasional anecdotal case reports of health professionals inhaling anaesthetic gases, of industrial solvent workers who abused solvents and so on.

When it became widespread among young teenagers it provoked lurid reports in the popular press, but little in the way of systematic research so that comparatively little is known about this form of drug abuse. Specifically, and partly because of the large number of chemicals involved, there is scant information about the development of tolerance and dependence. Although the panic of the 1970s has subsided, solvent abuse persists, especially among teenagers, and there are sporadic reports of 'outbreaks' of this form of drug abuse in different countries.

Typically, in the UK, if glue sniffing occurs in a particular locality, it is a group activity, more popular among boys than girls. The majority will experiment with it for a short time and then stop, with about one-tenth continuing to sniff in groups for a few months. A small number will continue solvent sniffing for many years, usually in a more solitary fashion and it is in this group that serious consequences, including fatalities, are more likely to occur. Chronic solvent abuse is associated with factors such as low socioeconomic status, disorganized families, unemployment and parental absence and is often seen in groups that are marginalized by the rest of society. In this situation, encouraged by peer pressure, solvent abuse becomes normalized and loses its deviant status. It is perhaps not surprising, given the subcultural context of solvent abuse, that it is associated with a higher incidence of delinquency and sociopathy, although the nature and direction of causality is not known.[70,71]

The substances that have been abused include a wide range of commercial and domestic products, such as glues (containing toluene and related hexanes), nail varnish and removers (amyl acetate and acetone), gas lighter fuel (butane) and cleaning fluids (trichloroethylene). The active constituents are volatile hydrocarbons which evaporate at room temperature, giving off fumes that can be inhaled. Aerosol products are also abused for the sake of the propellants they contain – substances such as butane or chlorinated fluorocarbons. It is obvious that all of these products are widely available and fairly cheap so that any youngster who wants to abuse them can obtain them easily.[71]

Methods of administration

The usual method of sniffing is to put some of the chosen product on to a piece of material, or into a paper or plastic bag (often a potato crisp bag), which is then held over the mouth and nose while deep breaths are taken. If air is exhaled into the bag, the carbon dioxide content of the air and vapour mixture increases, enhancing the drug experience. Where sniffing is a group activity, the same bag may be passed around the group. A very dangerous practice, with a high risk of death by suffocation, is to pour some of the solvent into a large plastic bag which is put right over the head so that air is excluded completely and the vapour is more concentrated.[71] Aerosols may be sprayed directly into the mouth.

As the subject breathes in and out, the solvents are rapidly absorbed through the large surface area of the lung and enter the bloodstream. Most are highly lipid soluble and are rapidly distributed throughout the nervous system where they depress many vital functions and produce the desired 'high' within a few minutes. Many are excreted, unchanged, through the lungs producing a characteristic odour on the breath, but others are metabolized and excreted in the urine. It is difficult to test urine for solvent abuse because of the wide variety of substances involved.

Effects

The desired effect of solvent abuse is euphoria, which may be achieved within a few minutes after just a few breaths. It is similar to being intoxicated with alcohol, but the intoxicated condition can be attained much more rapidly by using solvents. Like alcohol, most solvents act as central nervous system depressants, but because the higher centres of the brain that control behaviour are depressed first, the apparent initial effect of solvent abuse is of stimulation and of disinhibition. There may be feelings of omnipotence and recklessness so that dangerous behaviour of an impulsive or destructive nature may ensue.[70]

Other effects vary according to the solvent being inhaled, the amount being taken and the method and duration of inhalation, as well as the previous habits of the individual. They include giddiness, ataxia (unsteadiness), slurred speech and impaired judgement, associated with dullness, apathy and confusion. Some subjects experience hallucinations which are usually visual and often frightening. Other physical symptoms include nausea and vomiting, sneezing, coughing and diarrhoea. These effects wear off quite quickly, usually in less than an hour, leaving the user feeling drowsy.[72] Repeated inhalation, which is a common practice, may result in disorientation, fits and eventual unconsciousness with depression of respiration and heart rate.

A glue-sniffer's rash, although uncommon, has been described, believed to be due to the repeated application of a plastic bag containing solvent over the mouth and nose. The rash is symmetrical in distribution and consists of red papules and pustules extending from each nostril up the nasal fold and across the bridge of the nose.

As well as the dangerous consequence of suffocation if a plastic bag is placed right over the head, asphyxia may also occur due to inhalation of vomit during unconsciousness. Deaths have also been reported due to cardiac arrhythmias, which seem to occur most frequently if aerosol propellant gases are sprayed directly into the mouth. It has been suggested that many solvents sensitize the heart muscle, so that it reacts abnormally to stress by beating irregularly.[73] It may, therefore, be important not to startle an individual who is intoxicated with solvents. Fatal accidents sometimes occur during solvent intoxication; they may be the consequence of bizarre behaviour due to disorientation and hallucination, and are particularly likely if inhalation takes place in a dangerous situation – near a canal, for example, or on a roof-top.

Over the last decade there has been a steady upward trend in the number of deaths attributable to solvent abuse. Lighter fuel now accounts for 40–50% of these deaths because, when sprayed directly into the mouth, rapid cooling causes mucosal tissue in the airways to swell, leading to obstruction and suffocation due to laryngeal spasm.[71]

The toxic effects of many solvents are well known, particularly from experience in industrial medicine, and there is no doubt that some substances are very toxic and can cause severe tissue damage. However, the relevance of findings from chronic, low-dose exposure of factory workers to the repeated, acute, high-dose exposure of the adolescent solvent abuser is not clear. The chronic effects reported include liver and kidney damage, bone marrow depression, anaemia, encephalopathy and neuropathy. Many long-term effects are reversible if solvent abuse is stopped. Permanent brain damage seems to be rare although it can occur, particularly after long-term abuse of solvents. Computed tomographic scanning may then show widespread cerebral and cerebellar atrophy, with enlarged ventricles and widened sulci.[74] Chromosome damage has also been reported as well as blood abnormalities, but these effects of solvent abuse have not been conclusively proven.

Tolerance

It appears that tolerance to the effects of a particular solvent can develop if abuse persists over a long period – say of 6–12 months. Some individuals may then be abusing several pints of solvent each week.

Dependence

There is no doubt that psychological dependence on solvents develops in many young abusers who find it very difficult to reduce their consumption or stop altogether. True physical dependence with a defined withdrawal syndrome probably does not occur, although 'hangover' effects (headaches, nausea, drowsiness, etc.) may be prominent in heavy abusers. It is not clear whether these are the residual effects of the abused solvents or a 'withdrawal' syndrome due to absence of drugs from the body.[70]

Designer drugs

The term 'designer drugs' is used to describe clandestinely produced substances pharmacologically similar to drugs of abuse that are already strictly controlled by national and international law; so-called designer drugs are subtly different in chemical structure so that they remain out of reach of the law. They are in fact drug analogues deliberately synthesized to produce the euphoria or 'high' of controlled drugs, but able to be manufactured, sold and abused without risk of penalty.

The idea of producing analogues of a parent drug is neither new nor rare. Indeed, pharmaceutical companies perpetually try to produce analogues and have synthesized many. However, it was first done for the purpose of avoiding the law in the 1960s when hallucinogenic amphetamine analogues of mescaline were synthesized. Since then analogues of phencyclidine and methaqualone have been produced and, more recently, analogues of opioids have been identified. These are usually derivatives of either fentanyl or pethidine and are substituted for heroin. They are easy to produce and inexpensive, yet very potent and so are a source of considerable profit to the producer. Because of their potency they are taken only in very small doses and are therefore very difficult to detect by routine chemical analysis.

Fentanyl itself is a very potent synthetic opioid analgesic widely used during operative anaesthesia. A number of clandestinely produced analogues have been identified, some of which are 250 times as potent as heroin. This means that 1 g of the analogue can produce 500 000 doses to be traded on the street as 'heroin' or 'China white'. Because of their potency, these analogues carry a high risk of fatal overdose.

Analogues of pethidine are also more potent than the parent drug, but the clandestine production of one such analogue, MPPP, yields a number of impurities including a neurotoxic by-product, MPTP. This damages dopamine-containing neurones in the nervous system, causing a severe, irreversible neurological condition resembling Parkinson's syndrome and characterized by tremor, muscular rigidity, slowness of movement and speech, and a mask-like, expressionless face. This occurred, tragically, in several young people who had self-administered intravenously MPPP/MPTP that had been purchased as heroin. Another pethidine analogue, PEPAP, may contain a similarly neurotoxic by-product known as PEPTP. It is possible that more intravenous drug abusers who have been exposed to MPTP or PEPTP in the past, may develop Parkinson's syndrome at a later stage.

Ecstasy

Another important group of designer drugs derive from the hallucinogenic amphetamines. MDMA (3,4, methylene-dioxymethamphetamine), known as 'Ecstasy', and MDE are analogues of the controlled drug methylenedioxymethylamphetamine (MDA). Like the parent compound, these new drugs induce a state of altered consciousness, enhance visual, auditory and tactile perceptions and produce mild intoxication. They are also thought to damage serotonin-containing neurones in the nervous system.[75]

In the UK, the use of Ecstasy is intrinsically linked to a particular music scene that involves energetic dancing at parties and in clubs. Large numbers of young people 'go clubbing' regularly and drugs such as MDMA are often sold within the clubs themselves or are taken in by the young people, to be consumed in combination with alcohol and/or other drugs. Ecstasy tablets may also contain LSD, amphetamines, etc.[76] (Appendix 1).

The use of Ecstasy on a recreational basis is now believed to be very common in the UK and some other European countries, and a number of deaths associated with its use are reported each year, often receiving national attention. Death usually appears to be related to dehydration, hyperthermia and rhabdomyolyis leading to multiorgan failure. There have also been reports of spontaneous intracerebral haemorrhage following the use of Ecstasy, probably caused by sudden severe hypertension.

Those who wish to promote the drug as harmless often try to attribute serious side effects and death to the presence of contaminants, rather than to Ecstasy itself, or to its mode of use in crowded, hot venues. They also emphasize that successive doses are reported as less pleasurable than the initial dose with briefer and less intense psychological effects and conclude that long-term heavy use is therefore unlikely. However, it is clear that some individuals do take Ecstasy for long periods and there is some evidence of associated cognitive impairment, although establishing causality in polydrug abusers is not easy.[77]

MDMA has been widely abused in the USA and has been openly promoted as a legal euphoriant, thus illustrating the problem posed by designer drugs.[78] Because drug control laws usually define drugs in terms of their chemical structure, it is easy to side-step these laws by slightly changing the chemical structure of the drug. If the cumbersome process of changing the law is initiated so that the new drug is included, it is very easy to redesign the drug so that the new analogue remains out of reach. The difficulty of controlling these dangerous substances is compounded by the problems of identifying them in very low concentrations and then of describing them, ensuring that legislation cannot keep up with the constantly changing drug scene. This problem has been countered in the USA, where designer drugs have caused most trouble, by new legislation which makes it an offence to manufacture and distribute designer drugs (defined as a substance, other than a controlled substance, with a structure substantially similar to controlled drugs or designed to produce an effect substantially similar to that of a controlled drug). This law, which shifts the emphasis away from the actual substance of abuse and towards the process of manufacture and distribution, will obviate the need for new legislation to be passed to cope with the ever-changing chemical repertoire.[79]

In the UK, action has been taken against designer drugs in anticipation of future problems. Carfentanil and lofentanil, which are analogues of fentanyl, are now included in Class A of the Misuse of Drugs Act, as are any analogues of fentanyl and pethidine which may appear in future as drugs of abuse. This means that they are subject to the strictest controls and that the penalties for their misuse are severe (see Chapter 12).

Steroids

Anabolic steroids are drugs or hormonal substances, chemically and pharmacologically related to testosterone, which promote muscle growth. They occur naturally in the body, playing an important role in the development and functioning of the reproductive organs. They are 'anabolic' because they increase the retention of nitrogen in the body, a basic constituent of protein, thus promoting the growth and development of muscle tissue. They have limited medical use but are taken, inappropriately, by individuals for whom increased body size or increased muscle power is perceived as important – individuals such as bodybuilders, bouncers, doormen and even policemen, as well as weightlifters and athletes. Others may use steroids to increase their self-esteem, or to improve their appearance when stripped for the beach, etc.[80]

There is no accurate information about the extent of nonmedical steroid use in the UK but it appears that the majority of users are males aged 17–35 years, while there is some evidence of its growing popularity among younger teenagers too (mostly boys). In the USA, it has been estimated that there are 2–3 million people abusing these drugs, including half a million teenagers. Attention has focused on their use by sportsmen and women who believe that these drugs will make them stronger, faster, more competitive and more aggressive.

Not surprisingly, accurate data relating to the effects of steroids relates to their medical use for patients rather than their unsupervised use by athletes. However, it is generally accepted that they can increase muscle strength if they are used during periods of intense training and in conjunction with a carefully controlled high-protein diet. Used in isolation they may increase muscle mass but not strength.

A wide variety of anabolic steroids is available for nonmedical use. Most are manufactured in underground laboratories, but some intended for veterinary use have been diverted for human consumption. They are available in both oral and injectable forms and different steroids may be used simultaneously ('stacking'). It appears that they are often taken in a cyclical fashion with rest periods in between. During a cycle, the dose of steroids may be gradually increased during the first part of the cycle, and then tapered down near the end of the cycle; this pattern of dose management is called a 'pyramid'.

Adverse effects

Anabolic steroids may cause abnormalities of liver function tests although these usually return to normal when drug-taking ceases. They can cause facial acne and, if taken by children, may stunt growth.

More serious complications may also occur; these include a rare form of hepatitis and liver tumours. Steroids may also cause hypertension and have been implicated in coronary heart disease. They affect sexual function and when taken by women can cause virilization.[81,82] Adverse psychiatric effects, including confusion, sleep disorder, depression, hallucinations and paranoid delusions, can also occur, albeit rarely. A corollary of the desired effects of increased competitiveness and aggression is that users may become irritable, short-tempered and potentially violent: the so-called "roid rage".

Where steroids are taken by injection there is the possibility of syringes and needles being shared and a consequent risk of HIV infection. Indeed at some needle exchange schemes, steroid users account for a significant proportion of attenders; this appears to reflect the popularity of bodybuilding and the difficulty of obtaining suitable injection equipment for oil-based steroids.

Unlike most of the other substances that are frequently misused, steroids do not have an immediate psychoactive effect and they do not have reinforcing properties. In the UK, they are Prescription Only Medicines, covered by Schedule 4 of the Misuse of Drugs Regulations 1985 (see Chapter 12). They can only be sold by a pharmacist working in a registered pharmacy, but it is not illegal to possess or import them for personal use. Nonmedical steroid use is therefore different in many ways from other forms of substance misuse: it is not illegal (although nonmedical use is banned by the various sports authorities); most steroid users are health conscious, welcoming health checks and the opportunity to obtain sterile injection equipment; and they rarely misuse other drugs although there are some reports of amphetamine use. Nevertheless, it *is* a form of substance misuse; it is carried out secretively; and it is easy to understand that an athlete who achieves success while taking steroids may develop great faith in their effects and become psychologically dependent upon them. The relationship between steroid misuse and other forms of substance misuse is highlighted by experience in the USA, where anabolic steroids were made controlled drugs in 1991. Since then, 185 investigations of major dealers have been reported and 6 million dosage units and $2.5 million have been seized. Most cases have involved international trafficking with steroids originating from all over the world. It has also been found that many traffickers are involved in drugs other than steroids, most notably cocaine.

Over the counter medicines

Most drugs of abuse or those with dependence liability are controlled under the Misuse of Drugs Act 1971 and come within the scope of the Misuse of Drugs Regulations 1985 (see Chapter 12), requiring a doctor's prescription before they are dispensed. However, there are many other medications with a potential for misuse which are available from a pharmacist, 'over the counter', without the need for a doctor's prescription. For example, there is a range of cough mixtures and treatments for diarrhoea that contain codeine or similar drugs with opioid-like effects while the familiar remedy of kaolin and morphine mixture contains a dilute tincture of morphine itself. Similarly, there are nasal decongestants containing stimulant-like drugs (ephedrine, pseudoephedrine) and a range of antihistamines which are predominantly sedative in their effects.

These drugs are a cause for concern for a variety of reasons. Firstly, drug-dependent individuals are well informed about them and may use them deliberately to supplement other sources of supply. While most are formulated in such a way that they are not suitable for injection, there have been reports of users trying to extract active ingredients for this purpose. Secondly, many are compound preparations, containing more than one active ingredient. If the drug that the user wants is present only in low concentration, large quantities of the compound will be taken, perhaps resulting in toxicity from the other constituents.

Another important area of concern is that some individuals may take these drugs regularly over many years in an inappropriate fashion. Uninformed self-medication, however well intentioned, can lead to dependence upon the drugs with attendant risks to personal health. The extent of this type of use is, of course, unknown. However, it has been estimated that there are more than a quarter of a million analgesic abusers in the UK. They buy, over the counter, from pharmacists, supermarkets, newsagents and even slot machines, compounds containing aspirin and other 'minor' analgesics. Taken in excess for a prolonged period, these may cause serious renal damage and have been implicated as a cause of renal tumours.[83] In response to these concerns, restrictions have been introduced on the quantity of over the counter medicines that can be sold in shops other than pharmacies.

Herbal preparations and 'natural' medicines

In recent years there has been burgeoning interest in so-called natural remedies and foods because of a belief that herbal preparations, vitamins and minerals can only be beneficial and lack the side effects of modern, synthetic drugs. In fact, many modern drugs are derived originally from plants and are carefully formulated, under very strict controls, to ensure consistency of ingredients and dose. In contrast, natural preparations are not subject to the same controls and, despite an often blind trust in their safety, may cause serious side effects if taken in excess. Some may have mood-altering effects: for example in the USA, some herbal tea bags, popular because they were caffeine-free, in fact contained about 5 mg cocaine per bag. Similarly, so-called Asthma cigarettes contain stramonium leaves with hyoscine as an active ingredient, which may cause hallucinations.

Self-medication with herbal laxatives, such as preparations of senna or ipecac, may cause serious complications if doses are excessive. This may occur in association with eating disorders such as bulimia and anorexia, when there may be profound and life-threatening electrolyte disturbances. Another group of natural remedies with a long history of self-medication are the aphrodisiacs. Prolonged use of ginseng, for example, is said to cause a 'ginseng abuse syndrome', with hypertension, oedema, diarrhoea, skin rashes, insomnia and depression.

The combined use of drugs and alcohol

Despite considerable evidence that alcohol and drugs are used and misused concurrently, services for substance misusers and research into substance misuse usually focus either on drugs or on alcohol with little interaction between the two areas. With the behaviours overlapping, and the substances themselves interacting, it seems appropriate to consider, albeit briefly, the particular problems associated with the combined use of drugs and alcohol.

For example, epidemiological research shows that in the UK, cigarettes and alcohol are the first and second drug tried by schoolchildren. Thus it is not surprising that patients seeking treatment for drug abuse commonly give a history of alcohol use too. Indeed, recent evidence suggests that the prevalence of combined use in a population of alcoholics and/or drug addicts ranges from 29% to 95%. One study in the USA reported that, out of 298 drug abusers seeking treatment for cocaine abuse, 29% could be described as dependent on alcohol while about 62% met the criteria for having been dependent on alcohol at some previous time. Similarly, in another study, this time of clients in alcohol treatment agencies, the percentage using alcohol with drugs ranged from 57% for methadone to 95% for speed and amphetamines, while other drugs reported to have been used included crack, cocaine, heroin, sedatives and hallucinogens, as well as codeine and other opioids. Similar findings have been reported from other countries; in Australia, for example, there was a 45% prevalence of combined drug and alcohol use in a sample of 313 heroin users, while in Canada 20–45% of a sample of 427 patients meeting DSM-III criteria for alcohol abuse or dependence reported combined use of benzodiazepines and alcohol.[84]

The reasons for combining different substances vary from person to person. Sometimes they may be combined in a search for enhanced effect, as for example when cocaine abusers also use alcohol to potentiate cocaine euphoria.[85] Interestingly the same drug combination has been reported to have been used so that alcohol would counteract the negative acute effects of cocaine. Among alcoholics, the use of benzodiazepines is associated with a tendency to self-medicate for anxiety, while there is evidence that some injecting drug users use alcohol to enhance sexual activities and pleasure.

When different substances are taken simultaneously, they can interact in a number of different ways. Firstly, of course, they may act independently of one another so that the observed effects are no more and no less than if they were taken separately. Alternatively they may have a summative or additive effect, or work synergistically or, indeed, have an antagonistic effect. The underlying mechanisms for such interactions are usually not clear, although a possible mechanism for drug–alcohol interaction has now been described: at low blood alcohol concentrations, alcohol is mainly metabolized by alcohol dehydrogenase, leaving the microsomal ethanol-oxidizing system free to metabolize other drugs. At high blood alcohol concentrations, the latter system is utilized for alcohol metabolism so that the metabolism of other drugs is slowed and their effects are prolonged. This would explain why alcohol can enhance the psychomotor deficits associated with psychoactive drugs such as benzodiazepines, and perhaps why drug abusers who are involved in the combined use of drugs and alcohol report more severe drug dependence. However, it must be remembered that many other factors, such as the dose-time response, may also be important.[84]

In practice, although antagonistic effects are possible, the behavioural effects of combined use are similar to those commonly associated with either alcohol or illicit drugs, but are elevated. Thus the combined use of alcohol and cerebral depressants usually include impaired performance on driving and similar skills. Impairment of reaction time, attention and alertness have all been reported and it seems likely that they contribute to the causation of incidents such as traffic accidents, fires, falls, etc.

The combined use of drugs and alcohol has several implications for treatment. Firstly, a longer course of treatment may be needed as a result of the need to avoid possible harm arising from the interaction between drugs administered in treatment and the drug combination taken by the patient. More specifically, alcohol detoxification may be necessary before treatment for the drug problem can be initiated. In more general terms and in view of the prevalence of combined drug and alcohol use, the second major implication for treatment services is that there is a clear argument for combining the services offered to drug- and alcohol-dependent individuals.

Alcohol

Introduction

Other chapters in this book deal with general issues that are relevant to all psychoactive substances, including alcohol. Alcohol, however, occupies a unique place in many societies as a psychoactive substance that is legally available to large numbers of people, which can be produced domestically and bought without a prescription, not from a pharmacist, but in bars, shops (off-licences) and supermarkets. Its consumption forms part of the social fabric of many societies, where it can play an integral role in social occasions and where the alcohol industry can be integral to the economy of the country as a whole.

For all of these reasons alcohol is quite different from the other substances of abuse and dependence discussed in this book and this chapter focuses on those issues that are alcohol specific and that are not covered elsewhere.

Definitions

Unit of alcohol

Because alcohol can be purchased (or made) in many forms and in different strengths, it can be very difficult to assess consumption. To simplify this, a system of 'units' of alcohol has been devised, with one unit equal to 10 ml or 8 g of absolute alcohol. A half-pint (284 ml) of beer, a glass (125 ml) of table wine, a glass (50 ml) of fortified wine and a single measure (25 ml) of spirits each contain approximately one unit of alcohol, although this simplification ignores the different alcohol concentrations that occur in different beers and wines, for example.

The exact number of units of alcohol in a particular drink can be accurately calculated by multiplying the volume of the drink to be consumed (in millilitres) by its percentage alcohol content by volume (ABV, stated as a percentage figure on the bottle or can), multiplying again by 0.8 and then dividing by 1000: e.g. half a pint of 4% ABV beer contains $284 \times 4 \times 0.8/1000 = 0.9$ units; and 440 mls of premium lager with 5% ABV contains $440 \times 5 \times 0.8/1000 = 1.8$ units.

'Safe' limits and sensible drinking

Alcohol is a psychoactive substance and the notion of 'safety' is therefore related to the particular circumstances when it is consumed. For example it is not safe to consume any alcohol at all if it is important that judgement is unimpaired – for example when driving or operating any potentially hazardous machinery. 'Safety' is also related to alcohol's capacity to cause tissue damage in particular circumstances. Thus it is not safe for a pregnant woman to drink alcohol because it can damage the fetus, nor is it safe for someone with liver disease to drink alcohol because their ability to metabolize it is impaired. However, recognizing that (in some societies) the majority of people consume alcohol in moderate amounts, with only a minority drinking excessively in a way that damages their health, attempts have been made to identify a level of consumption that is of low risk. There is now a general consensus that for men, drinking up to 21 units of alcohol over a 7-day period is associated with a low risk to health, and that the equivalent figure for women is 14 units.[1]

This clear advice on limits for weekly consumption that are of low risk has been clouded by conflicting advice on daily consumption, which state that regular consumption by men of 3–4 units per day, and by women of 2–3 units per day, is of low risk.[2] However, most studies in the UK are based on the previously recommended, low risk limits for weekly consumption (21 units for men and 14 units for women). It is worth noting that an emphasis on 'safe' levels of consumption carries the disadvantage that it may encourage those who formerly drank less than this (or indeed nothing at all) to increase consumption, particularly when recent research has demonstrated that moderate alcohol consumption has a cardioprotective effect on middle-aged men and postmenopausal women.[2] Therefore, it is preferable to avoid the term 'safe' in favour of 'low risk'.

Harmful drinking and alcohol misuse

Men who drink more than 50 units per week and women who drink more than 35 units per week are at high risk of developing alcohol-related disease and this pattern of drinking is therefore described as harmful or alternatively as alcohol misuse.

Hazardous drinking

Drinking is described as hazardous when it exceeds safe limits but does not reach harmful levels. The term therefore describes intake of alcohol of 22–50 units per week by men and of 15–35 units per week by women and is related to an increased risk of alcohol-related harm.

It should be noted that the terms 'hazardous drinking' and 'harmful drinki to describe particular levels of consumption are purely arbitrary and ref

relative risk; thus a hazardous level for a healthy adult may be very harmful for an elderly person or an adolescent or indeed, very harmful if the healthy adult then drives a car.

Problem drinker

A problem drinker is an individual who is experiencing alcohol-related harm, regardless of their individual level of consumption. This usually occurs when consumption exceeds safe limits.

Alcohol dependence syndrome

The clinical features of the alcohol dependence syndrome were first described in 1976.[3] It is a clustering of signs and symptoms and can be of varying severity. It is diagnosed if three or more of the following conditions are fulfilled:

- A strong desire or compulsion to drink;
- Difficulty controlling the onset or termination of alcohol consumption or the level of use;
- Physiological withdrawal syndrome – or the use of alcohol to prevent its onset; Increasing tolerance to alcohol;
- Progressive neglect of other interests;
- Persisting use of alcohol despite evidence and awareness of alcohol-related harm;
- Reinstatement after abstinence.

It will be noted that these criteria are very similar to those described in Chapter 1 in relation to a more general description of the dependent state.

Extent and nature of the problem

In the UK efforts to control alcohol consumption entail licensing regulations that are perceived by many as byzantine in their complexity, inconsistent and intrusive on personal freedom.[4] Despite these laws, public disorder and drink/driving offences related to alcohol are frequent occurrences. These receive considerable media attention leading to a perception that excessive consumption is widespread and increasing and that the UK is somehow 'worse' at handling alcohol than other industrialized countries. It is therefore interesting to compare alcohol consumption in the UK with that in other European countries although it is difficult to obtain the accurate information on which to base such comparisons. For example, in addition to 'recorded' consumption – i.e. recorded for the purpose of taxation – there is also 'unrecorded' consumption. This includes domestically produced alcohol which, although ostensibly prepared for personal use may also be distributed illicitly, as well as alcohol smuggled in from abroad.

Despite these potential inaccuracies, it has been estimated that annual consumption in the UK is about 8 litres of pure alcohol per head of the population. This places the UK in the 20th position for European alcohol consumption which varies from 0.87 litres per capita in Turkey to 12.7 litres per capita in Luxembourg with France, Germany and Belgium close behind.[5] However, there are interesting trends in consumption almost everywhere, with marked reductions occurring in France, Italy and Spain and smaller reductions in Iceland, The Netherlands, Norway, Portugal, Slovakia and Switzerland. Some countries, such as Greece, Iceland and Luxembourg, are reporting increasing consumption while in others (Denmark, Sweden, Turkey, Finland and the UK) the position appears fairly stable.[6]

Apart from differing levels of consumption, there are also major differences between countries in their drinking habits and specifically in the preferred alcoholic beverage. Thus, in France, Greece and Portugal it is wine, in Denmark, Norway and The Netherlands it is beer, while in Iceland and Poland it is predominantly spirits. These differences reflect the different role of alcohol in different countries. For example, alcohol (as wine) is drunk every day as the expected accompaniment to meals in Southern European wine-producing countries whereas, in Northern Europe, drinking alcohol (as beer) is seen as a form of entertainment in its own right and integral to male bonding, as well as the almost inevitable accompaniment to major sporting events. It should also be remembered that it is possible for all of these occasions to occur without the support of alcohol. In Islamic countries where consumption of alcohol is forbidden, there is near-complete abstention. Illicit domestic production and consumption – where it exists – is on a small scale, partly for fear of the consequences if found out, but also because of the community's attitude towards alcohol.

Whatever the favoured drink, consumption by populations as a whole has a very similar pattern. There is a continuous spectrum of drinking behaviour with the majority of people drinking moderately and a small percentage drinking very heavily – although this small percentage accounts for a large number of people, nation-wide. Because there is no sharp delineation between moderate and heavy drinkers, it is difficult on the basis of population studies to be specific about harmful drinking at an individual level. However, using the definitions above, it is estimated that in the UK about 1.4 million people have harmful levels of alcohol consumption (>50 units/week for men, >35 units/week for women) and that 7 million people drink more than recommended 'sensible' amounts (21 units/week for men, >14 units/week for women).[7]

Within these very large figures about the incidence of harmful levels of drinking, there is particular concern about the number of young people in the UK who drink at harmful levels, with the age group of 18–24 years recorded as having the highest mean consumption and the highest percentage of heavy drinkers. Even more worrying is the evidence that across Europe as a whole, the age at which young people start to drink is falling.[6] In the UK for example, the number of regular drinkers aged 11–15 years increased from 13% in 1988 to 20% in 1996 and the average number of units consumed per week by this age group is also increasing.[8] There is some evidence that youth drinking is more common in the UK than in other parts of Europe with 15 year olds in Wales consuming significantly more alcohol than people of the same age in other parts of Europe.[6] The long-term effects on their health of excessive alcohol consumption by young people are not known. At the other end of the age spectrum, over the last 10 years there has been a 50% increase in the number drinking over a safe level in the 65 + age group.

Another worrying trend is the growth in alcohol consumption by women, both in terms of the average quantity consumed and the number of women drinking at hazardous levels. Thus women's average drinking per week increased from 5.4 units per week in 1992 to 6.3 units per week in 1996, although men's consumption remained steady over this period. Similarly, the percentage of women drinking above 'sensible' levels (i.e. > 14 units per week) increased from 9% in 1984 to 14% in 1996.[7] Although it is possible to explain such changes in terms of greater equality of opportunity for women (employment, earning power, recreation, etc.), it is a cause of particular concern, given the differences in alcohol metabolism in men and women which make the latter more susceptible to the adverse effects of alcohol. Furthermore, alcohol use disorder in a woman of child-bearing age risks the development of the fetal alcohol syndrome (see below).

Recognition of problem drinking

As with any other substance use disorder, making a diagnosis of alcohol use disorder (AUD) can be difficult because, for a variety of reasons, patients do not always volunteer an honest history of their alcohol consumption. A drinking history will explore issues such as the frequency of drinking; how much is consumed on a typical day, and in what form; the number of days in the previous month when consumption has exceeded 10 units; alcohol-related problems in the previous year, at home, at work, with the law, affecting health; alcohol-related injuries (self or others); the use of alcohol to resolve problems. If there is evidence of hazardous or harmful drinking an assessment of dependence should be made by asking whether the patient has difficulty controlling or cutting down the amount drunk and exploring the presence/absence of withdrawal symptoms and/or the use of alcohol to control them.

Although, as always, a careful history and physical examination form the basis of diagnosis, there are a number of biochemical and haematological investigations

Table 4.1 Methods of screenings for alcohol use disorder (AUD)

	Sensitivity	Specificity	Duration
Aspartate amino transferase	30–50%	80–86%	1–2 months
Alanine amino transferase	30–50%	80–86%	1–2 months
Gamma glutamyl transferase	50–70%	75–85%	1–2 months
Mean cell volume	25–52%	85–95%	1–2 months
Carbohydrate-deficient transferrin	40–70%	80–98%	1–3 months
AUDIT questionnaire	92%	93%	1–3 weeks

Source: Drummond C & Ghodse H.[12]

that can improve the accuracy of diagnosis and the subsequent management of the condition. In addition, methods of screening for AUD in primary care and in a general medical setting have been devised (Table 4.1). The criteria for diagnosis in accordance with ICD-10 and DSM-IV are described in Chapter 5.

Questionnaires

CAGE is one such screening test, comprised of only four questions (Do you have difficulty **C**utting down? Are you **A**ngry because someone criticized your drinking? Do you feel **G**uilty about drinking? Do you take an **E**ye-opener – morning drink to relieve withdrawal symptoms?).[9]

The Michigan Alcoholism Screening Test (MAST)[10] was another popular tool but both have now been overtaken by AUDIT, the Alcohol Use Disorders Identification Test, which was developed by the World Health Organization and which is now widely accepted as the standard tool.[11] It is short and can be administered by nonspecialist personnel and explores different aspects of Alcohol Use Disorders, including consumption, alcohol-related problems and dependence.

Biological markers

Liver enzymes

The effect of alcohol on the liver is well known and it is not surprising that this can be detected by abnormalities in liver enzymes, three of which are commonly used for screening for AUDs: aspartate amino transferase (AST), alanine amino transferase (ALT) and gamma glutamyl transferase (GGT). However, the amino transferases in particular are also found in many other body tissues (heart, muscle, kidney, brain) so that elevated levels are not diagnostic of liver disease. As ALT is more specific for liver damage than AST it is a more useful test of excessive drinking. GGT is mainly found in the liver and because its sensitivity and specificity for liver damage is higher than ALT and AST, it is the most useful widely available test for detecting AUDs; blood levels correlate with the quantity and frequency of heavy drinking and, like the other enzymes, its blood level normally returns to normal after 1–2 months abstinence.[12]

MCV

Excessive alcohol consumption is associated with macrocytosis (enlarged red cells) so that measurement of Mean Cell Volume (MCV) can be used for screening for AUDs. The mechanism of this effect is not known but chronic excessive alcohol consumption is associated with a number of vitamin deficiencies, including vitamin B and folate deficiencies which cause macrocytic anaemia. These and other conditions must be excluded before a diagnosis of alcohol misuse can be made.

Carbohydrate-deficient transferrin (CDT)

CDT is an enzyme which is relatively unaffected by liver disease. Currently it is available in only a few laboratories and is an expensive test in comparison with the more routinely available tests for liver enzymes; its main use is likely to be in the detection of relapse.[12]

Alcohol metabolism

Alcohol (ethanol) is consumed in a wide variety of drinks with widely varying alcoholic content. Whatever the source, it is rapidly absorbed from the upper gastrointestinal tract and is metabolized in the liver, mostly by alcohol dehydrogenase (ADH), with the microsomal ethanol oxidizing system (MEOS) and the catalase pathway playing a minor role. ADH converts ethanol to acetaldehyde which, in turn, is oxidized to acetate by acetaldehyde dehydrogenase (ALDH) and the acetate is then metabolized to carbon dioxide and water which are excreted.

ALDH is interesting because it can exist in a mutant, inactive form. This is rarely found in Caucasians but occurs in 40% of Orientals who inherit it as an autosomal dominant. Those with the inactive form of ALDH have a reduced ability to metabolize acetaldehyde which therefore accumulates in the body after the consumption of alcohol leading to a general vasodilatation and marked facial flushing.

If more alcohol is consumed than the liver can metabolize, a number of biochemical disturbances ensue, including hypo- or hyperglycaemia, lactic acidosis and ketoacidosis which contribute to the state of intoxication and the subsequent after effects. Chronic alcohol misuse leads to faster metabolism of ethanol because the MEOS becomes more active, accounting for up to 10% of ethanol oxidation.

Peak blood alcohol concentration is usually achieved approximately one hour after consumption, although this depends on factors such as the type of drink and its alcohol concentration, body mass and gender, speed of ingestion, the gastric emptying rate and on whether food was consumed at the same time. Peak concentrations are higher in women than in men (following a standard oral dose) because body water, in which ethanol is distributed, forms a smaller proportion of total body weight in women than men.

Alcohol is eliminated from the body at the rate of about 1 unit per hour although this too depends on individual variations such as body mass, gender and the development of tolerance to alcohol.

Adverse effects

Both acute and chronic alcohol misuse lead to a range of adverse consequences, although few of them are specific to alcohol. Therefore a high level of awareness and suspicion of alcohol as a causative factor aids the diagnosis of alcohol misuse and permits earlier therapeutic intervention.

All organs of the body are affected by excessive alcohol consumption so that the list of alcohol-related harms is very long and will not be described in detail here. It includes accidents and injury; oesophagitis, gastritis and pancreatitis; hypertension, cardiac arrhythmias, cardiomyopathy, cerebrovascular accidents; myopathy and neuropathy; specific neurological disorders; and liver damage. In addition there are a number of superficial physical signs that are highly suggestive of alcohol misuse and that should be specifically sought and recorded if this diagnosis is being considered, e.g. spider naevi, telangiectasia, facial mooning, parotid enlargement, palmar erythema, Dupuytren's contracture and gynaecomastia.[13]

Some of the harmful effects of alcohol are described in more detail below.

Liver damage

Excessive consumption of alcohol affects fat metabolism by the liver leading to the accumulation of fat in the liver cells. Although this is reversible if alcohol is withdrawn and is not in itself harmful, it reduces the liver's ability to metabolize other body toxins. Continued drinking leads to alcohol-induced hepatitis, an inflammatory condition of the liver which may be asymptomatic or may present with anorexia, fever and jaundice. The outcome depends on whether alcohol consumption ceases or continues. Cessation is likely to lead to recovery while continued consumption is associated with the development of severe hepatitis for which the mortality rate is up to 40%.

Cirrhosis is the most dangerous type of liver damage that occurs when liver cells have died and been replaced by fibrous scar tissue; it is more likely to occur in patients with severe hepatitis and women are more susceptible than men. Again, cirrhosis may remain asymptomatic for a long time and be diagnosed only incidentally. However, patients may present in liver failure or with bleeding from oesophageal varices due to raised pressure in the veins of the liver as they become involved in the fibrotic process. Hepatic carcinoma is more likely to develop in a cirrhotic liver.

Alcohol-induced liver disease is particularly important because of the association between alcohol misuse and the misuse of drugs by injection. Injecting drug users are at increased risk of developing hepatitis B and/or hepatitis C, the prognosis of which is significantly worse if the liver is also being damaged by alcohol.

Neurological syndromes

Chronic effects

Excessive consumption of alcohol over a long period has severe and lasting effects on the brain. A number of different pathologies and syndromes have been described, depending on which part of the brain is most severely affected by alcohol. For example, there may be atrophy of the cerebral cortex associated with impairment of intellectual capacity – the so-called alcoholic dementia. Similarly there may be atrophy of the cerebellar cortex which is associated with ataxia, predominantly affecting the trunk and legs rather than the arms. Both of these degenerative disorders may improve if there is a prolonged period of abstinence.

Wernicke–Korsakov syndrome

The Wernicke–Korsakoff syndrome occurs when there is excessive alcohol consumption by those who are thiamine deficient – a dietary deficiency which is not uncommon in those whose diet is dominated by alcohol. Wernicke's encephalopathy is the acute stage that develops over the course of a few days and is characterized by a confusional state, eye signs (nystagmus, ophthalmoplegia) and ataxia. It may be followed by Korsakoff's psychosis in which there is severe memory loss, involving both retrograde and anterograde amnesia but with other intellectual abilities remaining intact, perhaps accounting for the confabulation that often accompanies the amnesia. However, sometimes the amnesic syndrome occurs concurrently with the encephalopathy and sometimes the eye signs and ataxia do not occur.

Fetal alcohol syndrome

The consumption of alcohol during pregnancy has the potential to harm the developing fetus and, as animal research has shown, cause damage even at very low levels of consumption; there is no known 'safe' level of drinking in pregnancy.[14] Nevertheless, it is not surprising that the most serious damage to the fetus occurs in those whose consumption is at harmful levels, but the relationship between consumption and harm is not simple as some alcohol misusers produce children who are apparently normal.

The fetal alcohol syndrome encompasses several different features including growth retardation, both pre- and postnatal; central nervous system abnormalities such as microcephaly, learning disability, hypotonia, poor coordination and hyperactivity; a number of physical abnormalities such as congenital deformities of the eyes, ears, mouth, cardiovascular system, genitourinary tract and skeleton. Specific craniofacial abnormalities have also been described which include a short palpebral fissure with epicanthic folds, a short upturned nose, a thin upper lip and hypoplasia of the lower jaw. These, combined with microcephaly lead to a commonality of appearance which has been attributed to alcohol consumption and has been designated as a syndrome.[15]

Although alcohol-related damage may occur at any stage of the pregnancy, the most vulnerable period (as for most teratogenic substances) is from 4 to 10 weeks. Women are therefore advised not to consume any alcohol during the first trimester and then, if they wish to drink, to limit this to 1–2 units once or twice per week.

Management of problem drinking and its complications

Treatment of acute intoxication

The acute effects of excessive consumption of alcohol on the nervous system are well known to most people. Acute intoxication is characterized by impairment of cognitive function, motor coordination and sensory perception. The blood alcohol level at which this occurs depends on factors such as the rate of intake and on whether or not tolerance has developed. In nonhabitual drinkers blood concentrations of 30–70 mg/100 ml are associated with some impairment of cognitive functioning, etc. and there is obvious intoxication when blood levels of 150–250 mg/100 ml are reached. However, those who drink heavily and regularly become tolerant to some of the effects of alcohol and, with equally high blood levels, may show no sign of being drunk; however, despite this apparent normality, their judgement and coordination may be significantly impaired.

Although acute intoxication with alcohol may be summarily dismissed as mere drunkenness, it is in fact an overdose of a psychoactive substance and should be managed as such. Specifically, all of the usual precautions should be implemented when treating a patient rendered unconscious by alcohol in order to maintain an airway and to ensure that they do not inhale their vomit. While the majority 'sleep it off' without further intervention, there should be careful and regular observations in case respiratory depression ensues. Hypoglycaemia may also occur, manifested by sweating and lack of coordination – which are themselves symptoms of alcohol intoxication. Furthermore, there should be an awareness that there may have been simultaneous misuse of other substances which may interact with alcohol.

If young children have access to alcohol, they may drink it and become acutely and sometimes fatally poisoned. They are particularly susceptible to hypoglycaemia, which is more dangerous for them than for adults. Children with alcohol intoxication must therefore be monitored carefully for changes in blood sugar and liver function.

Alcohol withdrawal

The alcohol withdrawal syndrome occurs if an individual who has become dependent on alcohol suddenly stops drinking without taking substitute medication. This may occur if access to alcohol is denied – by admission to hospital for example, if the staff are unaware of the previous history of drinking – or if the person concerned decides that he or she wants to stop drinking and does so without seeking medical advice.

The severity of symptoms is related to the severity of the preceding dependence and to the quantity of alcohol habitually consumed. Minor symptoms may be intermittent and mild, starting 6–8 hours after the last drink and include anxiety, sweating, tremor, nausea, retching or vomiting, raised pulse rate and blood pressure. Because of the timescale of onset of symptoms, they are typically experienced first thing in the morning on waking. More severely dependent individuals may experience them within a few hours of drinking, during the day or night, if their blood alcohol level falls.

In severely dependent individuals sudden alcohol withdrawal may lead to the condition known as delirium tremens. This is characterized by clouding of consciousness, confusion, bizarre hallucinations affecting every sensory modality, and tremor. Visual hallucinations are common but do not always occur. Seizures (fits) occur in about 5–15% of alcohol-dependent individuals if they stop drinking. Prevention of these potentially life-threatening complications is the reason for managing alcohol withdrawal in a more structured way.

Detoxification

Detoxification may be managed in the out-patient setting by a very gradual stepped reduction in alcohol consumption. However, if attempts to reduce gradually have failed and/or if recent consumption exceeds 15 units per day, it is likely that medication will be needed to control withdrawal symptoms (anxiety, insomnia, nausea, tremor) and to reduce the risk of fits. A short-term, reducing course of chlordiazepoxide is recommended, starting with a dose of 20–30 mg three or four times daily and reducing to nil over five days. It is important that the patient does not consume alcohol if he/she is also taking chlordiazepoxide and, if there is

Box 4.1	Diazepam	Chlordiazepoxide
Day 1	15 mg four times daily	30 mg four times daily
Day 2	10 mg four times daily	30 mg three times daily
Day 3	10 mg three times daily	20 mg twice daily
Day 4	5 mg four times daily	10 mg twice daily
Day 5	5 mg three times daily	10 mg twice daily
Day 6	5 mg twice daily	10 mg at night
Day 7	5 mg at night	

concern that this advice will be ignored, medication should be issued on a daily basis and only after checks on blood, urine and breath for the presence of alcohol. Clomethiazole should not be prescribed at all for out-patient detoxification because of the potentially fatal interaction with alcohol if the patient continues drinking.

In-patient detoxification is indicated in most cases with serious comorbidity (whether physical or psychiatric), if there is a previous history of delirium tremens or fits or if there are early signs of encephalopathy. Lack of social support, including homelessness, and previous, unsuccessful attempts at detoxification in the out-patient setting are other reasons for admission for detoxification. Again, it involves the administration of sedative anticonvulsants, usually a benzodiazepine. An indicative regime is shown in Box 4.1.

Alternatively, benzodiazepines may be used on a 'symptom-triggered' basis, with, for example, diazepam 10–20 mg taken orally at 2-hourly intervals until agitation, sweating, tremor and tachycardia are adequately controlled, up to a maximum of 160 mg in 24 hours.[16] As a general principle, it is better to start treatment prophylactically, rather than waiting for 24 hours after the last drink, and to be sure that sufficient benzodiazepines are administered to control adequately withdrawal symptoms because adequate dosage reduces the risk of withdrawal seizures and delirium tremens. In this context it is clear that with very high levels of daily alcohol consumption, higher starting doses of benzodiazepines will be needed. However, doses of chlordiazepoxide in excess of 40 mg four times daily should only be prescribed where there is clear evidence of very severe alcohol dependence (e.g. more than 40 units of alcohol daily). Such high doses are rarely necessary in women and never in the elderly. They should never be given if there is evidence of liver impairment. It is worth noting that starting doses of benzodiazepines are likely to be higher in the not uncommon situation of dependence on both alcohol and benzodiazepines.

Impairment of liver function should always prompt particular care in managing detoxification because the liver's ability to metabolize drugs may be reduced, with an increased risk of drug intoxication. In this situation, smaller doses of a shorter-acting benzodiazepine should be given and this is usually undertaken on an in-patient basis where liver function can be closely monitored. Alternatively, chlomethiazole (chlormethiazole) 9 or 10 capsules daily in 3–4 divided doses may be used, but always in an environment of close monitoring. Clomethiazole is much less popular now than previously because of awareness of the potential for respiratory depression; it should rarely, if ever, be administered intravenously and, if it is given by this route, resuscitation facilities must be immediately available and the patient kept under close and constant observation because of the risk of severe respiratory failure and deep unconsciousness.

Delirium tremens

Early identification and correct management of alcohol withdrawal should prevent the onset of delirium tremens. However, it may occur despite careful management of withdrawal and patients may also present with delirium tremens following alcohol withdrawal outside hospital. If it occurs, the general principles of managing any disturbed and confused patient should be applied and a safe and well-lit environment with experienced staff who are able to remain calm is essential. If there is extreme agitation, physical restraint may be necessary as well as parenteral sedatives (e.g. intravenous diazepam 5–10 mg over 1–2 minutes, or intramuscular droperidol 10 mg). Intravenous chlormethiazole is effective but there is a risk of respiratory depression (see above). There should be regular monitoring of body temperature, fluids, electrolytes and blood sugar.

Withdrawal seizures

It is hoped that, with adequate preventative measures as described above, fits will not occur and they are unlikely if the patient is adequately sedated. If, despite best efforts, seizures do occur or if status epilepticus develops, a slow intravenous injection of diazepam or rectal diazepam should be given and the condition managed as for any patient with status epilepticus. If diazepam is given intravenously the risk of thrombophlebitis is minimized by using an emulsion. If fits persist following withdrawal, either phenytoin or carbamazepine are suitable anticonvulsants.

Wernicke–Korsakov syndrome

Because Wernicke's encephalopathy can arise very suddenly and without warning and because its early symptoms (ataxia and confusion) may be attributed to drunkenness, it is wise to give vitamin B$_1$ (thiamine) prophylactically to patients with a heavy alcohol intake because this may prevent the permanent brain damage that may follow undiagnosed (and therefore untreated) Wernicke's encephalopathy. Thiamine may be given orally (50 mg twice daily) but, because heavy drinkers have impaired absorption, parenteral administration is preferred, and is indicated for those who are perceived as particularly at risk, such as those with malnutrition, peripheral neuropathy or those with early signs of the syndrome. Pabrinex High Potency, which contains vitamins B and C in high dosage, should be given either intravenously or intramuscularly for 5 days, followed by oral administration. Because there may (rarely) be an anaphylactic reaction to Pabrinex, it should only be administered in the in-patient setting where resuscitation can be undertaken if necessary.

Relapse prevention

Brief intervention

It has been found that many people with AUD benefit from a short-term focused intervention in relation to their drinking behaviour, comprising an assessment of their alcohol intake, the provision of information about problem drinking and clear advice about reducing or stopping drinking. Such brief interventions may involve just a single patient contact although additional appointments may be offered. Relevant information includes leaflets, self-help manuals, advice about local and national support agencies, results of blood tests, etc. Primary care services are ideally placed to offer this sort of brief intervention and it has been found that this often reduces alcohol consumption and the proportion of the population drinking at hazardous levels. There are conflicting claims about the effectiveness of this approach with some studies suggesting that they are as effective as counselling carried out over a longer period or more specialist intervention. On balance it appears that brief interventions may help motivated people to reduce alcohol consumption to sensible limits but are probably not effective for those with established alcohol dependency.[17,18,19]

Motivational interviewing

The principles of motivational interviewing are outlined in Chapter 6 and this technique can be utilized during brief interventions. Indeed it can be particularly relevant in this situation where the patient's alcohol consumption has been revealed incidentally during the course of a consultation rather than being the specific reason for the consultation. At this point the doctor's (or other health professional's) view that the patient needs to change their drinking behaviour may not be shared by the patient him or herself – not least because they may never have considered this. The essential components of the motivational interviewing at this point are summarized by the acronym FRAMES:

Feedback about the risk of personal harm/impairment;
Responsibility: emphasis on personal responsibility for change;

Advice to cut down or, if necessary, stop drinking;

Menu of options for changing drinking;

Empathic interviewing;

Self efficacy: leaving the patient feeling able to cope with achieving agreed goals.

Abstinence or controlled drinking

The question of whether to advise a reduction in alcohol consumption or total abstinence is an important issue that is likely to arise at an early stage of any intervention and most patients will hope that they can achieve the former and be able to regain controlled social drinking. Notwithstanding this, abstinence is the preferred goal for older patients, for those who have previously tried and failed to achieve controlled drinking, those with serious physical dependency and for those with significant alcohol-related physical harm. The decision will be influenced by the family's views, if they are strongly opposed to attempting controlled drinking, also if the environment is such that relapse seems very likely if controlled drinking is tried.[20]

Conversely controlled drinking is likely to be a realistic goal if the problem is newly detected with no, or only minimal, signs of dependence and no major medical complications, if there is no history of psychiatric illness and no impulsive traits; if the patient is in a socially stable situation, is likely to comply with treatment and has had no previous experience of trying and failing to achieve controlled drinking. Both the patient and the partner/family should agree with this approach which should encompass a number of principles. Firstly, a drinking diary must be kept, recording all alcohol consumption; the maximum number of drinks permitted on any occasion should be agreed as well as the number of abstinent days. Controlled drinking includes drinking more slowly and/or reducing the alcoholic strength of drinks. The patient should be helped to develop an awareness of triggers for drinking excessively and assertiveness skills to refuse drinks as well as other ways of coping with triggers. A defined reward system for achieving goals should also be agreed.

Pharmacological approaches

Although there is no pharmacological 'solution' to alcohol dependence, two drugs have been licensed as adjunctive treatment, specifically for preventing relapse.

Disulfiram

Disulfiram acts by blocking the action of alcohol dehydrogenase, leading to an accumulation of acetaldehyde, which in turn causes unpleasant systemic effects if even small amounts of alcohol are consumed. Symptoms include flushing of the face, headache, increased heart rate and palpitations, nausea and vomiting, and these may be precipitated by the small amounts of alcohol that are present in many oral medicines. Large doses of alcohol taken after disulfiram may cause the potentially dangerous complications of cardiac arhythmias, hypotension and collapse. Disulfiram is usually given in a dose of 100–200 mg daily but satisfactory blood levels will not be achieved for a few days. The alternative approach to initiating treatment is to give 800 mg as a single dose on the first day, reducing over 5 days to the maintenance dose of 100–200 mg daily; this achieves satisfactory blood levels more swiftly but side effects (lethargy and fatigue, vomiting, unpleasant taste in the mouth) may be more troublesome.

Disulfiram can be helpful as a deterrent to taking the first drink and can be effective in reducing the number of drinking days and the quantity of alcohol consumed. However, it has not been shown conclusively to enhance abstinence.[18] Furthermore, because of the nature of the reaction that it causes, it is inappropriate for those with cardiovascular or respiratory disease, hepatic or renal impairment, diabetes or epilepsy, or for women who are pregnant or breastfeeding. Within these limitations, it appears to work best if the patient participates in the decision to use this medication and is therefore committed to it, and when there is adequate supervision to ensure that disulfiram is actually consumed. Above all it must be incorporated into a comprehensive treatment programme.

Acamprosate

Acamprosate is an analogue of gamma amino butyric acid (GABA) and, although its mechanism of action is not fully understood, it is thought to affect excitatory neurotransmitters in the brain. It appears to reduce craving for alcohol after withdrawal, thereby increasing the likelihood of continued abstinence[21,22] although, like disulfiram, it should be used as part of a therapeutic programme rather than in isolation. Unlike disulfiram, if the patient does return to drinking, there are no adverse interactions with alcohol. Acamprosate is prescribed in a dose of 666 mg three times daily for those weighing more than 60 kg; for those weighing less than this, the two later doses are halved (total dose 1332 mg). It should not be administered to those with hepatic or renal impairment nor to women who are pregnant or breastfeeding.

Other pharmacological approaches to relapse prevention include the opioid antagonist, naltrexone, in a dose of 50 mg daily.[23] It is suggested that this works by blocking or reducing the effects of alcohol on opioid receptor activity, making its consumption less pleasurable and thereby reducing its reinforcing effect. As with all other pharmacological approaches to relapse prevention, success depends on patient commitment and motivation.

Treatment matching

Finally it is worth emphasizing that, like all other forms of substance misuse, the matching of the treatment approach to the specific needs and situation of the individual is of paramount importance (see Chapter 6).[24,25]

Alcohol policies

Excessive alcohol consumption places an enormous burden on society – not just the personal harms outlined above, but also on family, friends and the wider community. The effects are obvious to everyone because of accidents and injuries, social disruption and law and order issues associated with drunkenness, family problems, absenteeism from work, impaired performance and unemployment, the impact on health services, premature death and so on. There have been no studies in the UK to calculate the financial costs of all such consequences but, drawing on research from other countries, it has been suggested that alcohol costs between 2% and 5% of the gross national product (GNP);[26] using the lower of these figures suggests that alcohol misuse in the UK costs the country more than £10 billion per year. For these reasons, although alcohol is used moderately by most of the population, it is not surprising that all societies have legislation controlling many aspects of its manufacture, distribution and trade.

Drink driving

Death and injuries in alcohol-related road traffic accidents are, rightly, a cause for public concern with hundreds of deaths and thousands of injuries each year caused by drivers who have been drinking. In response, in the UK, there is a permissible limit for alcohol consumption of 80 mg of alcohol per 100 ml of blood, with linked limits relating to breath and urine samples. However, a driver may only be tested if involved in an accident, if driving dangerously, or if the police suspect him or her of having been drinking. Until recently, a conviction for a drink-driving offence resulted in a ban of a minimum of 1 year and a reconviction within 10 years led to a 3-year ban. However, with growing public anger about the apparent leniency of sentencing in some cases and the rapidity with which known heavy drinkers resume dangerous driving, a new offence has been identified of causing death by dangerous driving. Furthermore, the maximum sentence for serious drink-driving offences has been doubled to 10 years and 'high risk' offenders are now required to take medical tests to prove that they are no longer heavy drinkers before regaining their licence. A 'high risk' offender is one who commits two or more drink-drive offences in a 10-year period or one who has a blood alcohol level greater than 200 mg.

What is interesting is that these increasingly draconian penalties, which would have been inconceivable 20 years ago, are now being introduced and imposed in response to public demand and opinion. This is reminiscent of the way in which severe restrictions on smoking in public places, which would once have been perceived as intolerable, are now permissible and accepted, and suggests that, for alcohol, as with smoking, public attitudes to excessive consumption may be beginning to change. In this emerging context it may become possible to set blood alcohol limits at a lower level than at present, drawing on experience from abroad. For example, in Japan and some Eastern European countries, the legal limit is zero; in Poland and Sweden it is 20 mg and in Australia, Belgium, Finland, Greece, Netherlands, Norway and Portugal, it is 50 mg. A lower limit is supported by experimental evidence showing that statistically significant performance impairment in laboratory tests occurs with blood levels of around 20 mg.[27] It has also been shown that a blood alcohol level of 60 mg is associated with an accident potential twice that at 0 mg; at 100 mg it is six times greater and, at 150 mg, it is 25 times greater. Conversely, there is a relatively small increase in accident potential with blood alcohol levels below 50 mg.[28] An additional measure could be to reduce the threshold for defining a 'high risk' offender from 200 mg to 150 mg, thereby ensuring that more people have to prove their fitness for relicensing.

Taxation

Governments have imposed taxes on alcohol for hundreds of years and the level of taxation nowadays may have a number of quite different objectives including income generation, encouraging employment and local manufacture, controlling the cost of living and inflation, and limiting the harmful effects of consumption. An important principle underpinning taxation decisions is the extent to which taxation affects price and the extent to which price affects consumption.

It is generally accepted that, as the real price of alcohol increases, consumption reduces and vice versa, although it must be acknowledged that this is a simplification of the relationship between these two factors and that other factors must be taken into account, such as disposable income. However, the relationship is important because research shows that the higher the average consumption of alcohol by a population, the higher the incidence of alcohol-related problems.[29] Therefore, using taxation to manipulate the price of alcohol to the consumer is potentially a powerful lever for changing consumption and the consequent impact of alcohol-related problems, although there is always the possibility that, if alcohol becomes excessively expensive, this might encourage domestic manufacture and/ or the use of illicit substances.

In practice, however, the potential flexibilities offered by manipulating taxation on alcohol in the UK are limited both by EU regulations and by other considerations. For example, because alcohol is consumed moderately by most people and plays an important part in social interactions, increasing taxation in an attempt to reduce population consumption is perceived as 'unfair' and is politically unpopular, as well as affecting the Retail Price Index. Also, differences in excise duty may contribute to big price differentials between countries, which in turn may lead either to an increase in smuggling or, for many UK residents, to frequent trips across the English Channel for bulk purchases of alcohol. This last point is important because income from excise duties is an important source of revenue for the government while the health of the alcohol industry – manufacture, distribution and sales – is also important because it is a major employer. Thus, despite well-articulated concerns about alcohol misuse, it is difficult for governments to balance the competing demands of minimizing excessive drinking while, at the same time, not undermining a profitable national industry. Market manipulation by varying the excise duty on different types of drinks is also difficult because EU regulations require that this should be linked to alcohol content. Thus, disproportionate increases in the tax on drinks favoured by young people (strong alcohol beer and lager, alcopops) in an effort to discourage under-age drinking, is impossible.

Licensing regulations

Another approach to controlling alcohol consumption is to regulate its sale – in terms of the places where it may be sold either for drinking on the premises (licensed) or for taking away ('off-licence'), the age at which alcohol may be purchased (and consumed in drinking venues) and the opening hours for such sales. Most countries regulate the sale of alcohol in some way but the restrictions vary from country to country, reflecting the varied drinking cultures that pertain in different areas. In Southern Europe, for example, with its vine-growing and wine-consumption tradition, the approach is far more liberal than in the north, with Spain having no licence requirements and no restrictions on hours of sale, whereas in Norway the sale of alcohol is limited to state-owned stores, which do not open on Sundays.

The approach adopted in the UK often seems illogical and out of step with modern lifestyles, both to tourists visiting the UK and to those who have travelled abroad and enjoyed a more relaxed approach. For example, although greater freedoms are now offered to those who wish to seek an extension of opening hours, the usual hours for on-licensed premises are 11 a.m. to 11 p.m. Another anachronism is that, with many supermarkets now staying open for 24 hours a day, the hours during which they may sell alcohol are different from those for other products in the same shop – leading to shoppers having to complete their purchases of alcohol by a certain time and, if necessary, resuming their shopping for other products when the alcohol 'deadline' has passed. There is therefore considerable demand for change and one argument put forward in support of a more liberal approach is that it would reduce the crowds of intoxicated drinkers emerging onto the streets when all on-licensed premises close at the same time – a phenomenon which does not occur, or which is much less marked, in those countries with a more relaxed approach to licensing hours. However, such arguments ignore the fact that the latter countries do not have the night-time culture of 'binge-drinking', with the specific aim of becoming intoxicated, which is particularly prevalent in the UK. It is therefore not clear whether more liberal or staggered hours would reduce disorder or would permit it to continue longer into the night.

The age at which young people are allowed to purchase alcohol is also a subject of much discussion because of concern that AUDs are increasingly being seen in teenagers. At present young people may purchase alcohol in a bar or off-licence from the age of 18 years. However, they may purchase alcohol with a meal (but not at a bar) from the age of 16. Youngsters are not allowed into bars under the age of 14 unless the licensee has a children's certificate that specifies the times and conditions when they may be present.

National and local strategies

It is clear that the manifold problems associated with excessive alcohol consumption require a range of responses at international, national and local levels. Firstly, such responses must be set in a strategic framework that encompasses health and community safety and that takes other substances of misuse into account. While national strategies are needed for issues such as taxation, advertising, licensing regulations and other legal matters, much of the preventative work and treatment services are best carried out at local level in a way that is sensitive to the needs of local communities. The latter is likely to involve a range of statutory and non-statutory agencies whose contributions must be coordinated so that they work in a synergistic and complementary fashion. In particular, given the evidence that there is widespread ignorance about 'safe' drinking levels and the consequences of misuse[30] there is clearly a need for public education campaigns on these topics. It is not easy to convey information about 'sensible' drinking because the issues are complex and this emphasizes the importance of local action that can be tailored to local circumstances.[31,32]

Assessment

Introduction

Careful, detailed and thorough assessment of individuals presenting with sub-stance-related problems is essential if they are to receive effective help. The purpose of the assessment is to identify the nature and severity of the drug-related problem; to understand why it arose, to assess its consequences and to establish the strengths and weaknesses of the patient and his or her situation. Armed with this information, it is possible to formulate and develop a treatment programme to help that particular individual to live a full life, integrated into society without the need for drugs.

The need for a very thorough assessment is crystallized by that last phrase, 'without the need for drugs'. While it is comparatively easy, in the sense of it being a straightforward procedure, to achieve drug withdrawal, continued abstinence ('staying off' i.e. relapse prevention) presents much more long-term and challenging problems. After all, having achieved abstinence, the substance-abusing individual usually finds him or herself in the same situation, with the same personal problems and the same personal resources – and with the same substances readily available on demand. Nothing will have changed except a temporary interruption of drug administration and it is perhaps only to be expected that the same behaviour should be resumed and often immediately. The key to staying off is change – in the individual, his or her life situation or the availability of drugs – and the whole point of the assessment procedure is to identify areas where change can be effected so that the need for drugs is reduced or, better still, eliminated.

It is not surprising that full assessment of the individual and all the antecedent and consequent problems is necessarily a lengthy procedure, and if the patient is referred to a specialist drug-dependence treatment unit (DDTU) it usually takes a couple of weeks. During this time the patient attends the specialist centre on several occasions and sees different members of the multidisciplinary team. Their enquiries may overlap to a certain extent, but gradually a picture is built up of the patient's drug/alcohol problem and how it has developed over the years, the family background, present social and financial circumstances and so on. These findings, together with the results of laboratory tests on blood and urine (and sometimes saliva or hair), are presented at a meeting of the multidisciplinary team and an individual treatment plan can be worked out.

A particular reason why assessment takes such a long time is that many patients attending specialist centres are, or claim to be, dependent on opiates and/or other drugs, and one of their reasons for attending the unit may be to obtain a prescription for drugs. Although this prescription may be the only way of retaining a patient in treatment, it is very important that it should not be handed out indiscriminately to everyone who claims to need it; a regular prescription for methadone, for example, could convert an occasional user of opiates into an opiate-dependent individual or it could be sold on the black market. Accurate diagnosis of dependence status is therefore very important.

The full assessment procedure is described below. It is intended only as a guide, to be modified according to the patient's needs, the presenting problem and the resources available to the professional who is being consulted.

Drug history

The purpose of this part of the history is to find out specifically and accurately about the patient's drug-taking behaviour, both at the present time and in the past, and to establish its importance in the patient's life as a whole. It must be appreciated from the beginning that the history given by the patient may be inaccurate and sometimes deliberately untruthful. The amount of drug taken may be understated, so that the apparent problem is minimized; alternatively it may be exaggerated in an attempt to get a larger dose prescribed. Illicit activity may be concealed. Truthful accounts are more likely to be obtained in a nonjudgmental situation and when confidentiality is assured.

It is first of all very important to establish why the patient is seeking help at this time and whether any specific event has precipitated their attendance. Information should be obtained about the first exposure to drug-taking and subsequent drug-taking should be similarly explored, ending up with recent patterns of abuse, including the methods and routes of drug administration. This part of the history-taking may be very complicated if the patient is or has been a polydrug abuser, and it is usually simplest to take each drug in turn, in chronological order of first use and to elicit all the relevant information for each drug separately. Specific enquiries should be made about amphetamines, methylphenidate (Ritalin), cocaine, cannabis, LSD, methadone, heroin, dipipanone (Diconal), barbiturates, methaqualone (Mandrax), benzodiazepines (diazepam, lorazepam, etc.) or other sedatives. A similar history should also be obtained about the use of tobacco or alcohol. The physical, psychological, social and legal consequences of drug use should be established and information elicited about previous attempts at seeking help and the other agencies with which the patient may have been in contact.

A format for obtaining all this information is outlined in Table 5.1. It suggests the most fruitful lines of questioning to elicit the maximum information, so that a full picture of the patient's drug-taking is built up. It is then possible to identify the main drug problem(s) for each patient, to find out if they are physically and/or psychologically dependent on drugs and to gain some idea of the severity of the drug dependence. The severity of drug dependence may be manifest in several ways, including duration of drug abuse, the quantity of drugs taken, the amount of drug-related activity compared with other activities in their life, the route of administration and the degree and extent of risk-taking behaviour.

A systematic assessment questionnaire, incorporating a scoring system for the severity of drug-related problems and the needs of the patient is included in Appendix 4 (St George's Substance Abuse Assessment Questionnaire). This is an excellent multidimensional assessment tool with rating of the level of problems and of the level of needs, scored by both patient and interviewer in each of the six problem areas. It is useful both for research purposes and for treatment planning.

Life history

Even a young drug abuser has a life behind him or her – a life history of many years, of which drug-taking forms only a part. Having explored, defined and understood the drug-taking, it is necessary to find out about all the other parts of the life history that provide the essential background to the foremost problem of drug abuse. It is said that to know all is to understand all; finding out about the life history of the drug abuser, about his or her environment, experiences and personality, aids the helper in understanding the whys and wherefores of the drug-taking. Reaching this understanding creates an empathy between the drug abuser and the professional helper that is the basis of any future therapeutic relationship.

The areas of the life history to be covered include the family history, which should specifically explore drug use by other members of the patient's family and their knowledge of and attitude towards the patient's drug-taking. Other import-ant information should be obtained about the patient's early history and academic record and, if there is any doubt, a specific enquiry should be made about the patient's ability to read and write. Their employment record should also be ascertained, but if it is impossible to enumerate all jobs or the number of jobs then the longest job held and the 'average duration' of jobs should be recorded. The marital and psychosexual history are of importance, as is the menstrual history if a

Table 5.1. Outline of drug history scheme

1. *Reason for referral*
   Type of help sought

2. *First exposure*
   Age
   Which drug
   Mode of administration
   Circumstances
      where
      who/how initiated
      source of drug
   Reaction to drug

3. *Subsequent use*
   Which drug(s)
      dose
      frequency of administration
      route
      date and age of becoming a regular user
      periods of heavy use
      maximum regular amount taken
      effects of drug
   Reasons for continuation
   Circumstances of drug-taking: solitary/with friends
   Preferred drug(s)
   Periods of abstinence:
      voluntary
      enforced
      reasons for relapse

4. *Recent use (last 4–6 weeks)*
   Drug(s):
      dose
      frequency
      route
   Any withdrawal symptoms
   Evidence of increasing tolerance; escalating dose
   Source of supply
   Price paid
   Continued use despite evidence of harm

Table 5.1 (*cont.*)

5. *History of self-injecting*
   Age first injected
   Duration of injecting
   Frequency
   Route: subcutaneous/intramuscular/intravenous
   Site

6. *HIV risk behaviour*
   Source of injection equipment
   Sharing of injection equipment
      last time shared
      number of others shared with
   Knowledge about sterilization procedures
   Knowledge about sources of clean equipment
   Heterosexual/homosexual risk behaviour
   Use of condoms
   Sexual behaviour when intoxicated
   Knowledge of HIV issues and transmission

7. *Consequences and complications of drug use*
   Physical illness: malnutrition; hepatitis; jaundice; abscesses; septicaemia; deep vein
   thrombosis; overdose; road traffic and other accidents; symptoms of abstinence syndrome
   Mental illness: episodes of drug-induced psychosis; intoxication leading to drowsiness and
   confusion; dementia
   Social problems: associated with drug use; amount spent weekly on drugs; source of that
   money; time spent on drug-taking; neglect of other activities
   Occupational problems: difficulties at work; suspensions, jobs lost
   Legal problems: drug-related criminal record; any pending court cases

8. *Contact with other treatment agencies or sources of help*
   e.g. DDTUs; doctors; probation services; local authorities; voluntary agencies, religious
   organizations, self-help groups, etc.

female patient is dependent on opiates; these drugs sometimes cause amenorrhoea and the early stages of pregnancy may not be diagnosed. It is also necessary to gain some idea of the patient's home circumstances, although a more detailed account will be elicited in the course of the social work assessment. An up-to-date account of the patient's legal history should be obtained and, perhaps most important of all, the patient's personality before drug-taking started should be explored. Here, information from parents or other friends or relatives may be very helpful, if the patient agrees to their participation in the enquiry.

A suggested format for establishing the patient's life history is provided in Table 5.2.

Table 5.2. Outline of life-history scheme

1. *Family history*

   Age and occupation of parents and siblings (if deceased: date and cause of death, together with patient's age at the time)

   Description of parents' personalities and their past and present attitudes towards patient

   History of illness or delinquency in family members

   Drug use (including alcohol, tobacco) by other family members

   Knowledge of patient's drug use by other family members, and their attitude towards it

   Relationship between various members of family

2. *Early history*

   Birth history

   Early development including time of milestones

   Childhood neurotic traits (bed-wetting, sleepwalking, tantrums, etc.) and periods of separation from parents

   Childhood illnesses

   Home life and atmosphere

3. *School*

   Schools attended

   Educational attainments

   Relationships with staff and peers

   Truancy

   Further education

   Vocational training

4. *Employment*

   Age of starting work

   Jobs held

   　dates

   　duration

   　wage

   　job satisfaction

   　reason for change

5. *Marital and psychosexual history*

   Date of marriage; spouse's name, age and occupation

   Children; names and ages

   General marital adjustment; any periods of permanent or temporary separation

   The same information should be collected for any further marriages or cohabitations

   Partner's drug-taking and knowledge of, and attitude to, patient's drug-taking

   Sexual inclinations and practices: masturbation; sexual fantasies; homosexuality; heterosexual experiences; contraception; sterilization

Table 5.2 (*cont.*)

6. *Menstrual history*
   Age when periods started
   Length of cycle
   Dysmenorrhoea
   Premenstrual tension
   Periods of amenorrhoea
   Date of last menstrual period
   Climacteric symptoms

7. *Previous illness*
   Physical
      major illnesses and accidents
      dates of admission to hospital
      accidental overdoses
   Psychiatric
      all psychiatric admissions and treatments
      attendance at psychiatric clinics
      suicide attempts; deliberate self-poisoning

8. *Home circumstances*
   Address; whom is patient living with
   Present income; its source
   Financial or domestic problems

9. *Legal history*
   Number of arrests, court appearances, convictions
   Periods in detention centre, Young Offenders Institutions, prison
   Periods of probation
   Nature of offences
   Outstanding court cases
   Disqualification from driving

10. *Previous personality (before drug use)*
    Interests, hobbies
    Social relations; family, friends
    Mood; mood swings
    Character: obsessionality, ambitions, future plans
    Religious beliefs and observances
    Evidence of personality disorder (ICD-10 F60)

Social work assessment

The patient (or client, when seen by a social worker) may be interviewed initially in the social worker's office or in a community venue, but a home visit, if the patient agrees, is often very helpful in permitting a first-hand appraisal of living conditions and lifestyle. In addition, information may be gathered from partners, relatives or a probation officer – but, of course, only with the consent of the patient.

It must be remembered throughout the assessment that many drug abusers and some individuals with an alcohol problem have been in conflict with the law and that they may have felt rejected by the caring professions in the past. They may still be involved in illicit activities which they fear may come to light in the course of a social enquiry. Thus, some abusers may be deceitful, devious and manipulative, and although they may have sought help voluntarily, they often remain suspicious of those who try to help them. To establish some degree of empathy with them, it is necessary to understand the motivation behind this behaviour, much of which is a learned response to pressures from peers, families and professionals. Only in an atmosphere of trust and confidentiality can the need, or otherwise, for social intervention be identified and the balance of positive and negative factors in the patient's environment and social networks be accurately assessed. The particular points to be addressed in more detail in the social work assessment are shown in Table 5.3.

Once the information in Table 5.3 has been elicited, a much clearer picture will have emerged about the patient's needs. Some patients, for example, may require assistance with problems relating to their material conditions. Practical advice and sometimes active intervention in difficulties related to housing, welfare benefits and debts may be welcomed, and some patients may benefit substantially from help in seeking training or in finding a job. Other patients require intervention on the ground that there is a risk of neglect or abuse to children living in the household (see Chapter 9), and sometimes there are particular family factors which warrant including one or more of the patient's family in the treatment plan. For example, it may be helpful to arrange for a preschool child to attend a day nursery or to refer a relative to a self-help support group. Sometimes a decision is made to involve the whole family in family therapy (Chapter 6). Finally, because many patients are already involved with other helping agencies, there may already be a professional worker taking an interest in their case, so that liaison is appropriate.

Perhaps the most important question to be addressed in the social work assessment is what sort of long-term help the patient will require. Because rehabilitation, the reintegration of the individual into society, is the statutory

Table 5.3. Outline of social work history scheme

---

1. Accommodation
  Locality
  Tenure
  Condition
  Whom the patient is living with

2. Employment
  Work experience and capabilities
  Need for vocational guidance and training
  Attitude towards work

3. Finances
  Income
  Benefits
  Debts

4. Social functioning
  How the day is spent

5. Social networks
  Friends and family
  Agencies
  Involvement with drug subculture
  Extent of loneliness and isolation

---

responsibility of the social services, the social worker is the key health care professional involved in this very long-term project and needs to assess what sort of therapeutic environment will be best for each patient. For example, for some patients complete removal to a drug-free therapeutic community may be the best way of achieving a permanently drug-free lifestyle. For others, this may be impractical or undesirable and placement in a hostel or day hospital may be more appropriate. Some, while remaining at home, may benefit from practical help and advice about changing their pattern of living in relation to work, leisure and social life, and some may benefit from individual or group psychotherapy.

These choices are made largely, but not solely, on the basis of the social work assessment, and the social worker is involved in their initiation if the patient is to be placed elsewhere, but more often their work involves seeing the patient on a regular basis for help, advice and counselling.

Family assessment

A more complete picture of the patient's drug-taking, lifestyle and background can be obtained if other members of the family are also interviewed. They may, for example, be able to confirm important details in the history and to elaborate upon them. However, a family assessment goes far beyond factual information gathering and seeks to explore the extent to which the drug-taking behaviour of the patient may have been, and still is being, affected by family attitudes and dynamics, and the effect of the drug-taking on the family. The fuller understanding of the patient's problem gained by such an assessment is of crucial importance in planning a treatment programme which is tailored to the individual's needs and is, therefore, more likely to succeed. In particular, it may indicate a need for family therapy and/or support for other family members.

The proportion of patients for whom a family assessment is considered appropriate and who give their consent for it is likely to be small, as the confidentiality of their consultation is often of paramount importance to substance abusers. Those who do give their consent can be divided into three groups:
- Patients in their late teens or early twenties, attending with their parents;
- Patients who attend with their nondrug-using partner;
- Patients who attend with their drug-using partner.

If the patient lives at home and attends with his or her parent(s), their knowledge of their child's drug-taking is assessed; whether, for example, they suspected the drug-taking themselves or were told by their child or by someone else. Their attitude towards the drug-taking is explored and, in particular, how they perceive their child's drug-taking in relation to their own use of drugs (tobacco, alcohol, prescribed drugs, etc.). It is important to establish the nature of drug-related family behaviour; whether, for example, family members collude to some degree with the patient's use, whether the patient splits the family, or if family members try to shield each other from the full knowledge of the patient's drug-taking. If, for example, there are secondary gains for the patient, vis-à-vis family dynamics, achieved by virtue of drug-taking, it may be extremely difficult, if not impossible, to eliminate this behaviour without some kind of family therapy. The assessment should also estimate the strength of the family unit and, in particular, of the parents' marriage, to see how much support they will be able to offer the patient during the very stressful situation of drug withdrawal; whether indeed the family wish to be involved in the treatment plan; and how much support they themselves may need too.

The assessment, if the patient attends with a nonusing partner, is in some ways similar to that outlined above. Again, it is necessary to gauge his or her knowledge and attitude towards the patient's drug-taking, and to assess the contribution of the dynamics of the relationship to maintaining drug-taking behaviour. The stability and strengths of the marriage or partnership must be explored, as must the partner's strengths and weaknesses, so that his or her need for support is fully understood. It may be helpful to find out if the partner was instrumental in bringing the patient to treatment, how this came about, and if there are any conditions attached to this situation.

When a patient attends with a drug-using partner, the assessment must address quite different problems, as it is necessary to establish the nature and severity of the partner's drug problem too, and his or her motivation to attend for treatment. The problems of uncoordinated drug withdrawal in couples should be discussed, together with the possibility of coordinated treatment. An important issue to be assessed is whether the using partner is likely to sabotage treatment or to encourage the abuse of prescriptions. Once again, the relative strengths of both individuals should be examined and any supports that they share should be identified.

Physical examination

Physical examination is an important part of the assessment procedure, permitting confirmation of details supplied in the history and sometimes providing new information. Objective signs of intoxication or withdrawal may contribute to the assessment of the severity of physical dependence, and sequelae of drug abuse that require medical intervention can be identified. The findings on physical examination vary according to the drug(s) of abuse and the method of their administration. No attempt is made in this brief account to cover all possible physical manifestations and complications of drug abuse, nor to deal with the differential diagnosis of unconsciousness due to drug overdose (see Chapter 8). Rather, it is intended as a guide to physical signs that may be recorded during the routine examination of a patient presenting with a drug problem, and offers some explanation as to how they have arisen.

General appearance

An appearance of general neglect coupled with poor nutritional state suggests a lifestyle that has become totally concerned with drugs, ignoring personal hygiene, food, clothes, etc. Marked weight loss is particularly seen with chronic use of stimulants such as amphetamines. Scars on the head may indicate injuries sustained during convulsions (usually in the course of sedative hypnotic withdrawal).

Gait

An unsteady gait (ataxia), often in association with slurred speech (an appearance similar to drunkenness), suggests intoxication with sedatives.

Eyes

Watering eyes occur during opiate withdrawal. Nystagmus is indicative of intoxication with sedative hypnotics. Pin-point pupils suggest the recent administration of opiates, while dilated pupils occur in the opiate abstinence syndrome. Dilated pupils may also occur following the use of amphetamine, cocaine, hallucinogens and anticholinergic drugs. Jaundice of the scleral conjunctivae suggests hepatitis, probably secondary to nonsterile injection or to the abuse of volatile solvents. Dilatation of conjunctival blood vessels results in red eye, usually due to cannabis abuse but sometimes to solvents. Jerky nystagmus may be seen in chronic barbiturate intoxication.

Nose

Congestion of the nasal mucosa (lining of the nose) occurs if drugs have been snorted. Ulceration or perforation of the nasal septum may occur, traditionally due to cocaine, but it also occurs if heroin is snorted. A runny nose (rhinorrhoea) is due to opiate withdrawal and leads to constant sniffing. A red, spotty rash around the nose and mouth may be due to solvent sniffing.

Mouth

There is a high incidence of dental caries in those who are dependent on opiates; this is attributable to poor dental hygiene and a predilection for sweet food. A particular type of carious lesion has been described which is larger than usual and found only on the labial and buccal surfaces of the teeth. Several teeth may have been lost in this way, or in the course of convulsions during the sedative hypnotic abstinence syndrome. Breath odour may indicate abuse of solvents or alcohol.

Skin

Because many people with a serious drug problem inject their drugs and do so repeatedly, the skin bears many marks (stigmata) of their drug-taking behaviour. Often these are due to the introduction of infection because of dirty injection techniques. Thus abscesses are common and there may also be the scars of healed abscesses.

Many drugs that are injected were manufactured and intended only for oral consumption; they have physical properties that render them totally unsuitable for injection and which can cause serious complications if they are administered in this way. Oral barbiturates, for example, when dispersed in water, are very acidic and highly irritant to the body's tissues. If injected subcutaneously (skin-popping), skin necrosis may occur, leading to shallow, sterile abscesses which heal leaving shallow, punched-out scars. These are frequently multiple and may be found anywhere on the body, but usually on the extremities.

Intravenous injection is, however, the preferred route of administration by most long-term, drug-dependent individuals, mainly because it provides maximum effect from the minimum amount of drug (and therefore gives best value for money). The veins of the arms are most accessible and stigmata of injection should be sought on the front of the elbows. Needle puncture marks may be seen in the skin overlying the veins which may be red and inflamed due to thrombophlebitis; there may be peripheral swelling (oedema) of the extremities due to the venous obstruction. This is particularly common if barbiturates are injected. Repeated injection leads to pigmentation of the skin over the veins (tracking) which may feel hard and stringy due to fibrosis after repeated thrombosis. When the veins of the arm can no longer be used for injection, others are used instead – in the foot, groin, neck – anywhere into which the frantic drug abuser can get a needle. Any of these sites may become thrombosed and infected, often by skin bacteria, because the skin is rarely cleaned before injection. Evidence of the use of neck veins, or of others even more extraordinary, indicates very severe dependence and this behaviour, repugnant even to other drug-dependent individuals, suggests a serious underlying personality disorder. Decorative tattoos may be placed to conceal evidence of drug injection.

Because of the progressive difficulty of intravenous injection, accidental injection into an adjacent artery sometimes occurs. If barbiturates are administered in this way they may cause acute arterial spasm which, if severe and prolonged, may lead to gangrene necessitating subsequent amputation. This is most frequently seen in the hand, where attempts to inject barbiturates into the small blood vessels have led to amputation of one or more fingers (or parts of fingers).

Gooseflesh (pilo-erection) is a well-known cutaneous sign of the opiate abstinence syndrome, while patients withdrawing from sedatives and alcohol may sweat profusely.

Cardiovascular system

Raised pulse rate (tachycardia) may be due to drug withdrawal (opiates, sedatives) or to intoxication with stimulant drugs, which may also cause irregularities of the heart (arrhythmias). High blood pressure may occur following the administration of amphetamine and similar drugs, while low blood pressure may occur following the administration of opiates and sedatives (although tolerance develops to this effect in chronic users). If the barbiturate abstinence syndrome is suspected, pulse and blood pressure should be measured with the patient supine and then standing; a fall in blood pressure (orthostatic hypotension) and an increase in heart rate of more than 15 is suggestive of barbiturate withdrawal.

A diagnosis of endocarditis should be considered in any drug abuser with a fever and a heart murmur and, as prompt treatment may be life-saving, a high index of suspicion should be maintained (see p. 283).

Respiratory system

Examination of the chest may be quite normal, although there may be signs of pulmonary embolism, infarction and of increased pulmonary blood pressure (pulmonary hypertension). Chest infections are common and there is a reported association between heroin use and asthma.

Abdomen

Enlargement of the liver (hepatomegaly) is common in those who inject drugs and is strongly suggestive of hepatitis. Because tolerance does not develop to the constipating effect of opiates, the colon (lower bowel) may be distended with faeces and easily palpable. In a female patient, the possibility of pregnancy should not be forgotten; it is not unknown for amenorrhoea to be attributed to drug abuse (opiates) and for pregnancy to be far advanced before it is diagnosed.

Neuromuscular system

Tremor and muscle twitching are signs of the opiate abstinence syndrome. Repeated intramuscular injection of some drugs, particularly pentazocine and pethidine, produces severe wasting of the muscle(s) into which the drug is injected; there may be fibrosis that entraps peripheral nerves and sometimes calcification. Peripheral nerves may also be damaged by accidental, intraneural injection of a drug.

Lymphatic system

Enlarged lymph nodes in axillae and groins are common if drugs are injected because of the repeated introduction of infection; they are usually bilateral, and if unilateral this indicates preferential injection on that side. Lymphadenopathy may carry a more sinister implication now as it also occurs in AIDS. Lymphatic obstruction due to repeated episodes of infection and inflammation may contribute to the development of chronically 'puffy' hands, with a characteristic, brawny oedema – typical of those who inject barbiturates into their hands and forearms.

Test of physical dependence on opiates (naloxone hydrochloride)

Physical dependence on opiates can be assessed using the opiate antagonist naloxone hydrochloride. Naloxone 0.4–0.8 mg (1–2 ml) is administered intramuscularly; this has no effect if the patient is not physically dependent on opiates. If the patient is physically dependent, the signs and symptoms of the opiate abstinence syndrome will become apparent within minutes of injection.[1] If unduly distressing, they can be relieved to some extent by giving morphine 15–30 mg; the patient should then be kept under observation for a couple of hours for signs of opiate intoxication because naloxone has a shorter duration of action than morphine. The patient's consent must always be obtained and the naloxone test should not be done if the patient is pregnant, as it may induce abortion.

Testing with naloxone is a procedure used more frequently by some treatment centres than others but it is rarely used in the UK. It can only assess pharmacological need and should never be the sole component of the assessment procedure. A recent development in naloxone testing, pioneered at St George's Hospital Medical School, avoids the potentially distressing systemic effects of the abstinence syndrome precipitated by naloxone and instead makes use of the local effect of naloxone on the pupil of the eye to assess opioid dependence status. The Ghodse Opioid Addiction Test relies on the observation that naloxone eye drops have no effect on the pupil of an opioid-naïve individual or on the pupil of the occasional user, but cause dilatation of the pupil if the individual is dependent on opioids. The test is carried out in a uniform light and, once the eyes have adapted to this, both pupils are measured. Naloxone eye drops are applied to one eye only and the pupils are measured again. If the pupil to which naloxone was applied is seen to be bigger than the control pupil, a diagnosis of opioid dependence can be made. This test is both sensitive and specific and can be carried out swiftly in the out-patient setting. Its main advantage is that it permits an accurate diagnosis of the dependent state to be made on a single visit, obviating the need for the prolonged assessment process outlined above which is very off-putting for many of those who would like to seek treatment. The test is facilitated by the use of a specially designed pupillometer to measure pupil size.[2–4]

Unfortunately, there is no similar test for the assessment of physical dependence on nonopiate drugs.

Mental state examination

Examination of the mental state is an essential component of the assessment procedure. Firstly, it may identify a coexistent psychiatric illness, such as depression, schizophrenia or agoraphobia, that requires treatment and which may be (or may have been) a contributory factor in the initiation and/or continuation of drug abuse. In addition, because most drugs of abuse have psychoactive properties, it is logical to seek the psychological consequences of their consumption. They may cause hallucinations or delusions, for example, or they may affect cognitive state, mood and thought. However, these symptoms and signs are not drug specific and cannot be diagnostic. Similar symptoms may arise during intoxication with one drug and in the abstinence syndrome of another. Their incidence and severity vary according to the dose consumed, individual sensitivity to the effect of the drug and the development of tolerance and physical dependence.

Nevertheless, the skilled interpretation of psychological signs and symptoms can make a significant contribution to the assessment of a drug-abuse problem, particularly when these observations are considered in conjunction with the history of drug-taking and the results of laboratory investigation. It should be stressed, however, that many patients – probably the majority – present with a perfectly normal and appropriate mental state. In addition, many of the drug effects outlined below are very subtle and are not easily discernible even by experienced observers.

As part of the examination of the patient's mental state, it is important to ascertain the degree of understanding and awareness of the extent to which his or her drug abuse is problematic and to establish whether the patient is able to attribute any abnormal psychic experiences, such as abnormal visual perceptions, to their use of psychoactive drugs.

Enquiries should also be made as to their motivation for seeking treatment at the current time, including external motivators such as forensic, employment or social factors, and intrinsic factors such as the psychological or medical sequelae of drug use. The patient's use of commonly employed defence mechanisms such as denial, minimization, rationalization and projection should also be explored and the interviewer should be alert to evasiveness and manipulative behaviour.

Finally, it is important to establish whether the patient is agreeable to treatment and the kind of treatment that they are requesting, which may, at times, differ from what the clinician feels is most appropriate.

General behaviour

Restlessness, anxiety and irritability may be caused either by intoxication with stimulants or hallucinogens, or by the withdrawal of opiates and sedatives. The latter may also be associated with muscle twitching and tremulousness. When due to stimulants, restlessness may be accompanied by repetitive behaviour patterns, incessant fiddling and picking at the skin. Restlessness and anxiety due to opiate withdrawal may be so severe that the patient cannot tolerate or endure the interview; there may also be repeated yawning. In contrast, quiet, withdrawn behaviour may follow consumption of sedatives or opiates which in higher doses cause drowsiness. General apathy follows stimulant withdrawal, and preoccupation with inner psychic phenomena after use of cannabis or hallucinogens may also lead to withdrawn behaviour. Hostile, aggressive behaviour, and sometimes violence, may occur with stimulant intoxication and also occurs as a paradoxical reaction in chronic intoxication with sedative hypnotics.

Talk

General talkativeness and pressure of speech is common in patients intoxicated with stimulants, who may flit from one topic to another. Cannabis too may induce chattiness. Lack of spontaneous speech and monosyllabic answers are common in those who have recently taken opiates and sedatives, but can also occur if the patient is preoccupied with the wretchedness of the abstinence syndrome of these drugs. Formal thought disorder occurs much less frequently in drug-induced psychosis than in other psychotic conditions (e.g. schizophrenia).

Mood

Changes in mood, which are often frequent and rapid (labile mood) are commonly associated with drug abuse. For example, elated mood with excessive cheerfulness, energy and confidence can follow stimulant abuse and may mimic mild hypomania. Abrupt withdrawal from stimulants in heavy users can precipitate sudden intense feelings of depression and anxiety ('the crash'), often with suicidal ideation; hypersomnolence may also be a feature. This is followed by a period of milder depressive symptoms characterized by apathy, anhedonia and anergia.[5,6] Alcohol and sedative misuse may be associated with depression of mood, which usually improves after a period of abstinence. Feelings of guilt, worthlessness and hopelessness are commonly expressed by chronically dependent individuals and it should be remembered that they have an increased risk of suicide;[7] the possibility of this should always be explored during a mental state examination.

A feeling of mental detachment, well-being and quiet euphoria is described by opiate users, while marked anxiety and depression are associated with withdrawal in dependent individuals. 'Bad trips', undesired and unpleasant drug experiences, associated especially with hallucinogens and stimulants, may result in marked panic attacks, depersonalization and feelings of extreme terror.

Thought content

A general suspiciousness of other people is a common consequence of regular consumption of stimulants and ideas of reference and paranoid delusions may be apparent. These may also occur after the administration of hallucinogens and cannabis.

Abnormal experiences and beliefs

Hallucinations are common after stimulants, hallucinogens and cannabis. Auditory and tactile hallucinations are typical of stimulant administration, and if the patient also suffers from delusions these are likely to be paranoid in nature. Paranoid delusions may also occur following cannabis consumption. The hallucinogens give rise to a wide variety of illusions and hallucinations; frank psychosis may ensue and flashbacks are common. Hallucinations and delusions may also occur in the course of sedative withdrawal. Abnormal beliefs in supernatural powers (e.g. the ability to fly) have been described during LSD use, sometimes with fatal consequences.

Cognitive state

A wide range of psychoactive drugs may impair the patient's general awareness and his or her ability to concentrate and attend to the interview. Disorientation and confusion may arise with stimulant or sedative intoxication. Withdrawal in heavy sedative abusers often produces a delirious state similar to alcoholic delirium tremens (see Chapter 4). Impairment of short-term memory and amnesic periods (memory blackouts) occur during periods of sedative and alcoholic intoxication.

Psychological assessment

Psychological assessment of the patient involves personality testing using standardized inventories to measure the patient's cognitive state, personality and social functioning and to identify specific deficits. In particular, the patient's suitability for different treatment options is assessed. For example, patients suffering from overwhelming anxiety may benefit from instruction in relaxation techniques; some patients may require social skills and assertiveness training; others, suffering from phobias, might benefit from desensitization. There is a wealth of psychological intervention which may be employed to reduce or eliminate the patient's need for psychoactive drugs, and psychological assessment aims to identify those patients to whom this may usefully be applied. In addition, psychological assessment may help to identify an individual's particular skills and aptitudes, facilitating more appropriate vocational guidance and rehabilitation.

Special investigations

Laboratory investigations may be helpful in assessing the general health status of the patient and in detecting adverse consequences of drug abuse, due either to the drug itself or to the methods of its administration, or to the lifestyle of the patient.

Haemoglobin

Venepuncture may be very difficult in chronic injectors because easily accessible veins are likely to be thrombosed. Haemoglobin and full blood count may provide evidence of nutritional deficiencies (iron, vitamins) that have led to anaemia. Anaemia can also occur if the bone marrow is depressed by solvent abuse and in the presence of chronic infection – in which case the ESR (erythrocyte sedimentation rate) will probably be raised too. A raised white cell count is common in drug abusers due to the frequency of infective complications of self-injection.

Urea

A raised blood urea suggests damage to the kidneys. This may occur in the course of solvent abuse, and may also be due to intravenous heroin use which can cause a nephrotic syndrome with protein in the urine. Renal damage is common and severe in those who abuse analgesics such as aspirin.

Liver function tests

These are often abnormal in those who inject drugs due to a high incidence of hepatitis. Typically, the liver enzymes (aspartate amino transferase, alanine amino transferase and gamma glutamyl transferase) are raised; bilirubin may be raised even if jaundice is not apparent clinically. Liver damage can also be caused by solvent abuse and by the adulterants of illicit drugs.

Wasserman reaction

In the midst of current concern about AIDS, the risk of syphilis in drug abusers who inject their drugs is rarely mentioned. However, syphilis is transmitted in exactly the same way as AIDS, so that those at risk of one are equally at risk from the other, and the Wasserman reaction (WR) test for syphilis should not be omitted.

Hepatitis

Over the last decade it has become apparent that infection with hepatitis C virus is very common within the injecting drug user population with high rates of detection of hepatitis C antibody among those tested. The patient should be counselled and consent given before testing (see Chapter 8).

Another variety of hepatitis common in injecting drug abusers is hepatitis B, which is detected in the body by various markers or antigens. Most tests for hepatitis seek to identify an antigen on the surface of the viral particle, named hepatitis surface antigen (HBsAg), formerly known as Australia antigen. This can be detected in the blood, not instantly after infection, but after a variable incubation period (2–6 months). The body responds to the viral antigens by producing antibodies (hepatitis antibodies) and their presence denotes prior infection with hepatitis virus. Any patient who has injected drugs should be tested for the presence of HBsAg and for its antibodies. Tests for other types of hepatitis – hepatitis A, and delta virus – are not done routinely, but are reserved for the investigation of a patient with a clinical diagnosis of hepatitis (see Chapter 8).

Test for HIV antibody

The test for HIV antibodies is available at most DDTUs and some patients may ask to have it done. Others, such as those who continue to share needles, patients with unexplained symptoms, and women who are pregnant or planning pregnancy, should be advised to be tested. The patient's consent must always be obtained and the test should never be carried out until the full implications of the result – whatever it may turn out to be – have been discussed with the patient at a special counselling session (Chapter 8).

Precautions for taking specimens from drug abusers

Because drug abusers who inject drugs are a high-risk group for HIV and AIDS as well as for hepatitis B and C, the clinical and laboratory workers who deal directly with them and/or their specimens (of blood, urine, etc.), have a potential occupational risk of becoming infected. In fact, there have been very few such cases, but if this good record is to be maintained, high standards of operational practice are essential to avoid inadvertent infection. As no cases of HIV infection have been attributable to air-borne droplet infection, precaution is concentrated on preventing accidental parenteral infection. These precautions apply when dealing with any drug abuser who self-injects, and not just to those known at the time to be HIV-positive or known to be carrying hepatitis viruses.

Particular care must be taken when needles, etc. are used for invasive procedures, which should be carried out by experienced staff wearing suitable protective clothing (e.g. gown, gloves, apron, as appropriate). The needle should not be removed from a disposable hypodermic syringe after use but both, together, should be placed in an appropriate, puncture-proof bin ('Sharps bin') for final disposal. Pre-existing skin wounds or abrasions should be kept covered.

Specimens of blood or urine should be placed in secure containers and then sealed in individual plastic bags before sending them to the laboratory. The accompanying request forms should be kept separate from the specimen containers and should indicate clearly that there is a risk (or suspicion of risk) that the specimens may be infected with HIV or hepatitis viruses. Any spillage of potentially infected body fluids must be dealt with straightaway, ensuring disinfection.

These procedures have received special emphasis since the advent of AIDS, although they are no more rigorous than those that should be employed to prevent contamination with hepatitis virus, which is much more infective and easier to transmit than HIV. They apply to all specimens obtained from high-risk patients, not just blood, and must be observed irrespective of the investigation for which the sample was taken.

Needle-stick injuries

Accidental puncture wounds (needle-stick injuries) should be treated promptly by thorough washing and encouraging bleeding, and should be reported. All hospitals have policies for dealing with such incidents, which may include prophylactic treatment such as immunization. Although full trials have not yet been carried out, it has been recommended that exposure to a known HIV-positive source should be treated immediately (within 1–2 hours) with triple therapy (i.e. combination therapy with three drugs) under the supervision of a specialist physician. Barrier contraception is advised for 3 months after the injury and blood donation should be avoided for 6 months. Staff working with injecting drug users should be encouraged to be immunized against hepatitis B. The risk of infection from a hepatitis C-positive patient following needle-stick injury is thought to be between 3% and 10%.[8]

In the UK, guidance has been issued about the action to be taken if a needle-stick injury is sustained in relation to a patient who refuses testing or who is unable to give consent to testing. If there is a good reason to suspect that the patient is suffering from a serious communicable disease for which prophylactic treatment is available (e.g. HIV infection) it is possible to test an existing blood sample taken for other purposes. However, this should only be done after consultation with an experienced colleague, the patient must be informed at the earliest opportunity and it is possible that the decision may be the subject of legal challenge.[9]

Chest radiography

Chest radiography should be carried out routinely. Radiographs may be completely normal, but following a period of unconsciousness (e.g. after an overdose) there may be evidence of aspiration pneumonia. In those who inject drugs, the signs of pulmonary embolism, infarction or hypertension may be apparent.

Bacteriological investigation

Swabs from all infected lesions should be sent to the laboratory for culture and sensitivity testing. Infection is often due to 'unusual' microorganisms, which rarely cause problems in those who do not inject drugs, but which gain access to the body by means of nonsterile injection techniques. It is important that they should be identified so that anti-infective treatment can be prompt and appropriate.

Laboratory investigation for drugs

The laboratory plays an important role in the diagnosis and management of many cases of drug abuse and dependence, often because the individuals concerned are not always truthful about their drug consumption and an independent, objective source of information is particularly useful.[10] However, all laboratory investigations, including tests for drugs, have their limitations, and the significance of the results can only be fully appreciated if these limitations are understood, and if the results are interpreted in the context of information gained from the history and examination of the patient.[11]

The choice of body fluid for drug analysis depends on a number of factors that are different for each drug, but the principal consideration is the distribution of the drug between the body fluids, notably blood and urine. This varies according to the length of time the drug has been in the body and the dose.

Once the drug has entered the body, whether by the respiratory system, the alimentary canal or by injection, it circulates in the blood, either as the free drug or bound to a protein. However, to produce its action on the body, the drug must pass from the bloodstream to the body cells and it is only the free, nonprotein-bound drug that can enter the body cells. The drug is rendered inactive and/or removed from the body by a variety of processes.

It may be combined (conjugated) in the liver with other chemical substances and the inactive conjugate subsequently excreted in the urine. Alternatively, it may be chemically altered (often in the liver) to produce pharmacologically active metabolites which, like the parent drug, may then undergo conjugation in the liver and excretion by the kidney. Damage to the liver (in hepatitis, for example) may reduce its ability to metabolize drugs.

The concentration of the drug in the blood at a particular time represents the amount of drug available to the body cells at the time the blood sample was taken and depends on the dose and on the rates of absorption and elimination. The time taken for the blood concentration to decline by 50% is known as the half-life of the drug. Drugs with a short half-life (e.g. heroin, cocaine) have blood levels that decrease rapidly with time, and that cannot easily be correlated with dose unless additional information is available.

Usually, urine samples are preferred for the analysis of drugs of abuse. Specimens are readily obtainable and, because the concentration of a drug in urine is much higher than in blood, it can be detected more easily and for longer after drug administration. A disadvantage of using urine is that some drugs are present only as metabolites which are common to a number of parent drugs; thus the detection of a particular metabolite may not identify exactly which drug was consumed. Blood has the advantage that the parent drug can be measured, but only if the sample is collected soon after the drug was taken. Another advantage is that tampering with a blood sample is more difficult than with a urine sample.

Testing for drugs, therefore, usually takes place on urine samples (hair and saliva may also be used), and it is, of course, essential to be absolutely sure that the urine specimen being tested has actually come from the patient being assessed – substitution of specimens is not unknown. Clearly, a single urine specimen cannot provide all the answers about an individual's drug-taking, but repeated tests can help to build up a more complete picture of drug-taking over a period of time.

Table 5.4. Drug distribution in blood and urine

	Blood		Urine	
	Half-life[a] (hours)	Blood level (μg per ml)[b]	90% excretion (days)[c]	Unchanged drug (%)[d]
CNS depressants				
Barbiturates				
Phenobarbitone	100	10–40	16	25
Butobarbitone	40	0.3–0.5	7	5
Amylobarbitone	24	0.3–0.5	6	1
Chlormethiazole	5	0.27–2.0		5
Benzodiazepines				
Diazepam	48	1.15–3.0	7	
CNS stimulants				
Amphetamines	12	1.01–0.1	3	3
Methylamphetamine	9	0.02–0.8	1.5	43
Cocaine	1	0.1–0.5	2	4
Narcotic analgesics				
Heroin	0.5			nil
Morphine	3	0.05	1	5
Codeine	3	0.01–0.1	1	
Methadone	15	0.05–0.07	2	4
LSD	3	0.004		1
Cannabis	30	0.007	12	

[a]Half-life: time in hours for the blood level to decrease by 50%.
[b]Blood level: the lower value is the likely blood level after a single, therapeutic (or usual) dose: the upper value is the likely value during chronic administration.
[c]90% excretion: time in days for 90% of the drug to be excreted in the urine.
[d]Unchanged drug: percentage of the unchanged drug excreted in the urine.
CNS, central nervous system.
Source: Bucknell P & Ghodse H.[19]

An additional benefit of urine testing is that it may have a significant deterrent effect on illicit drug-taking. If those attending for the treatment of a drug problem know that they may be asked for a urine sample, and know that a positive result will have adverse consequences, they may be less willing to risk illicit drug misuse. Random urine testing may thus help to prevent relapse.

Table 5.4 shows how different drugs are distributed in blood and urine. The figures in the table are only average values and will vary from patient to patient, as well as with the frequency of dosing and the dose of the drug.

Hair analysis

Techniques have now been developed to use hair samples to investigate an individual's consumption of drugs. It has been suggested that, because hair grows at a relatively constant rate of about 1 cm per month, the concentration of drugs at different points on the hair shaft can be used to measure the time that has elapsed since the drug was taken. Although there may be factors that limit interpretation, there is a theoretical potential for hair samples to be used for detailing an individual's drug history, and this has been used both in the clinical setting and in forensic casework.[12] It can be particularly useful to confirm or exclude retrospectively a period of claimed abstinence, where the patient or client in legal proceedings has not been monitored by regular urine testing.

Laboratory methods

Chromatography is a method for separating chemical substances that depends on differences between their rates of transfer between a moving stream of liquid or gas and a stationary material, usually a finely divided solid or film of liquid on the surface of such a solid. With thin-layer chromatography (TLC), the finely divided, solid stationary material is spread as a thin layer on a sheet of glass. In high-performance liquid chromatography (HPLC), the stationary material is packed into a steel tube and the moving stream of liquid is pumped through at high pressure, while in gas-liquid chromatography (GLC), a moving stream of gas is pumped through at high pressure.

Immunoassay depends on the interaction between the substance being measured and a specific antibody to that substance. The antibody is produced in animals (in the same way that antibodies are produced in humans during vaccination procedures) by previously injecting the chemical substance of interest, or a derivative, into an animal which responds by synthesizing the antibody. This is then isolated from the blood of the animal and can be used to detect the original chemical substance in other samples. The measurement of drugs using radio-immunoassay (RIA) or enzyme immunoassay (EMIT) relies on the use of reagents labelled with a radioactive marker or enzyme respectively.

Mass spectrometry, by accurate analysis of molecular weight can determine molecular structure and hence identify specific drugs.

The two screening methods that are used most commonly are TLC and EMIT. These methods can detect a wide variety of drugs including barbiturates, morphine, methadone and amphetamine. Confirmation of positive results is usually achieved by specific GLC or HPLC. In addition, specific immunoassay methods are available for some drugs and their metabolites. The most sensitive and specific method, available in some specialized laboratories, is GLC linked to a mass spectrometer.

Sophisticated equipment is needed to carry out these tests. As it is expensive to install and run, it is available only in specialized centres that provide a drug-screening service with a high level of expertise for surrounding hospitals, thus achieving economy of scale. This means, however, that there may be a delay of several days between sending a urine specimen to the laboratory and receiving a report on the drugs it contains.

Near patient testing

Near patient testing techniques have advanced in recent years. Initially EMIT technology and a small benchtop analyser was used but 'dipstick' methods are now more usual and kits are available for testing for a single drug or for several drugs simultaneously. The advantage of near patient testing is chiefly the rapid availability of a result, which may be useful in some clinical situations. However, the technique has limitations and potential pitfalls. The reliability may be affected by the competence of the staff undertaking the test who are often working in busy clinical settings, and positive tests may require laboratory confirmation. Also, the technique is not quantitative and cannot test for sample adulteration.

Interpretation of results

The interpretation of the results of analyses depends on the sensitivity and specificity of the analytical method used. Most laboratories use screening procedures for the common drugs that will only detect a single, minimum therapeutic dose for about 24 hours after administration. There are, however, large variations in drug metabolism and excretion between individuals so that the drug may be detected for less than 24 hours in some patients, but may persist for much longer in others. A negative result of a drug screen by these methods means only that the urine specimen contains less than the lowest amount detectable by the method. It does not necessarily mean the complete absence of the drug from the urine, nor that the drug has not been taken. Nevertheless, negative urine results may be very informative; for example, the repeated absence of opiates from the urine of an individual claiming to be dependent and seeking a prescription gives more precise information than a positive result which could mean either that the individual is dependent or that he or she is an occasional user.

Positive results must be interpreted in relation to the specificity of the method used. Identification of a drug solely by screening methods is fraught with difficulties and confirmation by a more specific method is essential for forensic work. However, due to constraints imposed by the pressure of work, time and money, many laboratories report results on the basis of screening procedures only. Thus, false positive results (a drug reported present when in fact it is absent) are not unknown. Awareness of this is very important because in attempting to assess the patient's drug consumption, excessive and misplaced reliance on the laboratory tests may be as misleading as unquestioning acceptance or automatic disbelief of the patient's account of his or her drug taking.

Drug-screening programmes

Following the lead of companies and corporations in the USA, there have been calls for drug-screening programmes in the UK for certain groups of individuals, and particularly for those whose mental impairment by drugs might put others at risk. Drug screening might involve either random testing or routine, regular testing, although neither is a foolproof method of detecting or preventing drug abuse. Leaving aside the important question of whether compulsory testing is an unacceptable infringement of individual rights, the usefulness of such a programme requires careful scrutiny. It has been claimed, for example, that drug testing may be beneficial because of its potential deterrent effect.

It has already been explained that negative results of urine testing for drugs do not necessarily mean that the individual concerned has not taken drugs. It might mean only that the dose was so small or had been taken so much earlier that the concentration of drug in the urine was too low to be detected by screening methods. Positive results too can be misleading. The available methods of screening urine are insufficiently accurate to be relied on and false positive results occur regularly. This problem could be overcome by the use of specific tests, but these are time consuming and expensive and therefore inappropriate for mass screening. Because of the limitations of drug-screening methods, the interpretation of the results is very important and this requires expert assessment of the history of drug use and the findings on clinical examination, which should be considered in conjunction with the result of the urine test.[13]

Given the very loose association between safety in the workplace and the use of drug screening, and the problems associated with the latter, introduction of such programmes is likely to remain controversial. However, in some countries screening for drugs has already become quite fashionable, generating an inappropriate demand for the service and increasing the likelihood of screening being imposed.[14] An alternative to screening is performance appraisal, carried out using computer/video technology to simulate real tasks for those whose impairment puts many others at significant risk. This approach seems preferable, because it emphasizes 'fitness to work', rather than querying drug abuse.

Summary

This chapter has been primarily concerned with the content of the assessment – what information to gather and, specifically, which questions to ask. The procedure that is outlined is not applicable to every situation in which a drug abuser seeks help: someone dropping in to an advice centre does not expect and is likely to feel resentful about detailed enquiries into their private life; a busy general practitioner may not have the time to explore the patient's background in the way that has been described. Clearly, it is up to the professional concerned to select appropriate areas and details of the assessment procedure, depending on the nature of the help that is required and the skills and resources available.

Specifically, because many substance abusers come into contact with the police, initial assessment may take place at a police station. This situation is discussed in more detail in Chapter 9, but it must be emphasized here that accurate documentation of the patient's physical and mental state is of particular importance in case the validity of statements is later challenged on medical grounds.

Although many of the questions and procedures described here may not be relevant to all professionals, the detailed nature of the elicited information emphasizes the complexity of drug abuse. It is not an isolated event in the person's life; many factors contributed to its developing in the past and many are contributing to its maintenance at the time that the individual asks for help. Undoubtedly, his or her drug-taking has had adverse consequences and these are probably continuing. In this complex situation it is not helpful, at any level of intervention, to jump to hasty conclusions about the nature of the problem or to offer ill-thought-out solutions. If drug abuse and drug dependence are perceived as ongoing interactions between the drug, the individual and society, then the purpose of the assessment is to tease out these interwoven threads, each of which is itself multistranded, to see how they are woven together.

For those with a long history of severe dependence, this teasing out is difficult and takes a long time, requiring all the approaches to assessment described in this chapter. Assessment comprises much more than information gathering, however. It is, after all, the time when the individual engages in, or is engaged in, treatment. Any such approach to any professional is difficult. Most patients, whatever their problem, are anxious in this situation, and when the problem is one of drug abuse or dependence the patient is likely to be very anxious indeed. It takes great courage to admit to a drug problem and to ask for help, especially if there have been previous attempts at dealing with it and previous failures. Anxiety may be disguised by hostile or aggressive behaviour; some patients, having taken drugs to give them courage to attend, may be intoxicated. Nevertheless, their seeking help is the all-important first step which they alone can take and which should be (must be) rewarded by positive responses from all involved in the assessment procedure.

A snappy telephonist, an off-putting receptionist, a doctor or nurse riled by an uncooperative patient can precipitate that patient's walking out, not to return or to try again – at least not for some time. Positive, friendly, non-judgmental attitudes are essential – exactly the responses, in fact, that any patient, regardless of ailment, is entitled to expect, but even more important for drug abusers who may have had many previous experiences of rejection. As their behaviour often elicits adverse responses in those whom they encounter, a high degree of professionalism is necessary on the part of all involved staff, who may require special training and support.

For many drug abusers and especially those with long and complex drug problems, the assessment procedure itself may be a therapeutic process. The telling of the 'life history' – some of it spontaneously, some in answer to direct questions – helps the patient, perhaps for the first time, to see his or her drug-taking in some sort of perspective. The account of the present social circumstances clearly identifies current problems and needs. This clarification to an outsider is, or can be, a clarification to the drug abuser too and what needs to be done, the way forward, can become apparent to both. Indeed the feedback to the patient, identifying their problems and planning subsequent care is of paramount importance. In particular, it offers a golden opportunity to engage the patient as an active participant in the treatment plan.

Assessment is not an end in itself. There is no point in defining the problem, understanding the antecedent circumstances and merely observing and recording the adverse consequences. The aim of assessment is to offer the patient an appropriate treatment programme. This will involve the drug of abuse certainly, but many other areas of the patient's life are likely to be affected too. Assessment should make apparent to both parties what changes are necessary, in which areas of the patient's life, and what the realistic expectations of such change are (although drug abuser and helping professional may not always agree). The skill of the helping professional lies in the accurate assessment of the problem and the accurate matching of the patient to treatment option.

Classification of substance-use disorders

There have been many approaches to classifying mental and behavioural disorders. The most widely used systems continue to be the World Health Organization's International Classification of Diseases and Related Health Problems, now in its tenth revision (ICD-10),[15] and the American Psychiatric Association's Diagnostic and Statistical Manual of Mental Disorders, third edition, revised (DSM-III-R),[16] and subsequently developed into DSM-IV.[17] Although the diagnostic criteria for substance dependence are fairly consistent across these systems, there are more discrepancies in the substance abuse and harmful use diagnostic categories. Nevertheless, both systems have reasonable reliability and validity.[18] This is very important because, with the huge amount of research being carried out internationally, it is essential to have common definitions of cases and conditions. In this context it is worth pointing out that the definitions of harmful and hazardous drinking described in Chapter 4 and widely utilized in the UK for public information purposes, are not fully consistent with these international classifications.

ICD-10

ICD-10 uses an alphanumeric coding scheme, based on codes with a single letter, followed by two numbers at the three-character level. Further detail is then provided by means of decimal numeric subdivisions at the four-character level. As it is designed to be a central ('core') classification for a family of disease- and health-related classifications, some members of the family of classifications are derived by using a fifth or even sixth character to specify more detail.

Within ICD-10, mental and behavioural disorders due to psychoactive substance use are classified within the block F10–F19. At this point it should be noted that the term 'disorder' is used throughout the classification, so as to avoid even greater problems inherent in the use of terms such as 'disease' and 'illness'. 'Disorder' is not an exact term, but in this context implies the existence of a clinically recognizable set of symptoms or behaviour associated, in most cases, with distress and with interference with personal functions. Social deviance or conflict alone, without personal dysfunction, is not included within this definition of mental disorder. Block F10–F19 contains a wide range of disorders of varying severity (from uncomplicated intoxication and harmful use to obvious psychotic disorders and dementia), that are all attributable to the use of one or more psychoactive substances (which may or may not have been medically prescribed).

The substance involved is indicated by means of the second and third characters (i.e. the first two digits after the letter F):

F10 mental and behavioural disorders due to use of *alcohol*;

F11 mental and behavioural disorders due to use of *opioids*;

F12 mental and behavioural disorders due to use of *cannabinoids*;

F13 mental and behavioural disorders due to use of *sedatives or hypnotics*;

F14 mental and behavioural disorders due to use of *cocaine*;

F15 mental and behavioural disorders due to use of other *stimulants* including *caffeine*;

F16 mental and behavioural disorders due to use of *hallucinogens*;

F17 mental and behavioural disorders due to use of *tobacco*;

F18 mental and behavioural disorders due to use of *volatile solvents*;

F19 mental and behavioural disorders due to multiple drug use and use of other
   psychoactive substances.

The identification of the psychoactive substance used may be made on the basis of
self-report data, objective analysis of specimens of urine, blood, etc., or other
evidence (presence of drug samples in the patient's possession, clinical signs and
symptoms, or reports from informed third parties, as described earlier). Objective
analysis provides the most compelling evidence of present or recent use, although
this information is of limited value in relation to past use. Whenever possible, it is
always advisable to seek corroboration from more than one source of evidence.

Although many drug users take more than one type of drug, the diagnosis of the
disorder should be classified, whenever possible, according to the most important
single substance (or class of substance) used. This may usually be done with regard
to the particular drug, or type of drug, causing the presenting disorder. When in
doubt, the code should be selected to identify the drug or type of drug most
frequently misused, particularly in those cases involving continuous or daily use.
Only in cases in which patterns of psychoactive substance taking are chaotic and
indiscriminate, or in which the contributions of different drugs are inextricably
mixed, should code F19 (disorders resulting from multiple drug use) be used.

Other points to be noted are as follows.

The misuse of nonpsychoactive substances, such as laxatives or aspirin, should
be coded by means of F55 (abuse of nondependence-producing substances), with
a fourth character to specify the type of substance involved.

Cases in which mental disorders (particularly delirium in the elderly) are due to
psychoactive substances, but without the presence of one of the disorders in this
block (e.g. harmful use or dependence syndrome), should be coded in F00–F09.
Where a state of delirium is superimposed upon a disorder in this block, it should
be coded by means of Flx.3 or Flx.4.

The level of alcohol involvement can be indicated by means of a supplementary
code (from Chapter XX of ICD-10): Y90 (evidence of alcohol involvement
determined by blood alcohol content) or Y91 (evidence of alcohol involvement
determined by level of intoxication).

The fourth character (after the decimal point) specifies the clinical condition
arising as a consequence of the use of a psychoactive substance. These are listed
below and should be used, as required, for each substance specified, although it
should be noted that not all four-character codes are applicable to all substances:

Flx.0 acute intoxication;

Flx.1 harmful use;

Flx.2 dependence syndrome;

Flx.3 withdrawal state;

Flx.4 withdrawal state with delirium;

F1x.5 psychotic disorder;

F1x.6 amnesic syndrome;

F1x.7 residual and late onset psychotic disorder;

F1x.8 other mental and behavioural disorders;

F1x.9 unspecified mental and behavioural disorder.

F1x.0 Acute intoxication

Acute intoxication is defined as a transient condition following the administration of alcohol or other psychoactive substance, resulting in disturbances in level of consciousness, cognition, perception, affect or behaviour, or other psycho-physiological functions and responses. This should be a main diagnosis only in cases where intoxication occurs without more persistent alcohol- or drug-related problems being concomitantly present. Where there are such problems, preced-ence should be given to diagnoses of harmful use (F1x.1), dependence syndrome (F1x.2), or psychotic disorder (F1x.5).

The following diagnostic guidelines are important.

Acute intoxication is usually closely related to dose levels. Exceptions to this may occur in individuals with certain underlying organic conditions (e.g. renal or hepatic insufficiency) in whom small doses of a substance may produce a dispro-portionately severe intoxicating effect. Disinhibition due to social context should also be taken into account (e.g. behavioural disinhibition at parties or carnivals). Acute intoxication is a transient phenomenon and its intensity reduces as time passes. In the absence of further use of the substance, the effects will eventually disappear and recovery is therefore complete, except where tissue damage or another complication has arisen.

It should be noted that the symptoms of intoxication need not always reflect the primary actions of the substance: for instance, depressant drugs may lead to symptoms of agitation or hyperactivity, and stimulant drugs may lead to socially withdrawn and introverted behaviour. The effects of substances such as cannabis and hallucinogens may be particularly unpredictable. Moreover, many psycho-active substances are capable of producing different types of effect at different dose levels. For example, alcohol may have apparent stimulant effects on behaviour at lower dose levels, may lead to agitation and aggression with increasing dose levels, and produce clear sedation at very high levels.

This diagnostic coding includes acute drunkenness in alcoholism, and 'bad trips' (due to hallucinogenic drugs).

The fifth character is used to indicate whether the acute intoxication is asso-ciated with any complications:

F1x.00 uncomplicated, this means that the intoxication is uncomplicated al-though the symptoms may be of varying severity, depending on the dose;

F1x.01 with trauma or other bodily injury;

F1x.02 with other medical complications, such as haematemesis or inhalation of vomit;

F1x.03 with delirium;

F1x.04 with perceptual distortions;

F1x.05 with coma;

F1x.06 with convulsions;

F1x.07 pathological intoxication. This grouping applies only to alcohol. It describes the sudden onset of aggression and often violent behaviour that is not typical of the individual when sober, very soon after drinking amounts of alcohol that would not produce intoxication in most people.

F1x.1 Harmful use

This is a pattern of psychoactive substance use that is causing damage to health. The damage may be physical (as in cases of hepatitis from the self-administration of injected drugs) or mental (e.g. episodes of depressive disorder secondary to heavy consumption of alcohol). The following diagnostic guidelines should be followed.

The diagnosis requires that actual damage should have been caused to the mental or physical health of the user.

Harmful patterns of use are often criticised by others and frequently associated with adverse social consequences of various kinds. The fact that a pattern of use or a particular substance is disapproved of by another person or by the culture, or may have led to socially negative consequences such as arrest or marital arguments is not in itself evidence of harmful use.

Acute intoxication (see F1x.0), or 'hangover' is not in itself sufficient evidence of the damage to health required for coding harmful use.

Harmful use should not be diagnosed if dependence syndrome (F1x.2), a psychotic disorder (F1x.5), or another specific form of drug- or alcohol-related disorder is present.

It is also worth noting that the term 'harmful use', as used in the various international classifications, is not equivalent to the term as defined at the beginning of this chapter, and does not specify any particular level of alcohol consumption.

F1x.2 Dependence syndrome

This is defined as a cluster of physiological, behavioural and cognitive phenomena in which the use of a substance or class of substances takes on a much higher priority for a given individual than other behaviours that once had greater value. A central descriptive characteristic of the dependence syndrome is the desire (often strong, sometimes overpowering) to take psychoactive drugs (which may or may not have been medically prescribed), alcohol, or tobacco. There may be evidence that return to substance use after a period of abstinence leads to a more rapid reappearance of other features of the syndrome than occurs with nondependent individuals.

A definite diagnosis of dependence should usually be made only if three or more of the following have been experienced or exhibited at some time during the previous year.

A strong desire or sense of compulsion to take the substance.

Difficulties in controlling substance-taking behaviour in terms of its onset, termination, or levels of use.

A physiological withdrawal state (see F1x.3 and F1x.4) when substance use has ceased or been reduced, as evidenced by the characteristic withdrawal syndrome for the substance, or use of the same (or a closely related) substance with the intention of relieving or avoiding withdrawal symptoms.

Evidence of tolerance, such that increased doses of the psychoactive substance are required in order to achieve effects originally produced by lower doses (clear examples of this are found in alcohol- and opiate-dependent individuals who may take daily doses sufficient to incapacitate or kill nontolerant users).

Progressive neglect of alternative pleasure or interests because of psychoactive substance abuse; increased amount of time necessary to obtain or take the substance or to recover from its effects.

Persisting with substance abuse despite clear evidence of overtly harmful consequences, such as harm to the liver through excessive drinking, depressive mood states consequent to periods of heavy substance use, or drug-related impairment of cognitive functioning; efforts should be made to determine that the user was actually, or could be expected to be, aware of the nature and extent of the harm.

Narrowing of the personal repertoire of patterns of psychoactive substance use has also been described as a characteristic feature (e.g. a tendency to drink alcoholic drinks in the same way on weekdays and weekends, regardless of social constraints that determine appropriate drinking behaviour).

It is an essential characteristic of the dependence syndrome that either psychoactive substance taking or a desire to take a particular substance should be present; the subjective awareness of compulsion to use drugs is most commonly seen during attempts to stop or control substance use. This diagnostic requirement would exclude, for instance, surgical patients given opioid drugs for the relief of pain, who may show signs of an opioid withdrawal state when drugs are not given but who have no desire to continue taking drugs.

The dependence syndrome may be present for a specific substance (e.g. tobacco or diazepam), for a class of substance (e.g. opioid drugs), or for a wider range of different substances (as for those individuals who feel a sense of compulsion regularly to use whatever drugs are available and who show distress, agitation, and/or physical signs of a withdrawal state upon abstinence).

F1x.2 (dependence syndrome) includes chronic alcoholism, dipsomania and drug addiction. The diagnosis of the dependence syndrome may be further specified by the following five-character codes:

F1x.20 currently abstinent;

F1x.21 currently abstinent, but in a protected environment (e.g. in hospital, in a therapeutic community, in prison);

F1x.22 currently on a clinically supervised maintenance or replacement regime (controlled dependence) (e.g. with methadone, nicotine gum or nicotine patch);

F1x.23 currently abstinent, but receiving treatment with aversive or blocking drugs (e.g. naltrexone or disulfiram);

F1x.24 currently using the substance (active dependence);

F1x.25 continuous use;

F1x.26 episodic use (dipsomania).

F1x.3 Withdrawal state

This describes a group of symptoms of variable clustering and severity occurring on absolute or relative withdrawal of a substance after repeated, and usually prolonged and/or high dose, use of that substance. The onset and course of the withdrawal state are time-limited and are related to the type of substance and the dose being used immediately before abstinence. The withdrawal state may be complicated by convulsions. The following diagnostic guidelines are important:

A withdrawal state is one of the indicators of dependence syndrome (see F1x.2) and this diagnosis should also be considered;

Withdrawal state should be coded as the main diagnosis if it is the reason for referral and sufficiently severe to require medical attention in its own right;

Physical symptoms vary according to the substance being used. Psychological disturbances (e.g. anxiety, depression, and sleep disorders) are also common features of withdrawal.

Typically, the patient is likely to report that withdrawal symptoms are relieved by further substance use.

It should be remembered that withdrawal symptoms can be induced by conditioned or learned stimuli in the absence of immediately preceding substance use. In such cases, a diagnosis of withdrawal state should be made only if it is warranted in terms of severity. It should also be noted that simple 'hangover' or tremor due to other conditions should not be confused with the symptoms of a withdrawal state.

The diagnosis of withdrawal state may be further specified by using the following five-character codes:
F1x.30 uncomplicated;
F1x.31 with convulsions.

F1x.4 Withdrawal state with delirium

A condition in which the withdrawal state (see F1x.3) is complicated by delirium.

Alcohol-induced delirium tremens should be coded here. Delirium tremens is a short-lived, but occasionally life-threatening, toxic-confusional state with accompanying somatic disturbances. It is usually a consequence of absolute or relative withdrawal of alcohol in severely dependent users with a long history of use. The onset usually occurs after withdrawal of alcohol but may, in some cases, appear during an episode of heavy drinking, in which case it should be coded here.

Prodromal symptoms typically include insomnia, tremulousness and fear, but the onset may also be preceded by withdrawal convulsions. The classical triad of symptoms includes clouding of consciousness and confusion, vivid hallucinations and illusions affecting any sensory modality, and marked tremor. Delusions, agitation, insomnia or sleep-cycle reversal, and autonomic overactivity are usually also present.

The diagnosis of withdrawal state with delirium may be further specified by using the following five-character codes:
F1x.40 without convulsions;
F1x.41 with convulsions.

F1x.5 Psychotic disorder

A cluster of psychotic phenomena that occur during or immediately after psychoactive substance use and are characterized by vivid hallucinations (typically auditory, but often in more than one sensory modality), misidentifications, delusions and/or ideas of reference (often of a paranoid or persecutory nature), psychomotor disturbances (excitement or stupor), and an abnormal affect, which may range from intense fear to ecstasy. The sensorium is usually clear but some degree of clouding of consciousness, though not severe confusion, may be present. The disorder typically resolves at least partially within 1 month and fully within 6 months.

The following diagnostic guidelines are relevant.

A psychotic disorder occurring during or immediately after drug use (usually within 48 hours) should be recorded here, provided that it is not a manifestation of drug withdrawal state with delirium (see F1x.4) or of late onset. Late-onset psychotic disorders (with onset more than 2 weeks after substance use) may occur, but should be coded as F1x.75.

Psychoactive substance-induced psychotic disorders may present with varying patterns of symptoms. These variations will be influenced by the type of substance involved and the personality of the user. For stimulant drugs such as cocaine and amphetamines, drug-induced psychotic disorders are generally closely related to high dose levels and/or prolonged use of the substance. A diagnosis of a psychotic disorder should not be made merely on the basis of perceptual distortions or hallucinatory experiences when substances having primary hallucinogenic effects (e.g. lysergide (LSD), mescaline, cannabis at high doses) have been taken. In such cases, and also for confusional states, a possible diagnosis of acute intoxication (F1x.0) should be considered.

Particular care should also be taken to avoid mistakenly diagnosing a more serious condition (e.g. schizophrenia) when a diagnosis of psychoactive substance-induced psychosis is appropriate. Many psychoactive substance-induced psychotic states are of short duration, provided that no further amounts of the drug are taken (as in the case of amphetamine and cocaine psychoses). False diagnosis in such cases may have distressing and costly implications for the patient and for the health services.

F1x.5 includes alcoholic hallucinosis, alcoholic jealousy, alcoholic paranoia.

The diagnosis of psychotic state may be further specified by the following five-character codes:

F1x.50 schizophrenia-like;

F1x.51 predominantly delusional;

F1x.52 predominantly hallucinatory (includes alcoholic hallucinosis);

F1x.53 predominantly polymorphic;

F1x.54 predominantly depressive symptoms;

F1x.55 predominantly manic symptoms;

F1x.56 mixed.

F1x.6 Amnesic syndrome

A syndrome associated with chronic prominent impairment of recent memory; remote memory is sometimes impaired, while immediate recall is preserved. Disturbances of time sense and ordering of events are usually evident, as are difficulties in learning new material. Confabulation may be marked, but is not invariably present. Other cognitive functions are usually relatively well preserved and amnesic defects are out of proportion to other disturbances. The following diagnostic guidelines are important.

Amnesic syndrome induced by alcohol or other psychoactive substances coded should meet the general criteria for organic amnesic syndrome:

memory impairment, as shown in impairment of recent memory (learning of new material), disturbances of time sense (rearrangements of chronological sequence, telescoping of repeated events into one, etc.);

absence of defect in immediate recall, of impairment of consciousness, and of generalized cognitive impairment;

history of objective evidence of chronic (and particularly high dose) use of alcohol or drugs.

personality changes, often with apparent apathy and loss of initiative, and a tendency towards self-neglect may also be present, but should not be regarded as necessary conditions for diagnosis.

Although confabulation may be marked it should not be regarded as a necessary prerequisite for diagnosis.

F1x.6 includes Korsakov's psychosis or syndrome, induced by alcohol or other psychoactive substances.

F1x.7 Residual and late-onset psychotic disorder

A disorder in which changes of cognition, affect, personality, or behaviour, induced by alcohol or another psychoactive substances, persist beyond the period during which a direct, substance-related effect might reasonably be assumed to be operating. The following diagnostic guidelines may be helpful.

The onset of the disorder should be directly related to the abuse of alcohol or a psychoactive substance. Cases in which the initial onset occurs later than episode(s) of substance abuse should be coded here only where clear and strong evidence is available to attribute the state to the residual effect of the substance. The disorder should represent a change from or a marked exaggeration of the prior and normal state of functioning.

The disorder should persist beyond any period of time during which direct effects of the psychoactive substance might be assumed to be operative (see F1x.0, acute intoxication). Alcohol- or psychoactive substance-induced dementia is not always irreversible; after an extended period of total abstinence, intellectual functions and memory may improve.

The disorder should be carefully distinguished from withdrawal-related conditions (see F1x.3 and F1x.4). It should be remembered that, under certain conditions and for certain substances, withdrawal-state phenomena may be present for a period of many days or weeks after discontinuation of the substance.

Conditions induced by a psychoactive substance, persisting after its use, and meeting the criteria for diagnosis of psychotic disorder should not be diagnosed here (use F1x.5, psychotic disorder). Patients who show the chronic end-state of Korsakov's syndrome should be coded under F1x.6.

Further specification of F1x.7 may be achieved by using the following five-character codes:

F1x.70 flashbacks, these may be distinguished from psychotic disorders partly by their episodic nature, frequently of very short duration (seconds or minutes), and by their duplication (sometimes exact) of previous drug-related experiences;

F1x.71 personality or behaviour disorder (meeting the criteria for organic personality disorder);

F1x.72 residual affective disorder (meeting the criteria for organic mood (affective) disorders);

F1x.73 dementia (meeting the general criteria for dementia);

F1x.74 other persisting cognitive impairment, this is a residual category for disorders with persisting cognitive impairment, which do not meet the criteria for psychoactive substance-induced amnesic syndrome (F1x.6) or dementia (F1x.73);

F1x.75 late-onset psychotic disorder.

F1x.8 Other mental and behaviour disorders

This diagnostic category is for any other disorder in which the use of a substance can be identified as contributing directly to the condition, but which does not meet the criteria for inclusion in any of the above disorders.

F1x.9 Unspecified mental and behavioural disorder

This category is for unspecified mental and behavioural disorder, induced by alcohol and drugs.

DSM-III-R

DSM-III-R, like ICD-10, acknowledges that no definition adequately specifies precise boundaries for the concept of mental disorder. However, each of the mental disorders is conceptualized as 'a clinically significant behavioural or psychological syndrome or pattern that occurs in a person and that is associated with present distress (a painful symptom) or disability (impairment in one or more important areas of functioning) or with a significantly increased risk of suffering death, pain, disability, or an important loss of freedom'. Whatever the original cause, a mental disorder is a manifestation of behavioural, psychological or biological dysfunction. It should also be appreciated that there is no assumption that each mental disorder is a discrete entity with sharp boundaries between the different disorders.

A major difference between the ICD-10 and DSM-III-R is that the latter is a multiaxial system, requiring cases to be evaluated on several 'axes', each of which refers to a different class of information. The entire classification of mental disorders is contained within Axes 1 (Clinical Syndromes) and 2 (Developmental Disorders and Personality Disorders) and multiple diagnoses are made when necessary to describe the current condition.

Diagnostic guidelines are provided indicating the number and balance of symptoms usually required before a confident diagnosis can be made. Statements about the duration of symptoms are intended as general guidelines rather than strict requirements so that clinicians should use their own judgement about the appropriateness of choosing diagnoses when the duration of particular symptoms varies slightly from that specified.

Mental disorders related to substance use are classified in two areas of DSM-III-R: Psychoactive Substance Use Disorders and Psychoactive Substance-Induced Organic Mental Disorders.

Psychoactive substance use disorders

This diagnostic class covers the symptoms and maladaptive behavioural changes associated with more or less regular use of psychoactive substances. These changes are perceived as undesirable in most cultures and the underlying conditions are described as mental disorders, distinguishing them from nonpathological psychoactive substance use (e.g. drinking a moderate amount of alcohol).

There are two main categories of substance use disorder and their diagnostic criteria are summarized below.

Criteria for psychoactive substance dependence

Dependence can be diagnosed if at least three of the following symptoms have occurred, some of which have persisted for at least 1 month, or have occurred repeatedly over a longer period of time:

1 Substance often taken in larger amounts or over a longer period than the person intended;
2 Persistent desire or one or more unsuccessful efforts to cut down or control substance use;
3 A great deal of time spent in activities necessary to get the substance (e.g. theft), taking the substance (e.g. chain smoking), or recovering from its effects;
4 Frequent intoxication or withdrawal symptoms when expected to fulfil major role obligations at work, school or home (e.g. not going to work because of a hangover; going to work or school while 'high'; intoxication while taking care of children), or when substance use is physically hazardous (e.g. driving while intoxicated);
5 Important social, occupational, or recreational activities given up or reduced because of substance use;
6 Continued substance use despite knowledge of having a persistent or recurrent social, psychological or physical problem that is caused or exacerbated by the use of the substance;
7 Marked tolerance; need for markedly increased amounts of the substance (i.e. at least a 50% increase) in order to achieve intoxication or desired

effect, or markedly diminished effect with continued use of the same amount. (The final two items listed (8 and 9) may not apply to cannabis, hallucinogens or phencyclidine.)

8 Characteristic withdrawal symptoms;
9 Substance often taken to relieve or avoid withdrawal symptoms.

Criteria for severity of psychoactive substance dependence

Mild. Few, if any, symptoms in excess of those required to make the diagnosis, and the symptoms result in no more than mild impairment in occupational functioning or in usual social activities or relationships with others.

Moderate. Symptoms or functional impairment between 'mild' and 'severe'.

Severe. Many symptoms in excess of those required to make the diagnosis, and the symptoms markedly interfere with occupational functioning or with usual social activities or relationships with others.

In partial remission. During the past 6 months, some use of the substance and some symptoms of dependence.

In full remission. During the past 6 months, either no use of the substance, or use of the substance and no symptoms of dependence.

Criteria for psychoactive substance abuse

Substance abuse can be diagnosed if all of the following criteria are fulfilled.

A maladaptive pattern of substance use indicated by at least one of the following:

(a) recurrent use in situations in which use is physically hazardous (e.g. driving while intoxicated);

(b) continued use despite knowledge of having a persistent or recurrent social, occupational, psychological, or physical problem caused or exacerbated by use of the substance.

Some symptoms persisting for at least 1 month or having occurred repeatedly over a longer period of time.

The patient has never met the criteria for Psychoactive Substance Dependence for this substance.

DSM-IV

Significant changes have recently been made in the diagnostic systems of the American Psychiatric Association, resulting in the development of DSM-IV, which has several important changes from the earlier DSM-III-R. For example, the stipulation in DSM-III that symptoms must 'have persisted for at least 1 month' is replaced with symptoms 'occurring at any time in the same 12-month period'. Broadening the dependence criteria will result in greater sensitivity of the dependence category, perhaps resulting in an increase in the breadth of individuals who are diagnosed with a disorder because it will no longer include only individuals who meet a significant number of criteria in a relatively short period of time. Another important change is grouping the criteria 'characteristic withdrawal symptoms' and 'substance taken to relieve or avoid withdrawal symptoms' into one category in DSM-IV, thus reducing the importance of physiological aspects of substance dependence by reducing the number of possible criteria. The criteria for substance dependence 'frequent intoxication or withdrawal when expected to fulfill major obligations at work, school or home or when substance use is physically hazardous' has been removed from DSM-IV, perhaps compromising the professional's ability to acknowledge the presence of impaired function in these locations; this may impair the diagnostic efficacy of the instrument.

It is acknowledged in DSM-IV that it is often difficult to determine whether presenting symptoms are indeed substance induced; i.e. that they are the direct physiological consequence of substance intoxication or withdrawal, medication use or toxin exposure. Two additional criteria have therefore been added to each of the substance-induced disorders, with the intention of providing general guidelines and of allowing for clinical judgement in determining whether symptoms are substance induced.

There is evidence from the history, physical examination, or laboratory findings of either:

(a) the symptoms developing during or within a month of substance intoxication or withdrawal;

(b) medication use is aetiologically related to the disturbance.

The disturbance is not better accounted for by a disorder that is not substance induced. Thus, if the symptoms precede substance use, or persist for more than a month after its cessation, or are substantially in excess of what might be expected, given the type, duration, or amount of substance used, this would suggest the existence of an independent nonsubstance-induced disorder.

The DSM-IV criteria for substance dependence and abuse, as well as those for substance intoxication and withdrawal are listed below.

Criteria for substance dependence

The essential features of substance dependence are a cluster of cognitive, behavioural and physiological symptoms indicating that the individual continues use of the substance despite significant substance-related problems. There is a pattern of repeated self-administration that usually results in tolerance, withdrawal and compulsive drug-taking behaviour.

Diagnosis of dependence should be made if three or more of the following have been experienced or exhibited at any time during the last year.

1. Tolerance defined by either:
   (a) the need for markedly increased amounts of substance to achieve intoxi-cation or desired effect;
   (b) a markedly diminished effect with continued use of the same amount of the substance.
2. Withdrawal, as evidenced by either of the following:
   (a) the characteristic withdrawal syndrome for the substance, or
   (b) the same (or closely related) substance is taken to relieve or avoid withdrawal symptoms.
3. The substance is often taken in larger amounts over a longer period of time than was intended.
4. Persistent desire or repeated, unsuccessful efforts to cut down or control substance use.
5. A great deal of time is spent in activities necessary to obtain the substance, use the substance, or recover from its effects.
6. Important social, occupational, or recreational activities are given up or reduced because of substance use.
7. There is continued substance use despite knowledge of having had a persistent or recurrent physical or psychological problem that was likely to have been caused or exacerbated by the substance.

It should be specified whether physiological dependence is present or absent (i.e. either 1 or 2, above, is present).

The course of the dependence should also be described using one of six defined specifiers.

Early full remission. No criteria for dependence/abuse for at least 1 month, but for less than 12 months.

Early partial remission. One or more criteria for dependence/abuse have been met for at least 1 month but for less than 12 months (but the full criteria for dependence have not been met).

Sustained full remission. No criteria for dependence/abuse have been met at any time during a period of 12 months or longer.

Sustained partial remission. One or more criteria for dependence/abuse have been met, but not the full criteria, for a period of 12 months or longer.

On agonist therapy. This term should be used if the individual is on a prescribed agonist medication, and criteria for dependence/abuse have been met for that class of medication for at least the past month (except tolerance to, or withdrawal from, the agonist). This specifier may also be used for those being treated for dependence using a partial agonist or agonist/antagonist.

In a controlled environment. This specifier is used if the individual is in an environment where access to alcohol and controlled substances is restricted and no criteria for dependence/abuse have been met for the previous month (e.g. in prison, therapeutic community, locked hospital ward).

Criteria for substance abuse

A maladaptive pattern of substance abuse leading to recurrent and significant adverse consequences related to the repeated use of substances, with clinically significant impairment or distress, as manifested by one or more of the following occurring at any time during the same 12-month period:

Recurrent substance abuse resulting in a failure to fulfill major role obligations at work, school, or home (e.g. repeated absences, poor performance, expulsion or suspension from school, child neglect);

Recurrent substance abuse in situations that are physically hazardous (e.g. driving, operating machinery);

Recurrent substance abuse-related legal problems;

Continued substance abuse despite having persistent or recurrent social or inter-personal problems caused or exacerbated by the effects of the substance (e.g. arguments and fights).

In addition, the symptoms should not have met the criteria for dependence on this class of substance.

Criteria for substance intoxication

The development of a reversible substance-specific syndrome due to the recent ingestion of (or exposure to) a substance.

Clinically significant maladaptive behavioural or psychological changes that are due to the effect of the substance on the central nervous system (e.g. belligerence, mood lability, cognitive impairment) developing during or shortly after use of the substance.

Criteria for substance withdrawal

The development of a substance-specific syndrome due to the cessation of (or reduction in) substance use that has been heavy and prolonged.

The substance-specific syndrome causes clinically significant distress or impair-ment in social, occupational or other important areas of functioning.

The symptoms are not due to a general medical condition and are not better accounted for by another mental disorder.

DSM-IV classification

In addition to the specifiers for substance dependence that have already been described, the following specifiers may also be utilized for substance-induced disorders:

with onset during intoxication (I);

with onset during withdrawal (W).

Within DSM-IV classification, the following substance-related disorders are separately enumerated.

Alcohol-related disorders

Alcohol use disorders

Alcohol dependence 303.90

Alcohol abuse 305.00

Alcohol-induced disorders

Alcohol intoxication 303.00

Uncomplicated alcohol withdrawal 291.80

Alcohol intoxication delirium 291.0

Alcohol withdrawal delirium 291.00

Alcohol-induced persisting dementia 291.20

Alcohol-induced persisting amnesic disorder 291.10

Alcohol-induced psychotic disorder 291.x

   with delusions 291.5

   with hallucinations 291.3

Alcohol-induced mood disorder 291.8

Alcohol-induced anxiety disorder 291.8

Alcohol-induced sexual dysfunction 291.8

Alcohol-induced sleep disorder 291.8

Alcohol-related disorder not otherwise specified (NOS) 291.9

Amphetamine (or amphetamine-like)-related disorders

Amphetamine use disorders

Amphetamine dependence 304.40

Amphetamine abuse 305.70

Amphetamine-induced disorders

Amphetamine intoxication 292.89

Amphetamine withdrawal 292.0

Amphetamine intoxication delirium 292.81

Amphetamine-induced psychotic disorder 292.xx

   with delusions 292.11

   with hallucinations 292.12

Amphetamine-induced mood disorder 292.89

Amphetamine-induced anxiety disorder 292.89

Amphetamine-induced sexual dysfunction 292.89

Amphetamine-induced sleep disorder 292.89

Amphetamine-related disorder NOS 292.9

Caffeine-related disorders
Caffeine-induced disorders
Caffeine intoxication 305.90
Caffeine-induced anxiety disorder 292.89
Caffeine-related sleep disorder 292.89
Caffeine-related disorder NOS 292.9

Cannabis-related disorders
Cannabis use disorders
Cannabis dependence 304.30
Cannabis abuse 305.20
Cannabis-induced disorders
Cannabis intoxication 292.89
Cannabis intoxication delirium 292.81
Cannabis-induced psychotic disorder 292.xx
    with delusions 292.11
    with hallucinations 292.12
Cannabis-induced anxiety disorder 292.89
Cannabis-related disorder NOS 292.9

Cocaine-related disorders
Cocaine use disorders
Cocaine dependence 304.20
Cocaine abuse 305.60
Cocaine-induced disorders
Cocaine intoxication 292.89
Cocaine withdrawal 292.00
Cocaine intoxication delirium 292.81
Cocaine-induced psychotic disorder
    with delusions 292.11
    with hallucinations 292.11
Cocaine-induced mood disorder 292.84
Cocaine-induced anxiety disorder 292.89
Cocaine-induced sexual dysfunction 292.89
Cocaine-induced sleep disorder 292.89
Cocaine-related disorder NOS 292.9

Hallucinogen-related disorders
Hallucinogen use disorders
Hallucinogen dependence 304.50
Hallucinogen abuse 305.30

Hallucinogen-induced disorders
Hallucinogen intoxication 292.89
Hallucinogen persisting perception disorder (flashbacks) 292.89
Hallucinogen intoxication delirium 292.81
Hallucinogen-induced psychotic disorder 292.xx
   with delusions 292.11
   with hallucinations 292.12
Hallucinogen-induced mood disorder 292.84
Hallucinogen-induced anxiety disorder 292.89
Hallucinogen-related disorder NOS 292.9

Inhalant-related disorders
Inhalant use disorders
Inhalant dependence 304.60
Inhalant abuse 305.90
Inhalant-induced disorders
Inhalant intoxication 292.89
Inhalant intoxication delirium 292.81
Inhalant-induced persisting dementia 292.82
Inhalant-induced psychotic disorder 292.xx
   with delusions 292.11
   with hallucinations 292.12
Inhalant-induced mood disorder 292.84
Inhalant-induced anxiety disorder 292.89
Inhalant-related disorder NOS 292.9

Nicotine-related disorders
Nicotine use disorder
Nicotine dependence 305.10
Nicotine-induced disorder
Nicotine withdrawal 292.0
Nicotine-related disorder NOS 292.9

Opioid-related disorders
Opioid use disorders
Opioid dependence 304.00
Opioid abuse 305.50
Opioid-induced disorders
Opioid intoxication 305.50
Opioid withdrawal 292.00

Opioid intoxication delirium 292.81
Opioid-induced psychotic disorder 292.xx
    with delusions 292.11
    with hallucinations 292.12
Opioid-induced mood disorder 292.84
Opioid-induced sexual dysfunction 292.89
Opioid-induced sleep disorder 292.89
Opioid-related disorder NOS 292.9

Phencyclidine (or phencyclidine-like)-related disorders
Phencyclidine use disorders
Phencyclidine dependence 304.90
Phencyclidine abuse 305.90
Phencyclidine-induced disorders
Phencyclidine intoxication 292.89
Phencyclidine intoxication delirium 292.81
Phencyclidine-induced psychotic disorder 292.xx
    with delusions 292.11
    with hallucinations 292.12
Phencyclidine-induced mood disorder 292.84
Phencyclidine-induced anxiety disorder 292.89
Phencyclidine-related disorder NOS 292.9

Sedative-, hypnotic-, or anxiolytic-related disorders
Sedative, hypnotic, or anxiolytic use disorders
Sedative, hypnotic or anxiolytic dependence 304.10
Sedative, hypnotic or anxiolytic abuse 305.40
Sedative-, hypnotic-, or anxiolytic-induced disorders
Sedative, hypnotic or anxiolytic intoxication 292.89
Sedative, hypnotic or anxiolytic withdrawal 292.0
Sedative, hypnotic or anxiolytic intoxication delirium 292.81
Sedative, hypnotic or anxiolytic withdrawal delirium 292.81
Sedative, hypnotic or anxiolytic persisting dementia 292.82
Sedative, hypnotic or anxiolytic persisting amnesic disorder 292.83
Sedative-, hypnotic- or anxiolytic-induced psychotic disorder 292.xx
    with delusions 292.11
    with hallucinations 292.12
Sedative-, hypnotic- or anxiolytic-induced mood disorder 292.84
Sedative-, hypnotic- or anxiolytic-induced anxiety disorder 292.89
Sedative-, hypnotic- or anxiolytic-induced sexual dysfunction 292.89

Sedative-, hypnotic- or anxiolytic-induced sleep disorder 292.89
Sedative-, hypnotic- or anxiolytic-related disorder NOS 292.9

Polysubstance-related disorder
Polysubstance dependence 304.80
Other (or unknown) substance-related disorders
Other (or unknown) substance dependence 304.90
Other (or unknown) substance abuse 305.90
Other (or unknown) substance-induced disorders
Other (or unknown) substance intoxication 292.89
Other (or unknown) substance withdrawal 292.0
Other (or unknown) substance intoxication delirium 292.81
Other (or unknown) substance persisting dementia 292.82
Other (or unknown) substance persisting amnesic disorder 292.83
Other (or unknown) substance-induced psychotic disorder 292.xx
   with delusions 292.11
   with hallucinations 292.12
Other (or unknown) substance-induced mood disorder 292.84
Other (or unknown) substance-induced anxiety disorder 292.89
Other (or unknown) substance-induced sexual dysfunction 292.89
Other (or unknown) substance-induced sleep disorder 292.89
Other (or unknown) substance-related disorder NOS 292.9

General measures of intervention

Introduction

Once assessment is completed, the crucial question of how to help a particular individual with their drug problem has to be answered. For some, the immediate response is pharmacological (see Chapter 7), although this is usually only a short-term measure and can only be one component of the total treatment response. But many who seek help have a drug problem with little or no physical dependence and for them there is no drug-specific treatment. For all drug abusers, therefore, it is essential to work out a long-term plan aimed at bringing about change in them and their lifestyle, so that they do not need to take drugs and can cope without them, even if they continue to be freely available.

A person's level of motivation for change is an important factor in determining the likely success of any intervention (and measurement of this will form part of the assessment interview). Of course, not every person presenting with a drug problem will be fully motivated to benefit from treatment, and a person's motivation for change will fluctuate depending on many factors. Most people have a degree of ambivalence, and a number of reasons for and against giving up or changing a habit, and the salience given to each of these can fluctuate even in a short time period. It may be helpful to think of motivation for change as a circle which the drug abuser may go round many times before achieving long-lasting change. The circle of motivation starts with the person not contemplating a change in their behaviour, either because of denial that a problem exists or because of a belief that the problem is unchangeable ('precontemplative' stage). The next stage is an awareness of the need and ability to change ('contemplative' stage) whilst nevertheless continuing with the behaviour. As individuals progress, they move on to the 'determination' stage, where the decision is made to take action and change. This is followed by a stage of active change, where the person's determination produces change-directed behaviour. The next part of the motivational circle is a 'maintenance of change' stage. If these efforts fail, a relapse occurs and the individual begins another cycle. One person may remain for several years at each stage, whilst someone else might experience all five on a daily basis.[1]

Each time the person goes around the circle, however, there is the possibility of gaining from the experience which may help future attempts. Rather than being a circle of change which includes, for some, relapse, it may be more accurate to think of this as a spiral of motivation, heading in the direction of eventual improvement. Several revolutions through the cycle are often needed to learn how to maintain change successfully.

The intervention offered will, to some extent, depend on the assessment of motivation for change, and it should not be assumed that everyone is at the active change state, nor that everyone will necessarily benefit from help directed at changing their behaviour. For most patients, however, some form of active-change treatment will be considered and a variety of treatment options are available. In virtually every case, if the treatment is to be of any value, it has to be on a voluntary basis and it is important that the patient participates in the choice of treatment option. Some treatments are directed at the underlying causes which may have initiated drug-taking and/or are contributing to its continuation. Some help to resolve the problems associated with or consequent upon drug-taking, and some deal more directly with the drug-taking behaviour itself, aiming to reduce or stop drug-taking, regardless of other problems or circumstances. Some treatments may be directed at helping the client's motivation for change, rather than directly changing the behaviour, while others are aimed at helping to prevent relapse in those who have achieved change. The setting for these treatment options is likewise varied, from a residential programme through hospital-based care, to self-help groups in the community. In recent years there have been considerable improvements in the provision of community treatments, often given by a multidisciplinary team seeing the patient at home or in another community venue.[2]

Not all interventions are suitable for every patient, nor are they mutually exclusive. A patient, for example, may attend for drug counselling, undergo vocational rehabilitation and go to a local self-help group while, at the same time, his or her daily dose of opiates is being gradually reduced according to a treatment contract drawn up on a contingency-management basis. It is perhaps unlikely that a single individual would be on the receiving end of so many interventions, but the important point is that treatment plans must be drawn up thoughtfully, according to the needs of the individual, utilizing, as appropriate, a single intervention or a 'mix' of interventions, or components of different interventions. There is no one approach that is 'right' or 'best'. If there were, the problems of drug abuse and dependence would be rapidly overcome and petty controversies between the advocates of different treatment modalities would disappear.

Because there are no hard and fast rules about management, much depends on the skills of professional health care workers in developing a treatment plan that meets the needs of the patient, and this in turn relies heavily on the findings of the assessment procedure. The key to successful intervention is to bring about change, and before that can be done, it is essential to know as much as possible about the existing situation.

The interventions that are briefly described in this chapter are mostly long-term measures, aimed at bringing about long-term and fundamental changes. They are often collectively described as 'rehabilitation', and the fact that in this book rehabilitative interventions are described before 'treatment' (i.e. detoxification, maintenance, etc.) emphasizes the fact that for most drug abusers, long-term change is more important than short-term intervention and that the two stages of response should be considered and often initiated concurrently.

Psychotherapy

It has been apparent for many years that classical, analytically orientated psycho-therapy is not suitable for drug-dependent patients. Early therapists emphasized the extreme difficulties encountered in trying to treat addicts, not least because it can be very difficult to engage them effectively in treatment and, if they do attend, their mental state may be adversely affected by drug use. In addition, such treatment is too time consuming and expensive to be a cost-effective option for treating the majority of problem drug users.

However, the term 'psychotherapy' embraces far more than classical techniques of psychoanalysis. In its broadest sense it is a treatment involving communication between patient and therapist aimed at modifying or alleviating the patient's 'illness', and any encounter between the patient and a health care worker thus offers an opportunity for psychotherapy. Awareness of the potential therapeutic value of this relationship and an appropriate structuring of the communication means that psychotherapy can become a component of an integrated approach to the treatment of drug dependence, rather than an alternative treatment strategy that is selected only occasionally.

Because many opiate-dependent individuals attend specialist treatment units regularly for long periods (months to years), possibly for opiate maintenance or for slow detoxification, long-term relationships can develop with clinic staff, which can be utilized to promote positive personality growth and psychological development. Similar opportunities arise with those who are dependent on seda-tive hypnotic drugs. It has been suggested that the supportive relationship that develops between patient and therapist becomes a substitute for drug use, just as drug dependency may be a substitute for certain aspects of important inter-personal relationships. A skilled therapist is unlikely to become a mere substitute for a drug, but having formed a good and supportive relationship with a patient is able to use it to identify and alter intrapsychic processes using techniques of insight, restructuring of belief systems, cognitive reframing and challenging of unhelpful beliefs, so that patients learn to see themselves and their problems more clearly and have the desire and the ability to cope with them.[3] This combining of psychodynamic approaches with cognitive therapy and training in skills using behavioural techniques has been developed in recent years into specialist psycho-therapeutic 'packages' for drug users, particularly those with personality disorders. Commonly, these two aspects of the programme (using the dynamics of a therapist–patient relationship and training in cognitive and behavioural skills) are delivered by separate therapists who work in close collaboration.

It should also be remembered that many drug-dependent individuals have significant psychiatric problems, especially in the areas of depression and anxiety. Drug use and abuse may result from attempts to medicate these problems and it is therefore not surprising that psychotherapy, which can often help to alleviate depression and anxiety, may indirectly cause a reduction in drug use too.

Supportive-expressive and interpersonal psychotherapy

As the name suggests, these are analytically orientated psychotherapies, in which the drug dependence is seen as intimately related to disorders in interpersonal functioning. Special attention is paid to the meanings that patients attach to their drug dependence, with the therapist taking an exploratory stance and using supportive techniques to help the patient identify and work through problematic relationships.

Group psychotherapy

Group psychotherapy is the technique of treating patients in groups rather than individually. The same group of individuals meets regularly, for example weekly or more often, with a trained leader who, depending on the type of group, may actively direct its focus. One of the aims might be to improve the ability of individual members to control their social behaviour – a skill in which some are deficient – and to this end the behavioural interactions between the members of the group are the subject of examination. Members of the group are confronted with observations about their own behaviour and become aware of their effect on others and of the effect of others on themselves. They learn to listen to interpretations of their behaviour and to deal with the resultant anxiety, which may be difficult and painful at first, so that techniques of circumvention are employed. If group membership remains stable over several months, the group becomes a cohesive structure and its members identify positively with each other and with the group. In this supportive environment, individual growth is possible and the experience gained within the group can be transferred to life outside the group.

Other groups focus on the belief systems held by different members, eliciting errors of thinking (e.g. 'I've made a mess of my life so far, therefore I will always be a worthless person') or unhelpful beliefs ('the only time I can ever enjoy myself is when I'm drunk'). With the help of the therapist, the group is able to challenge beliefs and restructure them, using a number of techniques. Other groups focus on behavioural and cognitive skills for managing emotional states, anger control, and skills for dealing with lapses and for avoiding relapse. These groups are sometimes run along the lines of educational courses, with behaviour rehearsal and group role-plays included among the techniques. 'Relapse prevention', on which some groups focus, is based on social-learning theory from psychology, and assumes that the road to relapse or continued abstinence follows a number of choice points; therapy in groups tends to include behavioural and cognitive techniques for dealing with the more common 'choice points', although a skilled therapist will be able to be flexible according to the needs of the group.

Superficially, group therapy is an attractive treatment option. This is firstly because the addition of the group dynamics to treatment techniques is potentially a powerful way of delivering therapy; and secondly because it seems to be a cost-effective method, compared with individual psychotherapy, of offering professional help to drug abusers. However, effective group therapy may require regular attendance by all members and drug abusers may be unreliable and not good at keeping regular appointments, often for legitimate social reasons. Furthermore, effective group therapy requires a high level of disclosure and some drug abusers, who may have been involved in criminal activities, may not be sufficiently reassured about the confidentiality of the proceedings to be frank and honest. Finally, it is easy for group therapy with drug abusers to degenerate into a complaints session about aspects of treatment policy and for the group to exert pressure for change in this policy. These factors, together with poor attendance rates, make it very difficult to direct the group into therapeutic interactions and a very skilful therapist is essential.

Group therapy for drug abuse is not a substitute for individual treatment but is an adjunct to it, aiming to foster individual development and growth. Those most likely to benefit from dynamic group therapy, and most suitable for it, usually have a long history of drug abuse, with only limited success in attaining periods of abstinence. They may also have interpersonal difficulties. In the UK many of these patients are on long-term (usually for a year) treatment contracts and receive maintenance prescriptions for opiates. However, membership of a group and attendance are voluntary (otherwise there is likely to be deliberate sabotaging of the group by the coerced members), and should not be made a condition of any treatment contract, and it is customary that the group therapist does not prescribe for the patients. Lack of motivation to achieve abstinence should not be a bar from the group. Although it is difficult to evaluate the effectiveness of group therapy, it has been found that cognitive-behavioural group therapy, emphasizing education and coping skill acquisition in the early after-care treatment of alcoholic patients, significantly reduced patient reports of drinking-related problems at 6-month follow-up. Interestingly, excessive stimulation of affect during interactional group therapy appeared to increase drinking-related complaints.[4]

Family therapy

The use of family therapy in the treatment of drug abuse is particularly appropriate because, as has long been recognized, the family as a whole may profoundly influence the behaviour of its individual members, including their use, or nonuse, of drugs. It is beyond the scope of this chapter to describe and discuss the underlying philosophy and nature of family therapy, but it is important to understand that the family is a relatively stable system that tends to resist change, and that drug abuse may have powerful adaptive consequences that help to maintain that stability.[5] For example, parents on the brink of divorce may remain united to cope with the recurrent crises of a drug-abusing child, and parents who cannot cope with the departure of their adolescent child from the family home may overtly or covertly encourage the drug abuse that keeps the child dependent on them.

Whatever the individual family scenario, the reaction of family members to the drug abuse of one of them often seems to be to maintain the drug-taking behaviour, whether or not they played a predisposing causal role in its initiation. Members of the family, albeit unconsciously, may actually encourage or reinforce drug-taking, and may seriously undermine any treatment programme, especially at the stage when the patient is showing progress and drug abuse is declining. Thus, in family therapy terms, the drug abuse of the patient is really that of the family as a whole, and it is logical to include the whole family in the treatment approach. Even when the drug abuser is a young adult who has left home, and even when that adult is married (with or without children), it is often the family of origin that continues to have a powerful influence on drug-taking and is the focus for family intervention.

The first problem is to persuade the families of drug abusers to participate in treatment. They may feel, for example, that being invited for family therapy implies that they are in some way to blame for the patient's drug problem. It is therefore essential to stress their potential helpfulness in the treatment process and it may be useful if they know in advance the period of treatment to which they are committing themselves. They may, after all, have had several previous experiences of 'failed' treatments and be unwilling to engage themselves in what seems like another gimmick.

In some types of family therapy the therapist will try to help the family to solve its problems and the individual family members to relate to each other in more positive and constructive ways. To do so, the therapist must 'join' the family group, initially by supporting the family and behaving according to its rules – adopting its style and affect. A new family system is thus formed, consisting of the old family plus the therapist who must establish a positive relationship with each member and establish a leadership within the family group. By joining the group in this way, the therapist can experience at first hand, and participate in, the behavioural interactions that have become the family's response to a particular problem. Often these habitual responses are maladaptive and a series of interventions may then be planned, using the therapist's skills to restructure the family's patterns of interactions, in order to implement change. Tasks may be assigned to individual family members to perform at home before the next session. This provides more 'practice' at better interpersonal relationships and increases the influence of the therapist, whose presence is felt in the family home even during everyday activities.[6]

Of course, a typical and understandable expectation on the part of the family is that it is the identified patient who should change or be changed by treatment. However, the drug-abusing individual does not live and behave in isolation, but interacts with the family group; his or her drug abuse is maintained because the family participates in maladaptive responses and interactions, and treatment is therefore targeted at the whole family. Nevertheless, it should be remembered that the goal of therapy is not the exploration of past events, but the alteration of the present situation. The symptoms of the identified patient should never be lost sight of, and the primary aim of treatment is to influence the rest of the family to help the patient with this problem. For adolescents it appears that family-based approaches are effective in engaging substance abusers in treatment and in reducing drug use.[7] However, the clinical significance of these changes, and whether they are maintained is less clear. Evidence for the effectiveness of family therapy for adult substance abusers is weaker.

A variation on family therapy is multiple-family therapy in which a number of drug addicts' families are treated conjointly. It is found that the families are able to support each other because of their shared experiences and that they learn to recognize and understand what is happening in their own family by observing similar phenomena in other families.[8] The support offered by the group is particularly helpful at the very difficult time when parents begin to detach themselves from the problems of their drug-abusing child. Another variant on systemic approaches is 'network therapy' in which family members and friends (where possible) are enlisted to provide ongoing support to promote attitude change. It uses psychodynamic and behavioural therapy while engaging the patient in a support network composed of family members and peers.

Drug counselling

Drug counselling at its simplest level is an advisory service. This deals with the realities of the patient's present situation, but the advice that is given is backed up by the practical help of a professional counsellor. Sessions occur regularly, by appointment, rather than on a casual, drop-in basis, and their frequency varies according to the particular needs of different patients. Counselling entails assessing the specific needs of individual patients and then providing or directing the patient towards the services that meet these needs.

Simply giving the patient time to talk about their problems can be, for some, a powerful technique in itself. The first step is to 'engage' the patient, and this is often best done using nondirective 'Rogerian' counselling. The key principles of this include taking a nonjudgmental approach, with the counsellor having an 'unconditional, positive regard' for the client; the essential skill is 'active listening', which will include summarizing and reflecting back to the client what he/she is saying. Once the counsellor has gained the trust and confidence of the client, and the client has been able to articulate his or her problems and concerns, then the counsellor will help the client to establish realistic goals, which may encompass not just drug-taking but also school, work, leisure-time activities, and relationships with family and friends. The available options are presented to the patient, who is helped to decide the best course of action – and then helped to follow the chosen course.[9]

It is important throughout that the patient perceives him or herself as having choices and is in the 'driving seat', accepting that any improvements or slips are due to his or her own efforts. The patient is essentially treating him or herself with the help of a counsellor, rather than being the passive recipient of treatment. Progress in achieving the stated goals is monitored by seeing the patient regularly, and problems can be appropriately dealt with as they arise by a counsellor who becomes well known to the patient and trusted.

Many kinds of problems are dealt with in counselling sessions. When appropriate, specific treatment options can be discussed, such as specific psychological techniques, in-patient, out-patient or community detoxification, maintenance treatment, drug-free therapeutic communities, etc., and the necessary arrangements for their implementation can be initiated. However, many areas of daily living may also be susceptible to advice and counselling. In particular, ways of avoiding encounters with other drug abusers and drugs should be explored so that essential changes in lifestyle are made. For some drug users, their whole role identity and personality may be as an addict, dealer or perhaps someone who commands respect in their community because of their drug use. Advice to avoid particular situations or a particular group of friends is unlikely to be effective by itself. There must, in addition, be practical help aimed at engaging the drug abuser in new ways of managing their time and developing alternative lifestyles. Similarly, it may be essential for some drug abusers to move house, away from their drug-taking environment, but again they may need positive help before this can be achieved.[10] Thus, drug counsellors often liaise with other agencies on the drug user's behalf and the value of this active, practical support should not be underestimated. This kind of work is sometimes referred to as the 'Community Reinforcement Approach'. This seeks to change the patient's social environment so that positive reinforcement is freely available without drugs. Emphasis is placed on developing rewarding employment, leisure activities and relationships that do not involve drugs, helping the patient to become more involved in what is more valued than drugs.

Counselling, insofar as it offers the drug abuser a supportive relationship with a trained counsellor, can of course be considered psychotherapeutic in its own right. Usually, however, no attempt is made to mediate intrapsychic processes or to engage in specific psychotherapeutic techniques.

Motivational interviewing

Motivational Interviewing (MI) or Motivational Enhancement Therapy is an approach to therapy which also draws on Rogerian, nondirective counselling models, but in addition incorporates Beck's model of cognitive therapy and elements of cognitive behavioural therapy. The therapist does not just reflect back the patient's words, but selects certain comments and through summarizing, affirming, reframing and questioning techniques, increases dissonance which is the vehicle for motivating change. As well as developing discrepancy in the patient's beliefs and behaviours, MI avoids argumentation and rolls with resistance, which among other things helps to keep the patient motivated for treatment. MI in addition helps raise the client's self-esteem, self-efficacy, and awareness of problems, it elicits self-motivational statements and pinpoints motivated behaviour. Importantly, it attributes responsibility to the client. Denial in this model is not viewed as a personality trait, but rather as an effect of the interaction between the person and those around him or her, and labelling is unimportant. Generally, MI will include feedback to the patient of the results of any investigations carried out, which are discussed in a nonjudgmental and empathic counselling style, getting the patient to draw their own conclusions where possible from the results. It is particularly helpful for patients who deny that they have a drug problem and are resistant to treatment. Although confrontational approaches have traditionally been used in this situation, they may actually increase resistance, rather than diminish it. Motivational interviewing techniques subtly encourage the patient to persuade the therapist that there is a drug problem and that change is necessary. This permits the introduction of various treatment options for discussion, with the therapist offering various strategies for change and helping the client to identify appropriate goals and ways of achieving them. In other words, the therapist is clandestinely directing the course of treatment, while at the same time letting the client believe that all the decisions have emerged naturally and are his or hers alone.[11,12]

Cognitive and behavioural techniques

A completely different approach to the management of drug abuse and dependence is the systematic application of cognitive and behavioural intervention techniques. These approaches focus on drug abuse as a disorder of behaviour, beliefs and core belief systems or cognitive schema, which therapy aims to modify. There is no attempt to identify the causes, which might or might not be amenable to treatment, nor to trace the history of the condition. Instead, current behaviour, emotions and beliefs, as they exist when the patient presents, are recognized as the pressing problem to be treated.

Drug abusers, however, often have other problems too, such as poverty, unemployment and homelessness, and it can be argued that it is pointless to try to deal with the drug abuse without first, or simultaneously, dealing with the associated problems – an approach that implies that these problems are the cause of the drug abuse. On the other hand, it can be argued that it is the drug abuse which has led to the other difficulties. If a cognitive or behavioural approach is adopted there is no reason to be concerned about cause and effect. The principle is to find out which behaviours and beliefs that might be changed are maintaining drug use, to decide what change is wanted and to devise a way of effecting this change. In more technical terms, before therapy can be initiated, a behavioural and/or cognitive analysis must be carried out so that current behaviours and ways of thinking are understood, goals are identified and the ways of achieving these goals are defined. According to the individual analysis, the resultant programme may be narrow, focusing only on the problem of drug abuse, or broad, encompassing a range of related problems and dealing with various aspects of the individual's behavioural repertoire and belief system.[13]

Behavioural therapies

The theoretical background to behaviour therapy comes from experimental work on theories of learning. There are many ways that learning takes place, and discovering the rules of these different learning theories has led to the development of various methods that can be clearly defined and that have specific goals which are measurable. These features make behaviour therapy open to testing to see if it works and what improvements can be made, which then in turn can be compared to discover which precise methods are the most effective. The first type of learning found to have implications for therapy was classical conditioning, first investigated by Pavlov. Operant conditioning and social-learning theories based on modelling are other examples. The term 'behavioural intervention' thus includes many different techniques, some of which are as old as the hills. Undoing learned associations by facing your fear ('climbing back onto the horse'), rewarding good behaviour, extinguishing bad, and making bitter medicine taste sweeter are all ploys that are used routinely, often automatically, in many therapeutic situations. What behavioural interventions have in common is a focus on changing behaviour in very specific ways. Their conscious and systematic application to all aspects of treatment, so that every therapeutic situation becomes a positive learning experience, is the basis of behavioural intervention.[14,15] Changing behaviour can lead to changes in thoughts and feelings and also to changes in relationships.

Cognitive therapy

Cognitive therapy is based on the recognition that thoughts and feelings are closely related. Our interpretation of ourselves, the future and those around us affect the way we feel and the way we behave. By focusing on our beliefs and patterns of thinking, cognitive therapists have found methods for helping people, including problem drug users, to change both feelings and behaviours. Cognitive therapy has developed from Beck's research and is an 'active, directive, time-limited treatment' that focuses on identifying a person's thoughts, beliefs, attitudes and assumptions that may be impeding positive behavioural change. Beliefs and assumptions that the person holds may be distorted (during childhood and learning experiences as an adult) and, as a result, the person may have negative beliefs which predispose, for example, towards low self-esteem, depression or anxiety, or the continued use of substances. Patients can learn, with the help of a therapist, to examine errors and distortions in thinking that lead to, or contribute to problematic behaviour. They learn to correct negatively biased attitudes and beliefs that are based on faulty assumptions and, as a result, learn to cope without drugs.[16]

Cognitive behavioural psychotherapy and relapse prevention

The principles of cognitive therapy can be applied in many interventions for substance abuse but are particularly helpful in relapse prevention where they are combined with behavioural therapies and referred to as cognitive behavioural therapy (CBT). CBT has two critical components, a functional analysis and skills training including cognitive techniques. Put simply, CBT helps patients recognize their risky situations, behaviours, emotions and beliefs, to avoid these situations when appropriate and to learn strategies for managing or coping with them when avoidance is not possible or desirable.

Relapse prevention

Relapse prevention programmes typically involve the identification of high-risk situations, when there is an increased likelihood of drug-taking behaviour. These may be caused by negative emotional states, interpersonal conflicts or direct/indirect social pressures, and the patient is encouraged to record their use of drugs, identifying the factors that may have triggered relapse. With the help of the therapist they can then analyse these situations and develop ways of dealing with them ('coping strategies') in future – perhaps by purposefully avoiding or preventing high-risk situations, or by using structured problem-solving techniques together with role-playing. Some approaches advocate graded exposure to environmental cues; others utilize rapid exposure (flooding), with or without the use of beta-blockers to alleviate the inevitable symptoms of anxiety that ensue. On those occasions when craving to take drugs develops, techniques such as 'urge-surfing' are advocated – allowing craving full rein, in the knowledge that it will, eventually, subside – or the 'Samurai' approach, in which the drug taker treats the urge to take drugs as an enemy that can be resisted by being prepared for the attack.[17,18]

An important element of relapse prevention may be the distinction between lapse and relapse, so that if resolution fails and drugs are taken, the individual does not feel that all is lost, but is able to regain control before relapse into full-blown problem drug-taking develops again. Interestingly, it has been found that opioid-dependent individuals who attributed to themselves greater responsibility for future relapse and who attributed relapse to personally controllable factors, were more likely to be completely abstinent, or to be able to prevent 'lapse' developing into relapse.[19]

Skills training

A relapse prevention programme may include several types of skills training, such as anger or sleep management, relaxation, problem solving or assertiveness training. Assertiveness training, for example, may contribute to the successful prevention of relapse by providing patients with skills for handling confrontations, dealing with unreasonable requests and asserting their own needs without dismissing or ignoring the needs of others. Skills training may provide alternative responses to the frustrations that so often precipitate renewed drug-taking. For example, patients may be helped to think through particular situations that they know are stressful and that have previously led to drug-taking, and then, with the therapist, discuss and role-play different ways of handling them, until they feel comfortable that they will have personal control of the situation. Similarly, assertiveness training may help patients develop refusal skills in situations where they feel pressured to accept drugs.

Contingency management

This is a procedure based on the principles of behaviour modification, or 'operant conditioning'. The starting point is the principle that the consequences of a behaviour will affect the frequency and strength of that behaviour. If the consequence is positive, then the behaviour will increase in frequency and/or strength if it is received and decrease if it is not (positive reinforcement and extinction respectively). If the consequence is negative, then the behaviour will decrease if the consequence is received, and increase if it is not (punishment and negative reinforcement respectively). There are numerous complications to these simple rules, such as the influence of the frequency of the consequence occurring. Thus, positive reinforcement which is received every time leads to rapid conditioning which is then quickly 'unlearned' once the reward stops; paradoxically, positive reinforcement which is received intermittently leads to behaviours which take longer to get rid of. Other complications include the effects of the delay between the behaviour and the consequence, and the association of other stimuli or 'cues' with the behaviour. Complex 'stimulus-response' chains are present in all but the simplest of behaviours, and with the majority of human behaviours any one response is likely to be under the control of many interacting stimuli and reinforcers.

Translated into helping someone with specific goals around drug use, it is possible to have specified rewards and privileges which are made contingent upon continuation or initiation of agreed behaviour. This can be thought of as the modern application of the well-known 'carrot and stick' approach, but with several important differences, the main one being that the desired (target) behaviour is defined and explained first, together with the contingent reward, before the procedure is initiated, rather than the individual learning by trial and error what is expected and what the price of failure or success is going to be. Another difference is that the procedures are based on scientific theory which allows for clear predictions to be made, again as opposed to trial and error.

In practice, contingency management utilizes positive reinforcers which are both ethically acceptable and under the control of the therapist. Punishment and negative reinforcement are never used as part of a therapeutic programme, nor is it ethical to use positive reinforcers to which the patient has a right of access. In consequence, the therapist is restricted but, nevertheless, may have a variety of reinforcers that can be utilized for contingency management.[20] For example, with an opiate-dependent individual who is attending a clinic regularly and frequently for a prescription for methadone (or other medication), reinforcers might include methadone take-home privileges (rather than having to take the methadone under supervision at the clinic), frequency of clinic attendance, time of appointment, enhanced access to counselling and other 'helping' services, and advantageous holiday arrangements, all of which can be made contingent upon certain behaviours.[21] In practice, similar systems may already exist but in an informal and unrecognized way which makes consistency of approach unlikely. Thus, if patients ask for special arrangements to be made for opiate prescription while they are on holiday, their request is more likely to be granted if they have been 'doing well', i.e. attending regularly with no evidence of illicit drug abuse, etc. Planned contingency management, however, means that drug abusers learn much more directly and therefore more easily and more quickly, exactly what is expected of them.

One way of introducing contingency management into the treatment of drug dependence is to utilize a written contract between the clinical staff and the patient. This defines the drugs (if any) to be prescribed, the dose reduction schedule, the duration of prescribing, the frequency of attendance at the clinic, other treatment approaches in which the patient will participate, the consequences of nonattendance and, in particular, the consequences of abusing illicit drugs, etc. Usually, if patients fail to keep their side of the contract and particularly if they continue to abuse illicit drugs, the prescribed dose of drug is quickly reduced.

Although contingency management is theoretically simple, there are certain practical problems peculiar to its application to the treatment of drug abuse. For example, it is often quite difficult to find out quickly whether patients have been abusing illicit drugs, because the results of urine tests may not be available for several days, or even a week or more. The inevitable delay before contingent measures can be implemented unfortunately impairs their efficacy.

However, the use of positive reinforcement, as well as having a therapeutic effect on individual patients, may also have a wider effect on the social and therapeutic atmosphere of the whole clinic by reducing confrontation between staff and patients. Relationships between staff and patients at such clinics are often difficult – patients are often manipulative and threatening in their attempts to obtain their drug of abuse or larger quantities of it, and the staff, frustrated and disheartened by recidivism, develop coercive attitudes towards patients. It is all too easy for the clinic appointment, far from being a therapeutic occasion, to become little more than a time for bargaining about a prescription.[22]

The deliberate adoption of contingency-management procedures helps patients to achieve defined and realistic goals for which they can be rewarded, rather than being punished all the time for failure to make progress towards undefined targets. Equally, positive and nonpunitive attitudes on the part of the staff are more likely to attract patients to treatment and to retain them in it. Many clinics already have rules which effectively act as contingencies to control behaviour, although if they are not applied systematically, maximum benefit is not achieved.

It should be apparent that where drug abusers are resident, either in hospital or in a therapeutic community, many potential reinforcers can be controlled and made contingent upon desired behaviour. For example, access to additional recreational facilities, extra visitors, etc. can all be made contingent on a target behaviour identified both by the patient and the therapy staff. A further refinement is to develop this into a voucher or points economy system, whereby points are given to patients contingent on desired behaviour, and taken away contingent on maladaptive behaviour. These points can then be exchanged on the ward for a variety of goods and services. All of the transaction 'rates' are clearly defined at the start and are recorded in personal booklets. An advantage of this system is that while some components are applicable to all residents, others can be personalized for the specific treatment needs of individual patients. It is important to understand, however, that among the most potent reinforcers available to staff are staff attention and time, which tend to be contingent on problematic or undesirable behaviour and thus may, unwittingly, increase these behaviours. An awareness of this and their use in a structured behavioural programme has obvious benefits for overcoming these problems.

It has been suggested that contingency-management procedures are little more than 'training' and that their efficacy lapses when contingent rewards and punishments are discontinued. This can be avoided firstly by manipulating the schedule of reinforcement (gradually reducing the frequency of reinforcement), and secondly by replacing the 'artificial' reinforcers of the ward with the 'natural' reinforcers which maintain behaviour in the outside world.[23] However, although it is true that undesirable patterns of behaviour, including drug abuse, may recur when treatment stops, this should be seen as yet another instance of relapse due to the severity of drug dependence and not necessarily as a failure of treatment. Undoubtedly, contingency management, carried out in a structured, systematic and comprehensive way, provides a firm and consistent structure for the drug abuser's life, and it may be the first time, or the first time for a long while, that he or she has experienced this. It provides the patient with an opportunity to learn the boundaries of acceptable behaviour, and even if relapse occurs the learning experience will not have been wasted.[24,25] One way to improve the long-term efficacy of contingency management is to involve the family, because it may have in its control many social and material reinforcers which can be made contingent on desired behaviour long after the patient has stopped attending hospitals and clinics.

Other behavioural approaches

Contingency management is a very direct approach to the treatment of drug abuse. Other types of behavioural intervention may be appropriate in certain cases. Many individuals resort to self-medication with psychoactive drugs when they feel tense and anxious, and the relief that they experience reinforces this behaviour and may contribute to relapse. Teaching patients to be aware of the situations that induce these feelings and to recognize their own emotional reactions is the first stage of teaching them how to respond in a healthier way. Training in techniques of relaxation may be of long-term value to these patients, reducing nervous tension, providing a natural way of dealing with stress, insomnia and life's challenges and inducing a feeling of general well-being. Some individuals with specific fears or phobias may be helped by desensitization, and others may benefit from training in problem solving, in assertiveness or in social skills.[26] The need for these very specific kinds of behavioural intervention becomes apparent in the course of the assessment procedure, which should establish if there are underlying or associated psychological problems that are amenable to intervention and treatment.

Aversive conditioning

Aversion therapy involves the association or 'pairing' of the drug use or related cues with unpleasant events so that, later, any exposure to the drug or its cues leads to unpleasant reactions which counter the effect of craving. This approach is now largely of historical interest only, with little evidence of effectiveness and with ethical drawbacks. Learning theory predicts that aversion therapy might work in the short term but this learning will be quickly reversed as soon as drug use is not followed by an aversive event. In addition, unlike with positive reinforcement, there are few 'natural' punishments to take over from the one used in aversion therapy, and so generalization outside the treatment setting is unlikely. And of course it is difficult to explain from learning theory alone why illness following intoxication does little to prevent doing it again. The use of disulfiram for alcoholics is perhaps conceptually the nearest to aversion therapy. If the patient has consumed disulfiram, any subsequent consumption of alcohol leads to vomiting and a subsequent reluctance to drink alcohol. However, it has not been possible to identify drugs that interact with other substances of abuse so that the opportunities for this type of aversive therapy are limited. Techniques for covert aversion therapy (or covert sensitization) have been tried as an alternative, in which the unpleasant effects are imagined rather than real and are associated with imagined drug use. This approach has the advantage that the drug abuser avoids the risk of drug consumption but there is little evidence for its effectiveness. In summary, aversion therapy has not been widely accepted and this appears to be due to issues related to public, patient and clinical acceptability.[27]

Cue exposure

It has long been recognized that, in addition to the primary reinforcing and dependence-producing properties of many drugs, environmental stimuli associated with drug-taking may contribute to the continuation of drug-taking behaviour. Exposure to these stimuli – or cues – which cannot always be avoided in everyday life, may lead to a variety of physiological (increased heart rate, decreased skin temperature, other signs of autonomic activation) and subjective responses long after a drug user has become abstinent, and usually cause craving for the drugs. However, carefully planned and executed programmes of exposure to these cues, either in reality or via video- or audiotapes, under conditions of close supervision or in a protected environment with no access to drugs, diminish both the physiological and subjective responses to them (classical or Pavlovian extinction). In theory, therefore, a drug abuser who experiences severe craving at the sight of drug-taking paraphernalia such as syringes and needles can be helped to overcome this by being shown them in situations where he or she cannot then take drugs. Although extinction of conditioned responses has been demonstrated in opiate addicts, it is not yet clear whether this approach has a long-term clinical effect and actually helps to prevent relapse.[28]

Vocational rehabilitation

Vocational rehabilitation is a treatment modality aimed at helping patients to acquire job-related skills. These may be specific skills, related to specific jobs and/or the interpersonal skills needed to obtain and retain employment. It should be noted in passing that there is actually no firm evidence to relate vocational rehabilitation and its ultimate goal of employment with treatment outcome, although there is a widely and strongly held belief in the therapeutic efficacy of work. This can, of course, become a self-fulfilling argument if being employed becomes a measure of treatment outcome. On behavioural grounds it can be argued that because drug abuse is just one component of an individual's total behavioural repertoire, intervening to encourage and develop desirable behaviour (i.e. obtaining a job), may lead to reduction of the undesirable behaviour (i.e. drug abuse) by direct competition – a sort of 'Satan finds work for idle hands' theory.[29] Obtaining a job does of course in addition provide a legal and stable income which can help the person get out of the cycle of social exclusion, crime and economic deprivation which, for some, make illicit drug use the only alternative.

Whatever the theory, it is undoubtedly true that unemployment rates may be very high among drug abusers and particularly among young drug abusers, and that they may be very receptive to help in this area of their lives. Delinquent adolescent behaviour and drug-taking may have interfered with their basic education. They may have extremely limited vocational skills and may be saddled with poor employment records. At times of high unemployment, particularly, it may be impossible for them to get a job without specific intervention and help.

The first step is an assessment of the patient's motivation, expectations and goals and of his or her existing skills and qualifications. A vocational plan can then be drawn up, with short- and long-term goals including, as appropriate, remedial education and specific academic and vocational skills. Knowing how to complete application forms is also important and, in particular, how to handle sensitive information about drug-taking and criminal history and how to emphasize positive aspects of previous employment. In addition, the acquisition of interview skills is vital; this may include learning relaxation techniques to reduce anxiety before the interview, good entrance and exit techniques, general behaviour during the interview with positive presentation of self, and how to cope with hostile interviewers. Role-playing and the use of video cameras may be useful preparation for these occasions. In particular, the problem of whether or not to tell the truth about drug-taking needs to be discussed. There is considerable prejudice against abusers and some employers may specifically try to find out about drug abuse through questioning and/or urine tests. Big companies with a high turnover of unskilled staff are most likely to be tolerant on this point.

The fear and anxiety of being rejected must also be dealt with, so that self-esteem, which may already be low, is not further impaired if the job application is unsuccessful. If successful, however, the ability to retain the job becomes very important and may rest equally on the particular ability to do the job competently and the possession of the interpersonal skills necessary for the workplace.

Vocational rehabilitation therefore encompasses a whole range of coping skills which contribute to the individual's ability to go out and get a job and keep it. Many of the problems of drug abusers are no different from those of other long-term unemployed, and referral to professional agencies may be valuable. However, schemes for vocational rehabilitation can also be incorporated into residential programmes for drug abusers and can be located in out-patient clinics. Enhanced access to vocational counselling, which may be eagerly sought, can be made contingent on desirable behaviour, such as desisting from the abuse of illicit drugs, and vocational goals may be included in the treatment contract between staff and patient.

Therapeutic communities

It has long been recognized that detoxification does not solve drug dependence, that the severity of drug dependence often leads to relapse and that it takes time for drug abusers to learn to live without drugs. For many people, the necessary change in their lifestyle is difficult or impossible if they remain in an environment where drugs are easily available, where they are among old friends who continue to take drugs and where a moment's craving can be translated too easily into drug abuse and relapse.

Therapeutic communities developed as one response to this situation. They generally insist on their residents being drug free, although often for only a short period (24 hours), before admission and some provide medical supervision of detoxification. Some have a democratic structure, others are unstructured, offering accommodation and time for those who want to explore the options that are open to them. Programmes last for varying lengths of time (3–15 months or even longer); they may offer group or individual psychotherapy which may be compulsory. Some will accept residents who are on bail and conditions of bail; and some offer vocational training.[30, 31] There are two main types of therapeutic community, religious communities and concept houses.

Religious communities

Offering support to those in need is fundamental to all religions and it is therefore not surprising that many set out to help substance abusers who are so often marginalized by society. The regimes that they adopt are obviously influenced by the underlying faith but Christian-based communities emphasize the importance of divine intervention in bringing about change, and Christian worship and Bible study form an important part of their therapeutic programmes.

Concept houses

Perhaps the best-known type of therapeutic community is the concept house. The first of these was Synanon, which was established in California in 1959. Others followed (Phoenix House, Daytop Village, Odyssey House), differing in the details of their organization, the degree of professional involvement and the therapeutic techniques used, but with obvious similarities to each other.

All are drug-free communities and are residential, so that their inmates are within the therapeutic environment for 24 hours every day. At first, residents are completely isolated from their former life and are not permitted to have visitors, letters or telephone calls. Daily life within the community is very structured, with residents spending most of their time in organized group activities and with little opportunity for doing anything alone. This forces interaction with other residents and permits constant scrutiny of their behaviour by their peers, and appropriate outspoken criticism.

Concept houses have a rigid social hierarchy with an autocratic leadership. Newcomers have very low status – they have few privileges and may be assigned menial household tasks. Those who remain abstinent, participate fully in community life and show personal growth in terms of honesty and self-awareness, move up the hierarchy, assuming greater responsibilities and enjoying increased privileges, so that senior residents become models for new residents. There is also a defined system of rewards and punishments, 'good' behaviour being rewarded with greater privileges, while breaking any of the community's rules is followed by punishments such as severe verbal reprimands, job demotion and loss of privileges.[32]

A variety of group therapies may be employed, but the most important is encounter-group therapy. This involves a small group of community members meeting three times a week or more. The composition of the group changes from session to session so that there is no opportunity for tacit or deliberate collusion between any members, and to emphasize the need for all residents to communicate with all other members of the community and not just with the few in a static group. The group leader may be formally appointed, may emerge from the group or may be the most senior resident there. At an encounter group there are aggressive verbal attacks upon individuals to confront them with their observed behaviour and attitudes within the community, and sometimes complaints about an individual are submitted before the group meets. Total honesty is expected, both in the verbal attacks and the responses, and shouting and swearing, far from being discouraged, are seen as manifestations of basic and honest 'gut reactions' that cut through the usual, more intellectual, defences. Uninhibited responses such as these are only permitted within the encounter-group meeting; at other times or places in the community such uncontrolled behaviour would be punished. An encounter-group meeting may last for several hours; its violent, emotional assault can be very exhausting and supportive measures are often necessary afterwards for those who have been the focus of confrontation. In recent years, however, concept houses have become less confrontational and more benign with greater emphasis on mutual respect and care for the individual – a change in attitude that has perhaps been brought about by the advent of HIV infection and the need to care for residents who may be facing an uncertain future.

Selection of patients suitable for a therapeutic community

Residence in a therapeutic community may be a useful option for chronic drug abusers whose previous attempts at abstinence have failed. It is suitable for young people in whom there is room and time for personality growth and development, and many therapeutic communities have an upper age limit of 35 years. Those who lack social skills, including those who have problems of socialization and problems of assertiveness, are particularly likely to benefit from community life. The rigid, structured system of the concept house is often helpful for the development of impulse control in young, risk-taking addicts, but it is unwise to expose anyone with a history of severe personality disorder or psychosis to the intense emotional experience of the encounter group.

Evaluation of the effectiveness of therapeutic communities shows that there is a consistent time-in-treatment effect so that those drug abusers who participate in the programme for more than 6 months subsequently do well. They are likely to remain substance free and have much less criminal activity for months or years after leaving the establishment. It is not surprising, however, that many who enter concept houses cannot endure the lifestyle and there is consequently a high drop-out rate with fewer than 40% of patients staying for more than 3 months. Some houses therefore have a more flexible induction programme to encourage more residents to stay longer. Some of those who 'graduate' successfully from therapeutic communities and remain drug abstinent subsequently find work in services for drug abusers, if they still find it difficult to separate completely from the world of drugs and drug dependence. However, it should be remembered that residents of therapeutic communities usually have a long history of drug abuse and dependence and a correspondingly poor prognosis. The success rate of the therapeutic communities, however small, is therefore especially creditable and valuable.

Although therapeutic communities are expensive facilities, research in the USA shows that they are cost effective in terms of the reduction in illicit drug use and in social and criminal justice costs while drug abusers are resident.[33,34] However, a major disadvantage of therapeutic communities is that they can only treat a small number of individuals at any one time. Given the scale of substance misuse problems nowadays, many would argue that it is better to invest in 'cheaper' community services that can help a much greater number of substance abusers.[35]

Hostels

The risk of relapse is high if newly abstinent drug-dependent individuals return to their old haunts and lifestyles, and hostel accommodation provides the opportunity for them to consolidate the success of withdrawal. Many of the pressures of daily life are reduced by staying in a hostel, and help and counselling is readily available if problems arise. However, there is little direct supervision, so that the residents regain responsibility for conducting their own lives in preparation for living independently. Thus, hostels often act as a halfway house or stepping stone between more supportive, residential treatment and ordinary life in the outside world. It is essential that rules about not bringing drugs or alcohol into the hostel are strictly enforced, so that those who are still vulnerable to relapse into drug abuse and dependence are not exposed to increased risk prematurely.

Self-help groups

The concept of self-help, in the sense of mutual help within a community, is a traditional and valued approach to many problems. With the changing structure of society, due to increased mobility and the loosening of family ties, this type of community support seems to occur less easily and more rarely, and more formal self-help groups (SHG) have emerged to fill the void.

Nowadays, an SHG is a group of individuals with similar problems who meet together voluntarily to help each other to help themselves. In the field of substance dependence, the best known SHG is Alcoholics Anonymous (AA), followed by Narcotics Anonymous (NA) (founded in 1953). Since then, a host of other groups have been formed in response to a variety of drug problems, such as tranquillizer dependence, opiate dependence, solvent abuse and cigarette smoking. They aim to help the drug-dependent or drug-abusing individual become abstinent.

These groups often begin due to the energy and enthusiasm of one or two individuals in a particular locality, and sometimes because of the absence (whether real or perceived), inadequacy or irrelevance of professional services for the particular problem. There is often an underlying philosophy that it is impossible for the individual to overcome the drug problem alone, but that this can be achieved with the help of the group. The common theme of all SHGs is of mutual aid – of individuals helping each other by offering friendship and sharing common experiences. They provide group support, social acceptance and social identity for individuals who may have become very isolated because of their drug problem. Furthermore, an established group possesses a wealth of experience and develops skills and expertise that may be of genuine practical help to those trying to cope with a drug problem.[36] Because those who have come off drugs usually continue to attend the group for a while, new members are able to meet and identify with abstinent individuals. This, in itself, may be a novel and very valuable experience for those who have been involved in a drug subculture for a long time and they may, for the first time, become aware that recovery is an attainable goal.

Because SHGs often develop where and because professional services fail to meet the needs of drug abusers, it is easy to understand why some have 'anti'-professional attitudes. Equally, some professional health care workers feel very threatened by these groups, which sometimes attract a lot of attention from the media. However, there need not be and should not be any conflict between the two 'systems'. Professional health care and SHGs should not compete but should complement each other, and professionals should recognize the value of SHGs in their area and reinforce their activities. They should encourage patients with drug-abuse problems to attend them and should not hesitate to refer patients to them. However, it is essential that professionals should not become directly involved in SHGs; if they do, the groups are no longer 'self-help', but just another professionally organized service, with a consequent loss of their unique kind of support and help.

In addition to SHGs for drug abusers, there is a complementary range of SHGs for their parents and families. These meet a need which is largely ignored elsewhere, and help families to cope with the strains of living with a drug abuser. Particularly in the early stages of a drug-taking career, parents may want to keep the knowledge of the drug problem within the family, and therefore find it difficult to seek help. They may be frightened by unpredictable mental states and unpredictable, sometimes aggressive, behaviour. They may be anxious about their own legal status if drugs are being taken in their home. Living with a drug abuser can thus be a very stressful experience and the support of others in the same predicament is usually a great relief. As the strength of the family unit as a whole is a very positive asset for the drug-abusing individual, any support given to the family may beneficially affect the outcome of the underlying drug-abuse problem.

Narcotics Anonymous and Alcoholics Anonymous

Narcotics Anonymous (NA) and Alcoholics Anonymous (AA) are international fellowships or societies for recovering addicts who meet regularly to help each other to stay off drugs or alcohol. They are open to anyone with any type of drug/alcohol problem, and the only requirement for membership is the desire to stop using drugs/alcohol. The approach is grounded in the concept of addiction as a spiritual and medical disease, a disease that according to this approach can be controlled but never cured.

NA and AA have a 'Twelve Step' programme for achieving abstinence (Appendix 6). The 12 steps taken by every NA member include:

1 Admitting that one is an addict and powerless over one's drug-taking;
2 Acknowledging that only a power greater than oneself (God) can help, and turning one's life over to Him;
3 Making a fearless moral inventory, recognizing defects of character and asking God to remove them;
4 Admitting previously committed wrongs and trying to make amends for them;
5 Carrying the spiritual message of NA to addicts and practising its principles in all aspects of daily life.

In addition, the 'Twelve Traditions' of NA/AA safeguard the freedom of the group by outlining the principles that guide its organization and administration: The groups are autonomous and self-supporting and decline outside contributions; they are nonprofessional and do not become involved in any issue or enterprise that may divert them from their primary purpose. Above all, the rule of anonymity

is considered paramount because it ensures that principles remain more important than individual personalities.[37]

Members of NA/AA attend meetings regularly. There is often a discussion based
on the Twelve Steps and great stress is placed on complete openness and honesty
with other members of the group, the single, shared common problem creating
strong bonds between individuals. The composition of the group changes, often
from meeting to meeting, and the constant flow of new members is valuable
because the necessary reiteration of the basic tenets on which they are based is
reinforced for more long-standing members. New members are encouraged to
look for a sponsor within the group, a particular person to turn to at times of great
need, and the responsibility of being a sponsor can be rewarding and helpful for
the person concerned.

An important component of the NA/AA programme for staying off drugs/
alcohol is the adoption of limited objectives. It recognizes that it is difficult (and
sometimes impossible) for a drug-dependent person to envisage the rest of life
without drugs, and so the addict is advised to promise him or herself not to use
drugs just for 1 day – something that many have done willingly or unwillingly in
the past and is therefore known to be possible. Having abstained for 1 day, the
addict renews this short achievable contract on a daily basis. If a day is too long,
the promise of an even shorter time span without drugs (say 5–10 minutes at a
time) can prevent the first resumption of drug use that signals relapse. This
strategy focuses the addict's attention on the immediate problem of not taking
drugs and undermines the practised excuses and rationalization for drug-taking
offered by experienced addicts. In addition, attainable and attained objectives are
immediately rewarding and therefore reinforce the desired behaviour.

The strong spiritual component of NA/AA may be off-putting to some potential
members, but the assertion that divine help is always available is necessary to
counterbalance the admission, in the first of the Twelve Steps, that one is powerless over one's addiction. Those who are willing to 'try' NA/AA should be advised
and encouraged to go to as many meetings as possible and even to attend the
meetings of more than one group. Time spent at NA/AA is time spent in a
substance-free environment, away from all the secondary reinforcers of a sub-
stance-using lifestyle, and is positively therapeutic in its own right.

Families Anonymous

Families Anonymous (FA) is an organization allied to NA and aims to help the
relatives of drug-dependent individuals. FA meetings, like NA meetings, are based
on openness and honesty and provide an opportunity for the families of drug
abusers to meet others in the same situation as themselves and to share experiences which may never previously have been divulged. These meetings offer social

acceptance and, for many families, a relief from social isolation and the accumulated experience of the members means that they are able to offer constructive advice and help in dealing with particular situations and problems.

Attending FA meetings can help to heal the emotional damage inflicted on the families of drug-abusing individuals and in some relationships this may be crucial to the success of attempts at drug abstinence. For example, some family members may become accustomed to a particular role which they may be reluctant to relinquish when the drug taker becomes abstinent, and they may unconsciously sabotage any hope of recovery. FA helps its members to be aware of the changes that occur within the family and to understand their own responses and, in this way, may make a very positive contribution, albeit indirectly, to the recovery of the drug-dependent individual. Members of the family of drug addicts may attend FA meetings even if the drug abuser is not attending NA.

Other types of self-help

Narcotics Anonymous and Alcoholics Anonymous emphasize the powerlessness of the individual to combat addiction alone, the lifelong nature of addiction and the fact that abstinent addicts never fully recover but are always 'recovering'. Other SHGs adopt a very different approach, with acknowledgement of personal responsibility for recovery and offering the potential of permanent recovery, usually in a secular environment.

Effectiveness

The effectiveness of Alcoholics Anonymous, the 'parent' of all subsequent 'Anonymous' groups has been evaluated and it was found that many people (35–65%) drop out in the first few months. However, of those who remain to become active members, 65–70% improve to some extent – drinking less than formerly or not at all.[38] Unfortunately, there has been no such systematic evaluation of other anonymous groups, or of alternative SHGs, and any such evaluation is likely to be very difficult because many individuals are involved in a variety of different treatment modalities at any one time and it is difficult to separate their individual effects.

Supportive groups

In addition to SHGs and groups that are conducted according to group analytical principles, there are a number of other groups, primarily supportive in nature, for drug abusers with particular needs. They differ from SHGs in being organized and run by a 'professional', but otherwise offer a similar caring and noncritical environment. For example, there is an increasing number of drug-dependent individuals who are parents, and they and their children have special needs which can be catered for – to a certain extent – in an informal group setting. This facilitates mutual support between the members by providing them with a time and a place to meet. They can chat about general child-care matters and other topics, exchange and share baby clothes and equipment, and the children can play with toys provided for the occasion. Clearly this resembles the ordinary 'parent and toddler' playgroup meetings which are attended by many new parents and which provide them with much needed support. Drug-abusing parents need this support too – and perhaps more than those who do not abuse drugs – but may be reluctant to attend an 'ordinary' playgroup because of anxiety about their drug problem. Thus a family group may fill a void in their lives and relieve their very serious problem of social isolation. This in turn may have a beneficial effect on other areas of their lives, including their drug-taking.

A supportive group may also be helpful to those who have just come off drugs and who are still at risk of resuming drug use. Those who are near the end of a detoxification programme (e.g. taking less than 10–15 mg methadone daily) may also attend this group, and the example of those who have successfully become abstinent acts as an example and encouragement for members of the group.

Groups such as these are frequently organized as part of the total programme of services of a specialist clinic. In addition, they are often organized by voluntary agencies as one component of a community, 'street-level' response to a local drug-abuse problem.

Minnesota method

The term 'Minnesota method' is very misleading, implying as it does a distinct method or way of treating substance dependence that is different from other methods. In practice, the Minnesota method integrates many of the treatment approaches described in this chapter into a programme that is tailored according to individual needs. It involves a multidisciplinary team that includes doctors, nurses, social workers, counsellors, psychologists, etc. who can provide a wide range of professional services.[39–41]

Treatment may be as an out-patient or as an in-patient, and begins with a thorough assessment and detoxification, if necessary. An individual treatment plan is then developed. In-patient treatment, when deemed appropriate, lasts for 4–6 weeks. There are regular individual counselling sessions and group therapy twice daily. There is an education programme for patients, with lectures, giving advice about ways of achieving recovery, and organized exercise and relaxation sessions which improve general mental and physical health, as well as providing opportunities for social interaction. Families are also involved in the treatment process by family therapy or family counselling.[39]

Perhaps the unique feature of the Minnesota method, if there is one, is the integration into the individual treatment programme of the NA philosophy. Patients participate in NA self-help groups while in the primary stage of treatment, and continue to do so when discharged to after-care. Because many patients find the idea of God and divine intervention in their recovery off-putting, the spiritual component of the philosophy is stressed rather than the religious component. The 'higher power' can be interpreted as the collective power of the whole group, so that it is to the care of the group, rather than to God, that the patient surrenders his or her will and life.

After a period of in-patient treatment, some patients may be discharged home, but continue to attend NA meetings. Others may require several months in a more structured environment, such as a hostel, where counselling and group therapy can continue, and where integration into the wider community can be achieved gradually, while involvement with the local NA group is developing.

Making attendance at NA a regular component of the treatment programme right from the beginning perhaps increases the likelihood of long-term involvement, which in turn may be a significant factor in the reported success of the Minnesota method.

Crisis intervention

Crisis-intervention centres are usually staffed by nurses and social workers with a doctor on call for medical emergencies. They offer temporary shelter and social support to drug abusers at times of crisis, when they may be more receptive to help and more motivated to tackle their drug problem. Although individual centres usually establish their own criteria for admission, they usually require that the individual is in a state of some immediate risk, such as being homeless. In the past, the severe barbiturate abusers, who repeatedly overdosed or attended A & E departments in a state of chronic intoxication, were particularly targeted by crisis-intervention centres because these patients were not fit to be discharged but created problems of management for ordinary hospital wards due to their disruptive behaviour.[42] Although this patient population has almost disappeared, the increase in numbers of cocaine abusers as well as opiate abusers has maintained the need for the centres.

Crisis intervention provides a humane response at a time of great need. It is unlikely to have much rehabilitative value unless the staff succeed in referring the drug abuser onwards to a longer-term programme. In so doing, crisis intervention proves its value as an acceptable entry point into treatment for many people who would otherwise not be helped.

Compulsory treatment

Treatment and rehabilitation in prisons

Because of the frequency of drug-related crime, prison populations contain a large proportion of substance misusers and it is generally acknowledged that this leads to particular problems in relation to preventing drugs entering prisons, misuse within the prison itself and the spread of infections related to self-injection (HIV, hepatitis C). It is therefore particularly important that prison officers who are in daily contact with prisoners, often for long periods, are knowledgeable about drug problems and approaches to treatment so that they can play their part in taking advantage of the unparalleled opportunities offered by a prison sentence for providing treatment to many who may not previously have been in contact with any treatment services. It is worth noting that there is no evidence that compulsory detention alone is beneficial in treating substance abuse.[43] In other words, merely separating a drug-dependent individual from his or her customary drug-taking environment is insufficient to bring about a sustained change in behaviour. Given the complex nature of drug dependence and its causes, this is perhaps not surprising, but it emphasizes the need for an energetic approach to treatment in the prison setting.

Coerced treatment

Apart from a custodial sentence there are many ways in which the criminal justice system can influence drug-taking behaviour and these may involve various degrees of coercion, typically by diverting someone convicted of a drug-related crime away from prison and into some form of treatment and making attendance for that treatment a condition of a noncustodial sentence. A number of such initiatives have recently been introduced in the UK with the aim of reducing levels of repeat offending amongst drug-misusing offenders. For example police forces are being encouraged to achieve comprehensive coverage of custody suites by face-to-face arrest referral schemes, which will offer help to substance misusers at the time of arrest, when they may be more receptive of such approaches. Drug Treatment and Testing Orders are also being tried as an alternative to custody for those found guilty of drug-related offences (see Chapter 2).[44] While these initiatives may be perceived as much more constructive approaches than merely confining someone in prison, there are important implications for civil rights. Specifically, it is essential that confidentiality is guaranteed and that effective and ethical treatment is provided when individuals may have had little choice but to cooperate.[35]

Finally, it should be noted that varying degrees of coercion may also be exercised by families, friends and employers and that, in this situation, the individual concerned may have little real commitment to the treatment process.

In-patient care

A patient may be admitted for in-patient care for a variety of reasons:

- For assessment of the state of dependence;
- For stabilization on opiates;
- For stabilization and subsequent detoxification of opiates, barbiturates, benzo-diazepines or other sedative hypnotics;
- For detoxification of alcohol-complicated drug dependency;
- For treatment of the secondary complications of drug abuse; for example, abscesses, hepatitis, septicaemia, HIV infection, AIDS;
- For the general sorting out of the chaos that severe dependence on drugs can cause;
- For assessment of mental state.

A multipurpose drug-dependence in-patient unit is therefore likely to have, at any one time, patients with a wide range of problems and who present a number of different and often difficult problems of management. It is fair to say that this is not an 'easy' group of patients. Although they come into hospital voluntarily (drug abuse and drug dependence do not constitute grounds for compulsory admission), they do not always comply with the prescribed treatment regime and may often go to extraordinary lengths to obtain extra drugs. This apparently wilful behaviour should be recognized as a manifestation of the severity of their dependence and, indeed, as a group they are usually the most severely dependent, many with a past history of failed attempts at detoxification. Some patients have another condition that makes their drug dependence more difficult to manage (e.g. pregnancy, psychosis, brain damage), and many have severe disorders of personality. However, the difficulties should not be exaggerated. Many patients are well-motivated, comply with the treatment regime and successfully complete the detoxification schedule for which they were admitted.

Ideally, the in-patient unit provides a structured and therapeutic environment in which specific and general treatment interventions can be implemented. A variety of activities should be organized on a regular basis to form a well-balanced timetable of events in which the patients are expected to participate. These include various group sessions, some of which may be conducted on group analytical lines, or use motivational interviewing techniques. They may focus on relapse prevention and anxiety and anger management, while others deal with the practical problems and difficulties associated with drug dependency, and aim to improve social and life skills. The latter are primarily supportive, rather like SHGs, and may tackle issues such as the problems people have in relating to others, their attitudes, behaviour and responsibilities. Specialist speakers may be invited to talk about topics of special concern, such as AIDS, rehabilitation units, etc. There may also be a range of activities aimed at improving the patient's general health with sessions or classes in physiotherapy, relaxation, yoga, keep fit, etc. Recreational activities may be organized including different sports, games and arts and crafts.[40]

It is hoped that patients in hospital, in this therapeutic environment, will start to develop a way of life and a daily routine that is not centred on drugs and drug-taking, and which they find more fulfilling. It would be naive, however, to pretend that it is easy to bring about these changes in lifestyle and underlying attitudes.

The first essential is, obviously, that the ward should be drug free – except for medically prescribed drugs. Although patients are admitted voluntarily, their motivation may fluctuate or they may not be motivated for treatment but have sought admission for other reasons, such as avoiding or reducing the severity of a court sentence. To ensure a drug-free environment, an in-patient unit for drug abusers is necessarily often a locked ward; patients are only allowed to leave for therapeutic or recreational activities, if escorted, and visitors are restricted to a few named and trustworthy individuals for each patient. If drugs are still smuggled in, it may be necessary for all gifts to patients to be inspected by the nursing staff, and for gifts of food to be restricted to unopened cans and packets. These measures seem, and indeed are, draconian. They have to be enforced because if just one person succeeds in introducing illicit drugs to the unit, the temptation to share them may prove too great for other patients whose treatment regime is therefore sabotaged. Before admission, patients may be asked to sign a 'contract' indicating that they understand the rules of the ward and agree to comply with them.

Failure to keep to the rules usually means that the patient will be discharged, but this apparently straightforward consequence may be difficult to implement in every case. Sometimes there is no definite evidence that illicit drugs have been consumed – merely a strong suspicion on the part of the nursing staff. Confirmation of drug-taking by a positive urine test may take so long that the result is irrelevant and discharge merely punitive if in the interim period the patient has not taken illicit drugs and has participated fully in the treatment programme. In addition, there may be overriding medical reasons for not immediately discharging an in-patient who has been abusing illicit drugs if, for example, the patient is pregnant, or severely ill, or in the middle of a sedative detoxification regime and at risk of suffering convulsions.

Aggressive behaviour is another problem that requires careful and sensitive management. It is not, of course, confined to DDTUs, but is perhaps more likely to occur there than on some other wards because of the high incidence of 'personality disorder' among drug-dependent in-patients, and sometimes because of intoxication with drugs. Undoubtedly, many patients find it difficult to tolerate the environment of a closed ward, particularly if they cannot resort to drug-taking, as they would undoubtedly like to. They may express their frustration by verbal and/or physical aggression. It is to be hoped that the professional skills and expertise of the staff minimize the risk of this, but patients should understand, before they are admitted, that violent or aggressive behaviour will not be tolerated. If it arises, the patients concerned may incur loss of privileges and visiting rights, or may be discharged immediately. On some occasions, however, even if there are good reasons to discharge a violent patient, there may be overwhelming medical reasons for not doing so.

The difficulties faced in the management of illicit drug-taking and of aggressive behaviour highlight the problems of caring for drug-dependent patients. They undoubtedly require firm and consistent handling, and this is essential if they are to learn that manipulative behaviour is not useful. At the same time, the desire on the part of professionals to be firm and consistent should not lead to a stereotyped response for every deviation, or a punitive attitude towards the very behaviour for which the patient is seeking help.

Treatment matching

It is apparent from the summary above of the many different interventions available to substance misusers that there is a wide range of approaches, suggesting that there is no one 'method' that is 'best' and the need to draw up a treatment plan specific to the needs of the individual patient is emphasized. Developing from this is the treatment matching hypothesis which acknowledges that substance dependence does not have one single cause but many, and recognizes that the outcome of treatment is affected by the patient's individual characteristics as much as by the nature of the treatment itself. This explains why very different treatments, based on different philosophies, can have very similar outcome results and also why a particular treatment is effective for one type of patient but not for another, who may respond to a very different approach. According to the treat-ment-matching hypothesis, overall outcome results would be enhanced if patients were treated in a way that responded to their unique problems. While this may seem self-evident, it is difficult to evaluate and therefore prove because it is not clear which patient characteristics should be used for the matching process. For example, severity of dependence, associated psychiatric problems and personality type might all be relevant. Work with alcohol-dependent individuals is encourag-ing and analysis of pharmacotherapy–psychotherapy treatment interventions showed that lower levels of verbal learning were associated with poorer drinking outcomes for relapse prevention which requires more complex cognitive abilities; and also that patients with high levels of craving did best with naltrexone, which reduces craving.[45]

Specific methods of treatment

Opiates

By the time that they seek help for their drug problem, most of those who abuse opiates have an established dependency and are seeking some sort of pharmacotherapy. They may want to come off drugs but fear the abstinence syndrome too much to attempt it alone, or they may be hoping for a long-term prescription for opiates because they are finding it increasingly difficult to maintain their drug habit from illicit sources.

Before any decision is made about detoxification using opiates or long-term maintenance treatment, it is essential to be sure that the patient is indeed genuinely physically dependent on opiates. This diagnosis is based on information acquired during the assessment period (Chapter 5); it relies on the history of drug-taking, with attention being given to whether the financial means of the patient adequately account for the drug use claimed, and the patient's familiarity with the drug scene. A careful physical examination, looking particularly for signs of opiate withdrawal (Chapter 3) and of self-injection, and the results of several urine tests are also very important. If the out-patient assessment of physical dependence is equivocal, the Ghodse Opiate Addiction Test (Chapter 5) can be tried and/or the patient admitted to hospital for more careful observation.

Detoxification – opiate withdrawal

Detoxification is the process of coming off drugs, of ridding the body of the drugs by withdrawing them, usually by giving gradually decreasing doses. The final goal is drug abstinence and there are many ways of achieving it. Detoxification can be carried out in general practice, in a community setting or at hospital, whether as an in-patient or as an out-patient; it can take days, weeks or months; it usually involves the prescription of opiate drugs, but this is not essential, and other drugs and other treatment modalities may be helpful too.

The choice of detoxification programme depends on what has been found during the assessment period: the severity of physical dependence, the nature of drug-related problems and previous experience of detoxification are some of the factors to be taken into account. The aim is to match the patient to the most appropriate course of detoxification. For example, a long-standing addict may need a few months on a stable dose of methadone to permit a general sorting out of all drug-related problems before a very gradual reduction of dosage is made. At the opposite end of the spectrum, those with only minimal physical dependence may be able to tolerate detoxification without opiates, but using other drugs to alleviate the symptoms of withdrawal.

If a patient has been referred to a specialist treatment unit, the course of detoxification is decided after discussion by the multidisciplinary team. Whenever possible, they take into account and incorporate the patient's wishes and preferences for a particular way of coming off drugs, but because of the very nature of drug dependence, this is not always possible. It is because they are so severely dependent that for some patients the time may never be quite right to attempt detoxification; there seems always to be a reason (an excuse) for delay in starting to come off. In essence, they become trapped by denial and rationalization and, left to themselves, would continue to take opiates probably indefinitely, with a promise to initiate withdrawal always a few weeks away.

It requires patience and skill to cut through these defences, to bring the patient to an acceptance of the realities of the situation and to initiate detoxification. Anyone involved in the treatment of drug-dependent patients needs to be aware of these difficulties and must guard against being manipulated into providing indefinite opiate maintenance by default. Opiate maintenance may, on occasion, be necessary, but it should result from a positive decision that is right for a particular patient; it should not be allowed to develop from a situation of ever-postponed detoxification.

This situation illustrates the difficulty of treating drug-dependent patients. Their stated reason for seeking help, that they want to come off drugs, may be at variance with their behaviour, which is drug seeking; they seek help voluntarily but then reject the advice they are given, so that arguing and bargaining about treatment, almost unheard of in other branches of medicine, occur frequently in the DDTUs. Such behaviour should be interpreted as a manifestation of the severity of dependence and should be responded to appropriately.

Of course, the patient's treatment aims are not always at variance with those of professional advisers. Some are highly motivated to come off drugs, indeed some (although in practice a minority) may wish to do so far more rapidly than is considered wise or likely to be successful by the professionals. In this situation, where the patient actually wants less opiate than might be prescribed, the choice of detoxification can safely be left to the patient. Any attempt to come off drugs should be welcomed and encouraged, and the belief on the part of the patient that a particular treatment is right, may be crucial to motivation to succeed – if only to prove the professionals wrong. Even if the attempt fails, the patient can always try again and may then be more receptive to advice and counselling.

The opiate abstinence syndrome, which develops if opiates are not prescribed during detoxification, varies in severity according to which opiate has been taken, for how long and in what dose. It may vary from a mild, 'flu'-like illness to a condition in which the patient is very distressed and feels truly wretched. Undoubtedly, fear of the abstinence syndrome and consequent anxiety about it can make all the symptoms far worse. In addition, just as different people have different pain thresholds and experience pain differently, so opiate-dependent individuals vary in the way that they experience the abstinence syndrome, even with similar levels of physical dependence. Whatever the differences, fear of abstinence syndrome may be worse than the condition itself and may be a barrier preventing patients from attempting detoxification. All patients should be reassured that their drug withdrawal will be correctly managed to prevent or minimize the symptoms and discomfort of the abstinence syndrome. A confident approach on the part of all involved professionals is essential to allay anxiety and to reassure those who may have heard lurid tales of 'cold turkey'.

Because the symptoms of opiate withdrawal can be (and usually are) prevented by a schedule of gradual dose reduction, there is a tendency for health care professionals to be dismissive about detoxification: 'Coming off is easy; staying off is the problem' is bandied about. It is true that opiate withdrawal is a straightforward medical procedure and causes no life-threatening medical emergency, but for the person involved it is a difficult step to take and one which requires courage. This should be recognized and respected.

It should also be appreciated that detoxification may need to be repeated: some patients resume illicit opiate abuse while undergoing detoxification and others do so later. Such relapses are not inevitable, and should not be anticipated by a negative approach; nevertheless they do occur and repeated attempts at detoxification are often necessary. Rather than treating relapse as a failure, any worthwhile period of abstinence should be welcomed as a success and the patient's achievement recognized. A positive approach encourages cooperative rather than confrontational attitudes between patients and staff, and in this atmosphere more patients will be prepared to try again.

Finally, it is worth emphasizing that opiate detoxification does not necessarily require referral to a specialist unit and indeed may be managed with no medical supervision at all. The opiate-dependent individual may choose to reduce his or her daily dose gradually, on his or her own. The patient may even choose to stop taking opiates abruptly, thereby causing the dreaded 'cold turkey'. There is no doubt that many addicts do come off drugs on their own and that many may do so repeatedly, sometimes when forcibly detained by concerned parents. On humane grounds, no one would recommend this course of action, but there is no medical contraindication (except pregnancy) if the individual concerned is otherwise well. Certainly, this approach is reasonable for young users with a fairly short (6 months to 1 year) history of daily use, who take only small amounts of heroin. They can be cared for at home during the withdrawal period, as if they are suffering from 'flu', with simple analgesics such as paracetamol being given to relieve muscular aches and pains. The major drawback of 'going it alone' is the consequent lack of professional help, guidance and counselling and of the specialized treatments that can help to reduce the risk of relapse.

If general practitioners are asked to help in such cases, they may prescribe antispasmodics (dicyclomine hydrochloride, hyoscine) to relieve colicky abdominal pains, diphenoxylate or loperamide for diarrhoea, or neuroleptic drugs such as phenothiazines. If they find that they have insufficient time available to offer an appropriate level of counselling, a collaborative approach with a local drug advisory service or community drugs team may prove helpful.[1] The type of case that may be managed in a primary care setting, without referral to a specialist agency, includes young drug-dependent individuals, particularly those with only a short history of dependence, and who will have good support from non-using family and friends during the difficult early days of withdrawal. For these patients, there are substantial advantages to being managed in the community, with fewer opportunities for becoming enmeshed in the subculture of established users who attend the specialist agencies. (Conversely, some patients are not suitable for detoxification in a primary care or community care setting. These include older users with a long history of substance misuse, who often obtain their drugs from multiple illicit sources and who have unsettled or even chaotic lifestyles.)

Detoxification using nonopiate drugs

Detoxification using nonopiate drugs can be started before full assessment of all the patient's problems has been completed and without the need to establish a firm diagnosis of physical dependence. Assessment of related problems can then continue during the detoxification procedure. Being able to start treatment quickly may be very helpful in engaging the patient in treatment because many lose interest and motivation during a long period of assessment.

Indications

1 Some patients may request assistance with opiate detoxification but do not want to take opiate drugs any more.
2 These regimes may be useful if there is any lingering doubt about whether the patient is really physically dependent on opiates or not. It must be remembered that taking opiates regularly during stabilization and detoxification may be

sufficient to cause dependence in a casual, previously nondependent opiate abuser, and that nonopiate 'detoxification' is a safer alternative for these patients.

3 In many countries, doctors are not permitted to prescribe opiates in the treatment of drug dependence, not even temporarily for the purpose of detoxification. In this situation, nonopiate drugs are the only way to provide some symptomatic relief during opiate abstinence, although they rarely, if ever, successfully relieve the subjective distress of withdrawal or craving.

Choice of nonopiate treatment programme: general principles

There are a variety of treatment approaches, none of which is noticeably better than any other. Opiate abstinence is not a life-threatening condition and the choice of treatment can be made according to what 'suits' individual patients, their particular circumstances and symptomatology. As detoxification often has to be repeated, some patients find that certain symptoms are very distressing and that a particular treatment regime may be helpful.

Whenever possible, the drugs chosen to alleviate the symptoms of opiate withdrawal should have little or no dependence liability of their own. There is no point in treating one kind of dependence by creating another and the individuals concerned have a proven vulnerability to the dependence-producing properties of psychoactive drugs.

Patients should be warned not to abuse any other drugs while undergoing detoxification because of the risk of drug interaction. They should be told specifically not to increase the dose of the prescribed drug on their own initiative. As a group who are very used to increasing the dose of drugs to gain increased effect, they are likely to do so with the drugs prescribed for detoxification if they seem to be controlling the symptoms of opiate withdrawal inadequately. Patients should be told that in this situation they should return for further assessment and help.

Despite these warnings, patients may present in an intoxicated state during their detoxification programme. The response to this situation depends on the circumstances and, in particular, on why the patient resumed drug abuse. If drugs were taken because the symptoms of opiate withdrawal were intolerable, it may be appropriate to increase the dose of prescribed drugs, to prescribe an additional drug, or to introduce a different type of treatment. If this does not prevent further episodes of intoxication, or if drug abuse is occurring for other reasons, such as an inability to stay away from the black market, it may be wiser to taper off the dose of prescribed drugs more quickly than planned. This will reduce the risk of drug interaction and of further episodes of intoxication and may discourage the patient from abusing illicit drugs in future.

Nonopiate treatment regimes

Neuroleptic drugs

Neuroleptic drugs such as the phenothiazines are particularly suitable for the management of the opiate abstinence syndrome because they have antiemetic, sedative and anticholinergic effects; the latter help to reduce abdominal cramps which may be a very distressing symptom of opiate withdrawal. Phenothiazines should be avoided if the patient has hepatitis and used cautiously if liver function tests are abnormal in any way.

A suitable dose regime would be chlorpromazine 25 mg, three times daily or perphenazine 2–4 mg twice daily or haloperidol 2–4 mg twice daily. This may be taken for 1–2 weeks and the dose should be tapered at the end of this time. The patient should be specifically warned not to increase the dose of neuroleptics to obtain greater symptomatic relief because of the risk of extrapyramidal side effects.

Diphenoxylate, loperamide

Diphenoxylate and loperamide are very mild opioid drugs with low dependence liability, used for symptomatic relief during the opiate abstinence syndrome, and particularly if severe diarrhoea is a prominent symptom. Diphenoxylate is available in combination with atropine, in the mass proportions of 100 parts to 1 part respectively, as co-phenotrope (diphenoxylate hydrochloride 2.5 mg; atropine sulphate 25 μg). Two tablets should be taken four times daily for 3–4 days, and then the dose should be gradually reduced. The dose of loperamide is 2 mg four times daily. Both of these drugs can be used if necessary as an adjunct to other nonopiate treatment regimes, such as chlorpromazine or clonidine.

Beta-adrenoreceptor blocking drugs

The use of beta-adrenoreceptor blocking drugs in the treatment of opiate withdrawal was originally based on an observation that propranolol abolished the euphoric effect of heroin in dependent individuals and that it reduced craving after heroin withdrawal. Propranolol may be helpful for patients with a high level of somatic anxiety, manifested by raised pulse rate, high blood pressure, etc. The effect of propranolol should be monitored and the dose adjusted according to the patient's response. A daily dose in the range of 80–160 mg, in divided doses, is usually effective and may be prescribed for a 2–3-week period. Oxprenolol may also be used. Beta-blockers should be avoided if the patient suffers from asthma.

Clonidine

Clonidine is an α_2-adrenergic agonist drug that acts on the locus coeruleus, suppressing the withdrawal overactivity of noradrenergic neurones and therefore reducing the release of noradrenalin. Thus it effectively suppresses some of the autonomic signs of opiate withdrawal[2] but is less effective at suppressing the subjective discomfort of withdrawal.[3] Unfortunately, the partial symptomatic relief provided by clonidine carries undesirable side effects of sedation and hypotension, and detoxification using clonidine is best carried out in hospital where blood pressure (standing and lying) can be monitored regularly. Because of these side effects, clonidine treatment is unsuitable for patients with cardiac or renal problems, who should not be exposed to the risk of hypotension, nor should it be used for pregnant women (see Chapter 9).

In hospital, treatment with clonidine should start with 200–400 µg daily, in divided doses, increasing gradually to a maximum of 1.2 mg daily, in divided doses (three times per day). Many patients cannot tolerate such a high dose because of postural hypotension, and if the blood pressure is less than 90/60, administration of clonidine should be postponed until the blood pressure has risen to this level. Treatment should continue for 5–6 days for heroin users and for 7–10 days for methadone users. Because of the theoretical risk of rebound hypertension on sudden cessation of clonidine treatment, it should be withdrawn gradually.

Clonidine may be used on an out-patient basis if arrangements are made to monitor blood pressure every day, for carefully selected patients who can be relied on to take the drug strictly in accordance with medical directions.[2] In such cases, the maximum dose should not exceed 400 µg taken in divided doses (100 µg taken four times daily).

A new innovation is the introduction in the USA of clonidine patches, applied on a weekly basis and which permit transdermal absorption of the drug.

Lofexidine

A structural analogue of clonidine, lofexidine can also be used for the alleviation of symptoms in patients undergoing opiate withdrawal. It appears to act centrally in the same way as clonidine, reducing sympathetic tone. Although it may be less sedating and less hypotensive than clonidine,[4,5] it may also be less effective at suppressing the signs of withdrawal. The contraindications are the same as for clonidine but it is more suitable for community-based or outpatient treatment,[1] providing there are facilities for monitoring blood pressure and pulse during the course of treatment. Patients should be warned about the risks of concurrent use of alcohol and sedative drugs, the effects of which may be potentiated, leading to drowsiness and dizziness which may affect driving and the operation of hazardous machinery.

Treatment should be initiated with doses of 200 µg twice daily, increasing as necessary (for symptom control) in steps of 200–400 µg daily to a maximum of

2.4 mg daily. Treatment should continue for 7–10 days and then the dose should be gradually reduced over a period of 2–4 days.

Accelerated detoxification

Traditionally, the severity of the opiate abstinence syndrome has been minimized by withdrawing opiates gradually over a period of several weeks. This has the disadvantage that a proportion of patients fail to complete the programme and drop out of treatment. In response to the perceived need for shorter courses of treatment, accelerated detoxification has been introduced as an alternative approach which attempts to compress the abstinence syndrome into as short a time as possible on the principle that a short period of very severe symptoms may be less distressing or easier to cope with than a more prolonged period of milder symptoms.

One way of obtaining sudden intense withdrawal is to give an opiate antagonist drug, such as naloxone, which displaces opiates from the receptors by competitive antagonism. Intramuscular or intravenous naloxone is given repeatedly, at frequent intervals, for a few days, until further injections have no effect and the patient is then considered detoxified. The abstinence syndrome induced in this way can be treated with a variety of drugs including neuroleptics, propranolol and atropine. A number of different regimes have been tried but all require hospital admission because of the severity of the withdrawal symptoms.

Treatment regimes were then developed using opiate antagonists and clonidine.[6,7] An example of such a regime is:

day 1: clonidine 100 µg three times a day;

day 2: clonidine 200–300 µg three times a day (according to effect and blood pressure); naloxone 0.2 mg intramuscular, then 0.4 mg intramuscular 2 hourly for four doses;

day 3: clonidine – same dose as day 2; naloxone 0.8 mg intramuscular; five doses at 2-hourly intervals;

day 4: if necessary, the completeness of detoxification can be demonstrated by a naloxone challenge: naloxone 0.4 mg intramuscular should produce no effect; naloxone 0.8 mg intramuscular 1 hour later should not cause any withdrawal response either.

Alternatively, naltrexone, an opiate antagonist with a longer duration of action than naloxone, can be used in conjunction with clonidine. Following a naloxone challenge test (0.8 mg naloxone intramuscular), clonidine 100–300 µg is administered orally to relieve withdrawal symptoms. Naltrexone 12.5 mg is given later on the first day, followed by 25 mg on the second day, 50 mg on the third day and

100 mg on the fourth day. Clonidine 100–300 μg is given three times a day for the first 2 days, with a total dose of 300–900 μg per day which is reduced to 300–600 μg on day 3 and to 300 μg or less on day 4, all in divided doses. The dose of clonidine should be adjusted according to the intensity of withdrawal symptoms and any evidence of hypotension, and all patients must be carefully monitored for this side effect.

Ultra-rapid detoxification

A variation on the above is the use of naltrexone to precipitate withdrawal while the patient is anaesthetized or under very heavy sedation. Antidiarrhoea drugs (e.g. octreatide), antiemetics (e.g. odantreson), clonidine and benzodiazepines are also included in a very powerful cocktail.[8] It is easy to understand why an apparently 'quick-fix' solution to their problems is appealing to those who have struggled with dependence for many years. However, there is real concern about the safety and efficacy of this approach[9] and unexpected fatalities have occurred.

Sedative drugs

If opiates cannot be prescribed for the purpose of detoxification, severe symptoms due to the opiate abstinence syndrome can be treated by the administration of a sedative drug (e.g. diazepam, clomethiazole). It should be appreciated that this course of action is not the treatment of choice: sedative drugs do not relieve the distress of opiate withdrawal nor the craving for opiates, although they do reduce associated anxiety. A further drawback to their use is that they have a dependence-producing liability of their own which makes them unsuitable for administration to individuals who are vulnerable to drug dependence. However, in some countries, doctors are not permitted to prescribe opiates to dependent individuals, and in this situation sedatives may be helpful for those with a moderate or severe degree of physical dependence on opiates. A short course is all that is required and suitable dose schedules are shown in Tables 7.1 and 7.2.

Acupuncture

The use of acupuncture in the treatment of drug dependence is a comparatively recent innovation. It followed the incidental observation in 1973 by doctors in Hong Kong that electroacupuncture being employed for analgesia satisfactorily relieved the symptoms of heroin withdrawal.[10] At first the acupuncture needles were inserted in the ear, in two points near the wrist and in the hand, but the technique was modified, with no reduction in effectiveness, so that now only the 'lung' points of the ear are used. The needles are electrically stimulated for 40 minutes with a gradually increasing current (bipolar spike wave form, AC current, pulse width 0.6 ms, frequency up to 111 Hz or cycles per second). Comfortable

Table 7.1. Use of diazepam in opiate detoxification

Day	Dose (mg) administered orally	Frequency of administration	Total dose (mg)
1–3	10	Four times daily	40
4	10	Three times daily	30
5	10	Twice daily	20
6	5	Twice daily	10
7	5	Once daily	5
8	—	—	—

Table 7.2. Use of clomethiazole in opiate detoxification

Day	Dose capsules administered orally	Frequency of administration	Total capsules
1–3	2	Four times daily	8
4	2	Three times daily	6
5	2	Twice daily	4
6	1	Twice daily	2
7	1	Once daily	1
8	—	—	—

Note: Each capsule (192 mg clomethiazole base) =5 ml elixir (250 mg/ 5 ml clomethiazole edisylate). See page 155 for precautionary measures for clomethiazole.

detoxification can be achieved with acupuncture alone if treatment can be given more or less continuously for the first 3–4 days after drug withdrawal.[11]

According to traditional theories, acupuncture helps the process of detoxification by releasing blockages of energy flow (*chi*) induced by the suppressive actions of opiates.[10] The discovery of the endogenous opiate-transmitter system gave acupuncture some scientific respectability. For example, the reversal of acupuncture-induced analgesia by naloxone implies that endogenous opiates and opiate receptors are involved in acupuncture-induced analgesia.[12] It was also found that a strain of mice, deficient in opiate receptors, had a poor analgesic response to acupuncture. In addition, heroin-dependent individuals treated with acupuncture were found to have raised concentrations of an endogenous opiate met-enkephalin in the cerebrospinal fluid.[10]

Acupuncture appears to have no harmful effects and thus there is no reason to deny it to those patients who believe that it is the key to their successful detoxification. However, in the absence of carefully designed and controlled trials, its

usefulness remains unproven, so that it is a treatment only for those who specifically request it and who have great faith in it.

Neuroelectric treatment (NET)
Experimentation with different methods of electroacupuncture revealed that the
acupuncture needles were unnecessary and that electrical stimulation could be
transmitted adequately transcutaneously using blunt electrodes. This eliminates
any pain associated with skin puncture and the risk of infection by contaminated
needles. In addition, because the treatment can be self-administered, it can be used
much more frequently and even while the patient is asleep, so that withdrawal
symptoms can be effectively prevented.[13]

The electrodes are hoop-shaped and have a conducting area of diameter
2.5 mm. They are attached to a headset, worn either on top of the head or round
the neck, and are held on to the concha of the ear by tension. Electrode jelly
improves the skin contact. A neurostimulator has been developed which can
deliver a variety of wave forms and parameters of current. Opiate-dependent
individuals are said to respond best to square wave electrical stimulation with
pulse width 0.25 ms and within the frequency range 75–300 Hz, but the choice of
frequency depends on the drug of abuse: 2000 Hz is used for those dependent on
cocaine and amphetamine, and 30–49 Hz for those dependent on sedative hypnotics. The current is gradually increased, usually by the patient, until it can be felt
in the ears (approximately 1–2 mA). Side-effects (nausea, headache) are reported
only rarely and can be reversed by reducing the current or by having more
frequent short periods of treatment; polarity may also be important and the
negative electrode should be attached to the left ear. The patient may be treated
continuously for the first 3–5 days after drug withdrawal and then receives 2–5
hours treatment per day for the next 10–21 days.

Like acupuncture, the effectiveness of NET is unproven scientifically; nevertheless, it seems to help some patients when used in conjunction with other treatment
methods, and it may obviate the need for additional psychoactive drugs.

Alternative medicine
In common with other chronic conditions for which there is no obvious and
universally accepted 'cure', drug dependence has been (and still is) treated by a
wide variety of methods, some of which seem bizarre to those trained in scientific
medicine. These unconventional approaches, including herbalism, vitamin and
mineral supplements, bathing, breathing and exercise, are usually harmless, although megadoses of vitamins are not. They often have a holistic emphasis on
good health and a healthy lifestyle, both mental and physical, which can be very
therapeutic. As these treatment methods are unproven, doctors can hardly recom-

mend them to patients but, in the absence of a conventional 'cure' for drug dependence, the doctor need not attempt to dissuade a patient from pursuing an alternative approach. If a particular patient really wants to do this, the doctor should admit his or her own ignorance and advise the patient to consult a recognized practitioner in the chosen field. The patient's faith or belief in a particular approach may be just sufficient to spark and maintain the elusive quality of motivation, and achieving detoxification is more important than the route by which it is attained. Therefore, there should be no conflict or antagonism about the patient's choice of treatment, so that there is no barrier to the patient's returning to more conventional treatment if and when he or she wants and needs to.

Detoxification using opiates

If a diagnosis is made of physical dependence on opiates, and if the decision is taken to prescribe opiates, at least in the short term, in reducing dosage for detoxification, the first step is to stabilize the patient on a pharmaceutical preparation of an opiate.

Choice of opiate for stabilization and detoxification

On pharmacological grounds, the choice of opiate for stabilization and detoxification is theoretically unimportant. Because of cross-tolerance, any opiate will prevent or relieve the abstinence syndrome caused by the withdrawal of any other opiate. Whichever drug is chosen, the aim is to maintain the blood opiate level between the dependence level and the tolerance level (see Fig. 7.1). If the blood opiate level falls below the dependence level, the symptoms of the opiate abstinence syndrome develop. If the tolerance level is exceeded, the patient will experience euphoria. Between these two levels is a 'therapeutic' range for blood opiate level, in which the dependent individual feels well, appears normal and is generally considered 'straight'. The therapeutic range is not fixed, but varies according to the individual severity of dependence. It is different in different people and at different times in a drug-taking career, and this explains why the stabilization dose varies from patient to patient and must be assessed on an individual basis.

Methadone is an ideal drug for opiate stabilization. It has a long duration of action (24–36 hours) so that a single daily dose maintains blood opiate levels within the desired range.[14] The patient experiences neither euphoria nor the abstinence syndrome, but is maintained in a 'normal' physiological state. It can be taken orally so that the complications of injection are avoided, and when dispensed for oral consumption it is in the form of a syrupy liquid which, even if diverted to the black market, is not suitable for injection.

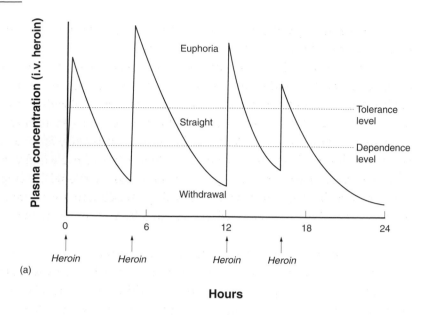

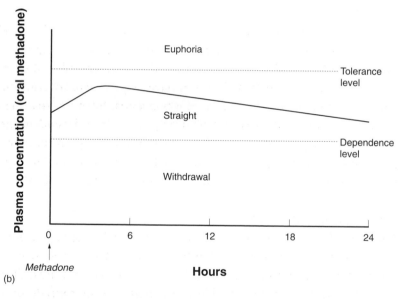

Fig. 7.1   Schematic diagram of (a) heroin and (b) methadone use.

These factors have led to its widespread acceptance as the drug of choice when opiates are to be prescribed to opiate-dependent individuals. Interestingly, when heroin syrup was compared with methadone syrup for stabilizing in-patient opiate addicts, the drugs were found to be equally effective on subjective and objective scores of withdrawal. Moreover, the addicts had a no better than random chance of identifying which opiate they had been given.[15] In the UK, methadone is prescribed as methadone mixture BNF (1 mg/ml).

Although much of the ensuing discussion focuses on the use of methadone for opiate detoxification and maintenance treatment, some doctors are unwilling to use it, often because of the strict legal requirements associated with its prescription (see Chapter 12). *Codeine* and *dihydrocodeine*, which are also opiates, offer an alternative that may be particularly suitable for the less severely dependent, with a fairly short history (less than 2 years) of daily use, but whose withdrawal symptoms are inadequately relieved by nonopiate drugs. It should be emphasized, however, that both of these drugs are widely abused and treatment regimens utilizing them should be managed just as carefully as those using methadone or heroin.

A total daily dose of 240–360 mg dihydrocodeine is adequate for most opiate-dependent individuals for whom this approach is suitable. This is equivalent to 8–12 tablets (each 30 mg) of dihydrocodeine, which should be taken in divided doses. Withdrawal is achieved by reducing the total dose by one tablet at agreed time intervals.

Some cough mixtures and other preparations that contain codeine in low concentration can be bought over the counter without prescription. Some non-medical agencies advise clients who do not wish to consult a doctor to achieve withdrawal using these medicines and have helped them to draw up their own detoxification schedule. In such cases it is essential to ensure that these drugs do not become just another source of supply for a drug-dependent individual. A further disadvantage of using these preparations, which are usually compound preparations containing other drugs, is that patients may develop dependence on the other constituents, making final withdrawal even more difficult.

Dose of opiate for stabilization

The dose to be prescribed is that which will adequately suppress the manifestations (signs and symptoms) of opiate withdrawal over a 24-hour period, but which does not produce intoxication (Appendix 7, 8). As most patients abuse illicit heroin of uncertain purity it is not possible to establish the appropriate dose from the history alone. Even for patients who abuse pharmaceutical opiates, it is unwise to prescribe the equivalent dose of methadone suggested by the history alone because of the uncertain reliability of this information. Thus, although a 'conversion' table is provided, giving the methadone 'equivalent' of other opiates (Table 7.3), it is much safer to establish the necessary daily dose of methadone on an individual basis by a formal stabilization procedure. Although the underlying principle is the same, the practical details of stabilization vary according to whether it is carried out on an out-patient, in-patient or day-patient basis.

Table 7.3. Opiate equivalents for withdrawal. Relative potencies for withdrawal protocols, equivalent of 1 mg methadone

Drug	Dose	Methadone equivalent
Codeine	15 mg	1 mg
Dextromoramide	0.5–1 mg	1 mg
Dextropropoxyphene	15–20 mg	1 mg
Dihydrocodeine	10 mg	1 mg
Dipipanone (Diconal)	2 mg	1 mg
Pharmaceutical heroin	1–2 mg	1 mg
Hydromorphone	0.5 mg	1 mg
Methadone linctus	1 mg/2.5 ml	1 mg
Methadone mixture	1 mg/ml	1 mg
Morphine	3 mg	1 mg
Pethidine	15 mg	1 mg
Buprenorphine[a]	40 µg	1 mg
Pentazocine[a]	10 mg	1 mg
Gee's linctus	10 mg (1.6 mg of morphine)	1 mg
J Collis Brown	10 ml (1 mg extract of opium)	1 mg

[a]Mixed agonist/antagonist.

This table can be used to convert the dose of other opioids into milligrams of methadone but, due to the different half-life of other drugs and their mode of administration, the conversion can only be a guide. Whichever drug of substitution is used, the dose should be titrated against the withdrawal symptoms and signs.

Out-patient stabilization

Out-patient stabilization is effected by daily appointments, with an incrementally increasing dose of opiate given under supervision and followed by a period of observation to ensure that intoxication does not occur (Appendix 9).

On the first day the patient is given 10–20 mg methadone, according to clinical judgement of the severity of physical dependence. This dose must be drunk in front of the doctor or nurse. It is very unwise to give more than 20 mg methadone as an initial dose, in case the patient has exaggerated the severity of his or her dependence and cannot really tolerate a high dose. The patient is then observed for 1 hour for any evidence of intoxication (especially drowsiness or pin-point pupils) but, if well, is permitted to leave.

When the patient returns, 24 hours later, he or she is assessed for any evidence of physical withdrawal such as feeling unwell, insomnia or muscle cramps, and objective signs such as pupil dilatation, yawning, sniffing, restlessness, gooseflesh, etc. If any of these symptoms or signs are present, even if only mildly, the daily dose of methadone should be increased by 10 mg, which is again consumed under supervision and the patient observed for the necessary 1 hour. This procedure is repeated daily until the patient no longer exhibits any evidence of the opiate abstinence syndrome. The dose prescribed on the previous day is then the baseline dosage which should be repeated daily thereafter.

The prescribing doctor should appreciate that there is no need to be excessively 'frugal' (or mean) about the dose of methadone. If the procedure described above is carried out, there is no risk that the patient will become intoxicated and the precise dose on which the patient is finally stabilized is unimportant as far as future management is concerned. Indeed, if the dose of methadone is not increased, because symptoms are felt to be 'too mild', it increases the likelihood of the patient seeking illicit opiates, thereby sabotaging the stabilization process and increasing the risk of intoxication.

The patient should be warned that the stabilization process will be adversely affected if he or she abuses illicit opiates during this period and that this leads to difficulty in assessing the correct dose. If opiates are taken illicitly, the following procedure should be adopted.

1 If there is evidence of the opiate abstinence syndrome at the time of attendance, the usual increment of 10 mg methadone can be made.

2 If there is no evidence of the opiate abstinence syndrome, the previous day's dose should be repeated. The patient can be told that if this is insufficient, leading to the emergence of withdrawal symptoms, he or she should attend again (on the same day) to receive a 10 mg dose of methadone, rather than seeking relief from an illicit source.

Patients therefore learn that the dose to be prescribed cannot be manipulated merely by their claiming that they had been forced to resort to illicit drugs. The daily dose of methadone will be increased only if there is clinical evidence at the time of attendance of the opiate abstinence syndrome.

In-patient stabilization

In-patient stabilization can be achieved more rapidly because the patient is under constant observation and supervision. After admission to hospital the patient is given no opiate until clinical observation reveals the symptoms and signs of the withdrawal syndrome. Methadone 10–20 mg is then administered and the patient is observed for evidence of intoxication. Methadone 10 mg is given as necessary through the day whenever evidence of the opiate abstinence syndrome recurs. The total dose of methadone required in the 24 hours from the onset of signs is thus calculated, and is the baseline dose which can be continued on a daily basis, usually divided between two doses per day.

One advantage of in-patient stabilization is its rapidity: patients quickly reach the baseline daily dose which ensures physical comfort. They are spared the early days of out-patient stabilization when the prescribed dose is small and when they may find it hard not to resort to illicit drugs. The indications for in-patient stabilization are:

1 If patients request it – usually because they feel that they would be unable to comply with the out-patient procedure.
2 If previous attempts at out-patient stabilization have been unsatisfactory due to noncompliance.
3 If out-patient assessment has been equivocal and the diagnosis of dependence is still uncertain.

Day-patient stabilization

Out-patient stabilization can be achieved more rapidly if it is possible for the patient to attend a day-care facility, hospital, clinic or doctor's surgery on a day-patient basis. In this situation, methadone can be administered as necessary, throughout the day, as long as the final dose is given no later than 1–2 hours before the patient leaves for home.

Alteration of stabilized dose

Once the baseline daily dose has been reached, either as an out-patient or as an in-patient, it cannot be increased merely at the patient's request. Occasionally, however, within a short period of stabilization, it may be necessary for an adjustment to be made, either increasing the dose if the patient is seen to be manifesting continuing signs of opiate withdrawal, or decreasing the dose if there is evidence of intoxication after the accumulation of several doses of methadone.

Dose reduction regimes

Detoxification using decreasing doses of opiates can be carried out as slowly or as quickly as desired. A general principle is that at higher dose levels, the daily dose reduction can be greater, because it represents a smaller percentage of the total, and that as the daily dose falls, reduction should be more gradual. For example, if the stabilization dose is more than 40 mg daily, the dose can be reduced by 5 mg daily until 40 mg/day has been reached; thereafter the dose should be reduced by 5 mg every other day. Alternatively, a patient who has been stabilized on methadone 60 mg daily could be detoxified in 30 days by reducing the dose by 2 mg each day. Detoxification in hospital can proceed more rapidly than on an out-patient basis.

Drug withdrawal can be carried out on a 'masked' or open basis. With the latter, the patient is aware of the dosage reduction schedule, but if withdrawal is 'masked', the reductions are made without the patient's knowledge; this may help patients whose anxiety about drug withdrawal makes the procedure more difficult than it need be. 'Masked' dose reduction regimes should only be conducted with the patient's consent. Sometimes patients prefer to prepare their own detoxification schedule, which should be discussed with staff and, if necessary, amended before the start.

Fixed-term opiate-treatment contract

A much slower and therefore more prolonged reduction of opiates may be appropriate for some patients. In this situation, opiates are prescribed for a predetermined period, usually of 6 months, but sometimes for 1 year. At the same time, the patient and the staff work towards attaining and maintaining a constructive and healthy lifestyle. A complete treatment plan is worked out describing the opiate dose regime, the treatment aims and the activities and treatment approaches in which the patient is expected to participate. This is formally presented to the patient as a contract, which is signed by the patient and the key health care professional, and which is filed in the case notes where it can be referred to if necessary. The contract is conceptually a contingency-management contract (see Chapter 6) and includes rewards for progress and sanctions for relapse and other undesirable behaviour. It provides a framework for the individual patient to take an active part in treatment, reduces dissent between patient and staff and ensures continuity of treatment even if staff change.

Because the expressed goal is to work towards abstention within a definite if prolonged time period, it is against the philosophy and purpose of the contract for it to be used as a form of indefinite opiate maintenance. The contract should not be renewed immediately or continuously if the patient relapses, although he or she may still be offered treatment. Similarly, extension of the contract should be occasional rather than customary, and should only occur after full review of the situation by the whole multidisciplinary team (if the patient is attending a specialist treatment clinic).[16]

It should be apparent that a contract such as this, in which opiates are prescribed for several months, is unsuitable for those whose dependence status is doubtful or who have only a mild degree of physical dependence. It should be reserved for those patients who have not been able to achieve long-term abstinence after several attempts at detoxification, both as an in-patient and as an out-patient. For many of these individuals, whatever the original cause(s) of their drug dependence, it seems to have become the core of their other problems, and they have a better chance of breaking into this cycle if they have a guaranteed supply of their drug. Freed from the need to seek and buy opiates illicitly, they can attempt to resolve coexistent problems, and the consequent reduction of stress may make it easier for them to give up taking opiates.

Opiate maintenance

An alternative to detoxification is maintenance treatment, which means the legal supply to the dependent individual of a daily dose of opiate sufficient to prevent the onset of the abstinence syndrome. Having achieved stabilization, the patient is subsequently maintained on the baseline daily dose of opiate for a prolonged period, and perhaps indefinitely.[17,18] This should never be offered as a first line of treatment, except perhaps for an elderly patient or for an individual with AIDS, but it could be considered for patients who have relapsed several times during or after detoxification. Thus it is suitable for those who can lead a more or less normal life when they take opiates in a stable and nonescalating dose, but who cannot do so if opiates are withdrawn.

To spare the patient the temptation of having large quantities of drug available for personal consumption or to sell, methadone should be made available in quantities sufficient only for 1 day at a time. If the patient cannot attend the clinic every day to receive and consume the drug under supervision, arrangements can be made with a local pharmacist for the prescription to be dispensed on a daily basis, with a double ration on weekends.

Supervised consumption, either at the clinic or at the local pharmacy, should be continued after dose stabilization and this can be reviewed in light of factors such as patient stability and compliance with treatment. Allowing the patient to collect methadone less frequently than daily should be the subject of careful consideration, taking into account the risks of accidental overdose and of diversion of methadone to the illicit market. Less frequent collection may be considered where the patient is stable and compliant and may be used as a 'reward' in the therapeutic contract.

The special arrangements and requirements associated with prescribing controlled drugs to addicts are described in Chapter 12.

Maintenance or withdrawal?

Undoubtedly, if the treatment regime is observed, methadone maintenance will keep the patient in a physiologically normal condition, able to work and earn a living. It removes the need to obtain drugs illicitly, it 'saves' the patient from the black market, it eliminates the need for injection, with all its potentially hazardous consequences.[19]

However, a serious cause for concern is that long-term opiate maintenance is not really treatment in any meaningful sense of the word. It offers no chance or hope of cure, but is only a way of maintaining the dependent state. It encourages drug-dependent individuals towards a passive acceptance of their condition, and for the thousands of young drug abusers of today it is a severe penalty for youthful errors.

A subtle implication of such a policy, if it becomes routine, is that it is so clearly the 'end of the road' that some opiate-dependent individuals may be unwilling to present for a treatment which is the final confirmation of the hopelessness of their condition and of the impossibility of change. Instead of coming forward for help at an early stage of their drug-taking career, they continue with illicit drug abuse and the advantages of early intervention are lost.

It is often suggested that drug withdrawal will only be successful if the patient 'wants' to come off drugs, and until that time arises, he or she should be provided with a maintenance prescription. Undoubtedly, motivation for abstinence is very important and may be crucial to the long-term success of detoxification. For some patients, motivation is triggered by the legal, social or medical consequences of their drug abuse and dependence; many patients, for example, have given up drug-taking because of fear of AIDS. For others, any latent motivation that they may have to become abstinent is counteracted by the profound psychological dependence induced by opiates, by their intense craving and need for drugs, which becomes more severe the longer they take opiates (illicit or prescribed). Thus, lack of motivation can be seen as a symptom and as an indication of the severity of dependence, and waiting for motivation to 'happen' may be a comfortable collusion with the patient that nothing can or should be done to interrupt their drug-dependent condition.

Of course, patients cannot be forced to accept detoxification, but if, when they seek help, this does not include the option of maintenance for which perhaps they had hoped, they may be persuaded by the positive attitudes of health care professionals towards attempting detoxification. If opiate maintenance is routinely available as a treatment option, it is understandable and to be expected that many will opt for it rather than face the anxieties of being without their drug, and the chance of achieving abstinence is lost – at least for a while.

In summary, therefore, long-term methadone maintenance should be regarded very much as the last resort in the management of opiate dependence, particularly for the young addicts of today. Withdrawal should be attempted and repeated, if only to establish that it cannot be tolerated or that the addict's life without drugs becomes increasingly chaotic. There are a few patients – and it is only a small proportion – who will do better if they receive a regular prescription for opiates; they will have a more stable lifestyle and will cease the use of illicit drugs. The decision about maintenance or withdrawal and short-term or long-term treatment needs to be made on an individual patient basis, taking into account the chronicity and severity of dependence as well as personal and social circumstances. There can be no absolutely rigid rules.

Oral or intravenous? Heroin or methadone?

The theoretical basis of opiate maintenance is simple – so simple that the practical problems of implementing it as a treatment modality may be overlooked by those who are unfamiliar with drug-dependent individuals and their lifestyle. Problems arise because a patient on maintenance treatment cannot be isolated from a world with a drugs black market, where opiates and injectable drugs command a high premium. This situation means that when opiates are prescribed to a patient either for stabilization or maintenance, every effort must be made to ensure that the legally prescribed, pharmaceutically pure drugs do not become diverted to the black market. The aim, therefore, is to prescribe the opiate with the least black market value and potential, and to prescribe the 'right' (minimum) dose, so that the patient has to take it all, personally, to prevent the onset of withdrawal symptoms and has no surplus to produce euphoria or to sell. Methadone mixture which has ideal pharmacokinetic properties for opiate maintenance fulfils these criteria too.

However, many patients want more than to be kept in a state of physiological normality by oral methadone. They crave the 'rush' or 'high' that follows injection and, rejecting methadone maintenance, turn to the black market for the heroin they prefer. Others accept the methadone and obtain illicit heroin as well. Many abuse a variety of other psychoactive drugs, according to availability and personal whim.

Self-injection may be an important component of this drug-taking behaviour. It may have started because the effect of injected drugs was preferred, but there are often sound economic reasons too: the cost of a drug habit increases in step with the increase in tolerance, and administration by injection delivers the whole dose directly into the bloodstream, for maximum effect without any waste. By association with the rewarding properties of the drug, injection acquires secondary reinforcing properties of its own and many addicts are reluctant to relinquish it. For some individuals (the true 'needle-freaks'), the act of injection is as important as any drug that they inject.

Of course, every effort should be made to persuade and encourage these patients to accept maintenance opiates in oral form. Some do settle down with an oral drug, provided a regular supply is guaranteed, but others remain unwilling to give up injection, often suspicious about the effectiveness of oral drugs.

Such behaviour can be interpreted as a manifestation of the severity of their dependence, and in this situation rigid adherence to a policy of only prescribing oral methadone effectively excludes the most severely dependent patients from treatment. It may therefore prove necessary to prescribe injectable drugs, trying after a few weeks or months to gradually change over to an oral substitute. For the transition period, patients may receive part of their opiate in injectable form and part in oral form.

The justification for prescribing injectable opiates is that for a certain small group of patients it may be the only way to engage them in treatment at all, and that without this 'lure' they will remain out of reach of all the interventions (counselling, psychotherapy, behaviour therapy, social work intervention, etc.) that make up the totality of treatment for drug dependence.

If injectable opiates are prescribed, methadone is still the drug of choice because once daily administration maintains the patient free from withdrawal symptoms, whereas heroin requires more frequent administration. In practice, the advantage of methadone over heroin is less clear-cut, because many who receive the former prefer to divide the dose and have several smaller injections so that they can experience the 'high' after injection more often. Injectable heroin is prescribed to some patients if it is felt that this is the only way that they can be engaged in treatment.

The prescription of injectable drugs to severely dependent individuals may also be a way of reducing the harm that these patients do to themselves. The black market heroin that they otherwise use is of variable and unknown purity, and the syringes and needles used to inject it are often scarce and are frequently shared. The user is at risk from infection, from overdose and from the effect of injected adulterants. In contrast, pharmaceutically pure opiates, injected in a known and appropriate dose using a sterile syringe, are much safer. Those receiving injectable drugs should be educated in the correct procedure for sterile injection and advised about the least harmful route for injection (subcutaneous or intramuscular in preference to intravenous), and the safest sites (arm, rather than jugular vein). Once again, however, the advantage of prescribed over illicit drugs is often more theoretical than real. For severely dependent patients, involvement in the black market becomes an integral part of their drug-taking life and lifestyle. It is not surprising, therefore, that buying and selling of illicit drugs does not always cease when, or because, the individual concerned is given a maintenance prescription for opiates; the clinic is just one source among several for obtaining drugs. In some cases therefore, opiate maintenance, even if injectable drugs are prescribed, fails to bring the promised order and stability to the lifestyle of the opiate-dependent individual. In this situation, it may be felt that prescribing injectable opiates is serving no useful purpose at all and a change is made to oral opiates; the knowledge that they may lose their guaranteed supply of pure opiate may encourage some patients to desist from black market activity and to participate fully in the treatment process.[20]

It should be noted that there is little research evidence supporting the effectiveness of prescribing injectable preparations to opiate-dependent individuals, nor has the long-term safety of this practice been fully evaluated. In the UK, uniquely, physicians' judgement on this issue is trusted whereas, in other countries, their practice is severely restricted in this area.[21]

High-dose methadone maintenance

A very different approach to opiate maintenance has been adopted at some centres in the USA, where the policy is not to give the minimum dose of methadone, but a high dose achieved by stepwise increments.[14,19]

The rationale is that at low doses of prescribed methadone the patient requires only a small quantity of 'extra', usually illicit, opiate to reach and exceed the blood opiate level at which euphoria is experienced. As the maintenance dose of methadone increases, the proportionate increase in the tolerance level is much greater and it takes proportionately more supplemental opiate to exceed it. With a maintenance dose of 80–90 mg it becomes pharmacologically impossible (it is said) for the patient to experience euphoria. However much illicit opiate is consumed, the patient does not get a 'high'. When taking these large doses the patient should not experience any craving for opiates, and even if illicit opiates are tried, their euphoric effects are blocked. Because they are no longer rewarding, opiate-seeking behaviour should cease because of extinction of a previously conditioned response.

A disadvantage of high-dose methadone maintenance is that unless methadone consumption is supervised every day at the clinic, there is a risk that part of the large doses prescribed may be sold on the black market and other drugs bought instead. In common with all maintenance programmes, it prolongs the state of dependence in individuals who might otherwise become abstinent. Finally, increasing the daily dose of methadone to this level worsens the severity of physical dependence on opiates, even if certain aspects of daily life, such as attending school, getting a job, desisting from crime, improve.

Levacetylmethadol (USA: laevo-alpha-acetylmethadol, LAAM)

A major concern about opiate maintenance treatment is that prescribed drugs may be diverted to the black market. One approach to this problem, adopted first in the USA, is that the patient attends the clinic daily and consumes methadone under supervision. This is inconvenient for the patient and time consuming for clinic staff, who have less time for counselling, etc. The use of levacetylmethadol (LAAM) is a way of reducing these problems because the patient only needs to attend the clinic three times a week.

LAAM is a synthetic opiate which suppresses the opiate abstinence syndrome for 48–72 hours. Its extended pharmacological action is due to its biotransformation to an active metabolite, noracetylmethadol. When administered orally three times weekly, LAAM provides safe and effective maintenance, with no evidence of the opiate abstinence syndrome despite the long gaps between treatment. Because patients attend for treatment less frequently, their lives can become less medication and clinic orientated. It is felt that they thus become less psychologically dependent on medication and identify more easily with a drug-free lifestyle.[22] However, although the risk of abuse is minimized by the gradual onset of effects after oral administration, LAAM does have potential for abuse.[23] Furthermore, there is some evidence that LAAM is less effective than methadone in relation to retention in treatment and discontinuation of treatment because of side effects.[24]

Because of its long duration of action, induction of treatment with LAAM and dose stabilization should be carried out slowly, starting with a dose of 20 mg, three times weekly and increasing by 10 mg every other dose, until the maintenance dose is achieved. Although the slower pace of stabilization may be difficult for a few patients, once it is achieved the smooth therapeutic action of LAAM eliminates the daily 'highs' and 'lows' that occasionally occur with methadone, so that patients feel healthier, more alert and 'normal' on LAAM. Some patients may require a slightly higher dose than usual at the weekend, so that they have no withdrawal symptoms during the 72 hours before the next clinic attendance. American studies have shown that the efficacy of LAAM is dose related, with higher doses blocking withdrawal symptoms more effectively and increasing abstinence from other opioids.[25]

Patients should be warned of the delayed onset of action of LAAM so that they do not take additional opiates (or other central nervous system sedatives) and precipitate a serious overdose. If this occurs, high doses of naloxone are required and may need to be repeated for up to 72 hours.

LAAM has recently (2000) been licensed for use in the UK for the treatment of adult opioid addicts who have previously been treated with methadone. It is not intended for take-home use and should only be administered under the supervision of a physician with experience in addiction treatment. It should be noted that there have been reports of severe cardiac side effects in some patients.

Buprenorphine

Buprenorphine has recently been licensed in the UK for the treatment of opioid addiction. Dosage is usually in the range of 8–12 mg daily. Because of its partial antagonist properties, the first dose of buprenorphine should be administered several hours after the last dose of heroin, in case it precipitates the withdrawal syndrome. Once-daily dosing is sufficient and, because it is readily dissolved and can thus be misused by injection, supervised consumption should be considered particularly because, in some parts of the UK, buprenorphine has been the most widely misused opiate. At present, there is only limited experience in the UK of the use of buprenorphine for opioid detoxification or maintenance, but it may be suitable for some patients, particularly where methadone prescription has been repeatedly ineffective. Efficacy in maintenance treatment, in terms of retention in treatment, reducing craving and reduction of use of illicit drugs, appears to be dose related.[26] Buprenorphine is regularly used for opioid maintenance in France and a new preparation has been formulated combining a high dose of buprenorphine with naloxone.[27] Theoretically, this should limit its potential for intravenous abuse because injected naloxone antagonizes the effect of buprenorphine.

Opiate antagonists

Once opiate detoxification has been achieved, the individual remains at risk of relapse for some time and may, if exposed to a situation previously associated with drug-taking, experience severe craving and even the symptoms of opiate withdrawal. He or she may then succumb to this need and take opiates, and in a similar situation is even more likely to take them again; he or she is then well on the way to relapse.

It has been argued that if opiates had no effect and specifically did not relieve the symptoms of abstinence, their use would not then be repeated; the individual would 'learn' that opiates were not useful. In more technical terms, opiates would have been robbed of their reinforcing effect and, eventually, opiate-seeking behaviour should cease as a result of extinction of a previously conditioned response.

The clinical use of opiate antagonists rests on these suppositions. They are drugs that block or counteract the effects of opiates so that if an 'ex-addict' – an opiate-dependent individual who has become abstinent – is maintained on an antagonist and then takes an opiate drug, he or she experiences none of its effects.

Naloxone is a pure opiate antagonist, but is unsuitable for relapse prevention because it has low oral efficacy and its short duration of action necessitates frequent administration. Naltrexone is more suitable; it can be taken orally and because it blocks the effects of opiates for up to 72 hours, it requires administration only three times a week. If naltrexone is given to an individual who is still physically dependent on opiates, it precipitates withdrawal symptoms which are protracted because of the long duration of action of naltrexone. It should not therefore be administered until 7 days after the last dose of heroin or 10 days after the last dose of methadone. It should be preceded by a naloxone challenge test: naloxone 0.4 mg is injected intramuscularly and the patient is observed for 1 hour for evidence of the opiate abstinence syndrome; if there are no symptoms, the injection is repeated once and observation continues. If withdrawal symptoms appear, they will be short-lived (2 hours) because of the short duration of action of naloxone, and can be relieved, if necessary, by opiate administration. If there is no evidence of the opiate abstinence syndrome after naloxone, it is safe to initiate treatment with naltrexone. The initial dose is 25 mg, and if there are no symptoms of withdrawal, a regime of 50 mg per day can be initiated the following day. However, because of the drug's long duration of action, administration three times a week is common, with 100 mg on Monday and Wednesday and 150 mg on Friday.

Although the use of opiate antagonists is theoretically simple, it requires a high degree of motivation on the part of the patient to take naltrexone regularly, because it has no reinforcing effect of its own and because it robs opiates of their pleasurable effects. It should be administered under supervision either by a close family member or at the clinic to ensure that it is taken. Those who do best on naltrexone form a fairly small group, usually with a history of stable relationships and employment. It may, for example, be particularly suitable for 'professional' (e.g. doctor) addicts. It is also useful in the management of female patients who have just given birth to a child whom they fear may be taken from them if they resume drug abuse and who are therefore highly motivated to remain abstinent. However, it should not be prescribed for those who are pregnant or breast-feeding.

To improve patient cooperation, external reinforcers such as payments have been tried and longer-acting antagonists, such as depot preparations of naloxone which extend opiate blocking for up to 60 days, are also being tested. These would have the practical advantage that once the injection had been given, patient noncompliance could not occur.

For individuals such as these, naltrexone provides not a cure but some protection against becoming dependent again, and this protective effect can be enhanced by concurrent psychotherapy, family therapy, behaviour therapy, etc. Indeed, naltrexone should only be considered an adjunct to other forms of support and treatment for patients who have recently come off opiates, rather than a treatment in its own right. There is a clear relationship between time spent on naltrexone and opiate-free status but, of course, naltrexone cannot provide permanent protection. Nevertheless, after cessation of treatment, it can be resumed if the patient relapses (but before dependence develops), or feels vulnerable to relapse, and may prevent occasional illicit use progressing quickly into regular and compulsive use.

Because there is concern that naltrexone, even in therapeutic dosage, may be hepatotoxic in some patients, it is only given to patients with normal liver function, and this should be monitored regularly throughout treatment. The long-term regular use of antagonists (i.e. for years) is not recommended because of potential adverse effects.

Patients should be warned that the blockade effect of naltrexone is competitive, and that although it is possible to overcome the block with very large doses of opiates, it is extremely dangerous to attempt to do so because of the risk of overdose. Patients on naltrexone should be given a 'caution card' issued by the drug manufacturers; this states the nature of their medication and explains that if they have an accident, for example, and require opiate analgesia, they will need much larger doses than usual. It should be made clear to the patient that naltrexone has no effect in preventing abuse of other classes of drugs.

Sedative hypnotic drugs

Sedative hypnotic drugs cause physical dependence and an abstinence syndrome which may be of life-threatening severity. Maintenance treatment, i.e. the legal prescription of the drug in sufficient dosage to prevent the onset of the abstinence syndrome, might therefore seem a reasonable treatment option. However, because tolerance to the effects of sedative hypnotics is limited, their continued consumption in high dosage keeps the patient in an unacceptable state of intoxication, often incapable of leading a useful life. It is for this reason that maintenance on sedative hypnotic drugs is not a helpful or practical response and should not be adopted.

Drug withdrawal

Patients who are dependent on sedative hypnotic drugs can generally be regarded as falling into one of two groups; those who are dependent on prescribed drugs, and those who obtain their drugs illicitly and who often abuse other drugs and alcohol too. The management of these two groups is different.

'Therapeutic' sedative dependence

Those who are dependent on prescribed sedatives (frequently benzodiazepines) have often been receiving long-term prescriptions from a single prescriber. The dose may be within or above the normal therapeutic range and may be a stable dose or one that has been increasing at a fairly gradual rate. These patients are not usually part of a drug subculture, they are not involved in other forms of drug abuse, nor are they dependent on drugs of other classes.

Many of these patients can be treated on an out-patient basis with a very gradual reduction of dosage over several weeks or perhaps even months – usually from the same, single prescriber. As a rule of thumb, benzodiazepines can be withdrawn in steps of about 1/8 (range 1/10–1/4) of their daily dose every fortnight. Patients who are taking short- or medium-acting benzodiazepines may find withdrawal particularly difficult because of the rapid alterations in blood concentrations that occur and the consequent variations in symptomatology. In such cases they should be transferred to an equivalent dose of diazepam, which should preferably be taken in a single dose at night (see Table 7.4). The dose of diazepam can then be reduced in fortnightly steps of 2–2.5 mg. If withdrawal symptoms occur, the dose should be maintained until they improve, when reduction can be resumed, if necessary in smaller fortnightly steps. In general, prescriptions should only be for 1

Table 7.4. Approximate doses of benzodiazepines equivalent to diazepam 5 mg

Drug	Dose
Diazepam	5 mg
Chlordiazepoxide	15 mg
Loprazolam	0.5–1.0 mg
Lorazepam	500 μg
Lormetazepam	0.5–1.0 mg
Nitrazepam	5 mg
Oxazepam	15 mg
Temazepam	10 mg
Triazolam	125–250 μg

week at a time because larger quantities, to last for a longer period, may prove too great a temptation for someone who is finding withdrawal very difficult.

Adjunctive treatment such as group or individual anxiety-management programmes can also be offered, but continuing psychological support is the most important element and the patient should be seen at least weekly. During withdrawal, and afterwards, the patient may attribute all untoward symptoms – both physical and psychological – to drug withdrawal, and may have unrealistic expectations about the outcome of treatment. Advice about nonpharmacological approaches to symptom management is therefore important and this can be helped by the patient keeping a diary of severe symptoms. Beta-blockers may lessen some symptoms but should only be tried if other measures fail, and never as the first response. Antidepressants should only be used if clinical depression is present.

Some patients may need or request in-patient withdrawal treatment, either because the prescribed dose is very high or because the patient prefers a more rapid detoxification which would be too risky on an out-patient basis.

Nontherapeutic sedative dependence

Sedative hypnotic drug abusers who are abusing drugs of other classes (polydrug users) and those who take sedatives obtained illicitly (sometimes obtained from several medical practitioners), are usually taking very high doses and are part of the addiction subculture.

Previously, this group mainly abused barbiturates, often intravenously. Nowadays, barbiturate abuse has lessened and has largely been replaced by abuse of benzodiazepines. These drugs are less toxic than barbiturates and there is a reduced risk of serious overdose necessitating intensive medical intervention. However, heavy sedative drug abusers continue to have serious legal, social and medical difficulties.

Out-patient detoxification is seldom appropriate for these patients, who are unlikely to comply with the planned programme and who are at risk of suffering serious withdrawal phenomena such as convulsions or toxic confusional states.[28-30] Very occasionally, an opiate-dependent individual who also takes a stable dose of benzodiazepine (within or near the therapeutic dose) may be suitable for out-patient withdrawal of sedatives with a fixed-term reduction schedule over 2–4 weeks.

In-patient detoxification is the treatment of choice and is strongly advised for patients who are dependent on sedatives. It can be divided into four phases:

1 Observation;
2 Stabilization on sedatives;
3 Detoxification; and
4 Postwithdrawal observation.

Observation

The patient is observed from the time of admission for signs of sedative withdrawal (such as tremor, agitation, tachycardia, postural hypotension). Sedatives are not given unless there is evidence of physical dependence. However, as the later signs of sedative withdrawal are dangerous, it is important that the earlier signs are not missed.

In the case of patients who are abusing long-acting benzodiazepines, signs of withdrawal may not appear for several days and it is necessary to be alert to the possibility that a patient may need to start a sedative schedule as long as 5–7 days after admission. Usually, however, evidence of withdrawal is obvious much earlier than this.

Stabilization on sedatives

If the patient shows signs of sedative abstinence, a suitable sedative drug should be administered. Theoretically, because of cross-tolerance, any sedative drug can be used, but it is customary to choose a drug from the same group as the patient's drug of abuse. Furthermore, long-acting drugs are preferable because the more stable blood levels prevent rapid swings in symptomatology. Thus, diazepam is prescribed for those whose principal drug of abuse is a benzodiazepine and phenobarbitone for those who abuse barbiturates; chlordiazepoxide or clomethiazole is prescribed to alcohol abusers (see Chapter 4).

The stabilization dose should be adjusted according to individual need. The history of drug consumption (which drug, what dosage) may be helpful but is not always reliable, so that safe stabilization relies heavily on careful observation of symptoms. The aim is to maintain the patient, temporarily, in a condition of very, very mild intoxication, manifest by slight sedation, so that the patient feels comfortable and there is no risk of serious withdrawal events. Stabilization regimes are described below for diazepam and phenobarbitone; that for diazepam is described in most detail, but exactly the same principles apply whichever drug is selected. It must be emphasized that these regimes are intended only as guidelines. Decisions about the frequency of administration of drugs and the necessary dose depend on clinical judgement of observed symptoms and signs. It should be remembered that lower dosages of drugs may be required in patients with severe liver disease.

Diazepam. If diazepam is chosen as the drug for stabilization, 20 mg is given orally and the patient is observed. If after 1 hour the symptoms of withdrawal persist, this dose may be repeated. Usually, however, and certainly after a total dose of 40 mg, symptomatic relief is obvious. Thereafter, observations continue and diazepam 20 mg is given if and when symptoms re-emerge. In any case, diazepam 20 mg should be given after 6 hours and repeated at 6-hourly intervals. However, care must be taken not to oversedate the patient; excessive drowsiness, confusion, ataxia, slurred speech and nystagmus are warning signs that the patient is becoming intoxicated, with a serious risk of respiratory depression.[28] If three or more of these symptoms are present, the next dose of diazepam should be omitted. Mild symptoms of intoxication can be managed by dose reduction rather than omission. In practice, most patients will be satisfactorily stabilized on diazepam 80–100 mg daily, in divided doses.

Rarely, the patient may be suffering nausea and vomiting as a result of drug withdrawal, or be so agitated that oral administration is initially impractical. In this situation 10–20 mg diazepam can be given intravenously, at a rate of 5 mg/min, until the patient is calm. This can be repeated if necessary after 30–60 minutes. Subsequent doses can then be given orally according to the clinical situation.

For patients with severe liver disease it may be more appropriate to select a different benzodiazepine, with a shorter half-life. Oxazepam (15–30 mg four times daily) or lorazepam (1–2 mg four times daily) are possible alternatives.

Phenobarbitone. The initial dose is 120 mg orally which can be repeated after 1 hour if necessary. This dose, equivalent to 1.8 mg/kg, is satisfactory for a patient of 'normal' weight (70 kg), but may require adjustment in obese or underweight patients. Phenobarbitone 120 mg should be administered 6 hourly unless clinical observation of intoxication suggests that a dose should be reduced or omitted (see above); if signs of withdrawal emerge, the dose may need to be increased. Phenobarbitone too, if necessary, can be given by intramuscular or intravenous injection (1.75 mg/kg).

Once the patient has been satisfactorily stabilized, this dose is maintained for 3–7 days. Three days is sufficient for those dependent on barbiturates, but those

Table 7.5. Benzodiazepine withdrawal schedule, showing dose of diazepam (mg) administered orally

Day	Time of dose administration				Total
	08.00	12.00	17.00	22.00	
1–7	20	20	20	20	80
8	20	10	20	20	70
9	20	10	10	20	60
10	10	10	10	20	50
11	10	10	10	10	40
12	10	5	10	10	35
13	10	5	5	10	30
14	5	5	5	10	25
15	5	5	5	5	20
16	5	—	5	5	15
17	5	—	—	5	10
18	5	—	—	5	10
19	—	—	—	5	5
20	—	—	—	5	5
21	—	—	—	—	0

who have been abusing predominantly long-acting sedatives, such as diazepam, should receive the full stabilization dose for 7 days before any dose reduction is initiated. Observation continues throughout this period of stabilization and appropriate adjustment of the dose may be necessary. If withdrawal signs re-emerge the dose should be increased, and if intoxication develops the dose should be reduced.

Some patients abuse a mixture of benzodiazepines, alcohol and barbiturates. The choice of detoxification agent is not critical in these cases, although it is probably better to use one with a greater anticonvulsant action. In all cases, only a single drug is prescribed.

Detoxification schedule

Daily incremental reductions of the dose are made over a period of 14–21 days. Larger incremental reductions can be made at the beginning of the detoxification schedule, when they represent a small percentage of the total daily dose, and smaller reductions at the end. Examples of typical withdrawal schedules are shown in Tables 7.5 and 7.6.

Table 7.6. Barbiturate withdrawal schedule, showing dose of phenobarbitone administered orally

| Day | Time of dose administration | | | | Total |
	08.00	12.00	17.00	22.00	
1–3	150	150	150	150	600
4	150	120	120	150	540
5	120	120	120	120	480
6	120	90	90	120	420
7	90	90	90	90	360
8	90	60	60	90	300
9	60	60	60	60	240
10	60	45	45	60	210
11	45	45	45	45	180
12	45	30	30	45	150
13	30	30	30	30	120
14	30	15	15	30	90
15	15	15	15	30	75
16	15	15	15	15	60
17	15	—	15	15	45
18	15	—	—	15	30
19	—	—	—	15	15
20	—	—	—	—	—

Adjustment of the stabilization dose or of the rate of reduction is made only on the basis of clinical indications to do so and not merely at the patient's request. The purpose of treatment is to withdraw the patient safely from a toxic agent rather than to perpetuate the use of drugs. Increasing the dose or slowing the rate of dose reduction according to the patient's whim undermines this philosophy, while accelerating the process increases the risk of withdrawal convulsions.

Postwithdrawal observation

After completion of sedative withdrawal, a minimum period of observation in hospital is recommended before the patient is discharged in case there are delayed manifestations of the abstinence syndrome, such as convulsions. Barbiturate-dependent individuals should stay in hospital for at least 2–3 days after completing drug withdrawal, but those dependent on benzodiazepines should stay for 7–10 days.

Patients should be strongly discouraged from discharging themselves during any phase of sedative withdrawal. If there is evidence of mental disorder at the time of threatened self-discharge, then consideration can be given to compulsorily detaining the patient for his or her own safety under Section 5(2) of the Mental Health Act 1983. Patients who refuse to continue with the detoxification schedule should be advised to remain in hospital for a minimum period of 2 days after the last dose, to minimize (though not eliminate)the risk of convulsions after leaving hospital.

Convulsions (during/after sedative detoxification)

If a sedative detoxification procedure such as that outlined above is adhered to, it is unlikely that convulsions will occur. However, although infrequent, they may arise even in the course of the best managed schedules, and sometimes even when the patient is being prescribed sedatives. If convulsions are severe or develop into status epilepticus, the emergency treatment is lorazepam or diazepam administered by slow intravenous injection. Lorazepam (4 mg) has a longer duration of antiepileptic action than diazepam and the latter is also associated with a higher risk of thrombophlebitis. This is reduced by using an emulsion and 10–20 mg should be administered at a rate of 0.5 ml (2.5 mg) per 30 seconds, repeated if necessary after 30–60 minutes. Facilities for resuscitation must be immediately available; if they are not, smaller doses of lorazepam or diazepam should be given intravenously. Alternatively, diazepam may be given rectally, as a rectal solution (absorption from diazepam suppositories is too slow for the management of status epilepticus). Sodium amylobarbitone 250 mg intramuscularly is an alternative treatment.

If convulsions occur during the periods of stabilization or detoxification, this suggests that the stabilized dose is too small or that the rate of withdrawal is too rapid, and an appropriate adjustment of the daily dose of sedative should be made. If they occur when withdrawal has been completed, sedatives should be reintroduced and withdrawn again at a slower rate.

It should be noted that phenytoin and other anticonvulsants are ineffective in preventing withdrawal fits and are not effective substitutes for gradual sedative detoxification. Phenothiazines and other drugs with epileptogenic properties should be avoided during sedative withdrawal.

Intoxication

If sedative intoxication develops while the patient is taking the standard stabilization dose, this may indicate that the initial diagnosis of sedative dependence was incorrect and that the patient has not developed tolerance to these drugs. Alternatively, it may suggest that the patient is simultaneously abusing illicit drugs. Whatever the cause, reduction of dose is necessary but careful observation should continue.

If intoxication develops during the period of drug withdrawal, this is probably due to illicit sedative abuse. Doses should be omitted while the patient is intoxicated, but otherwise the detoxification schedule should be adhered to.

LSD and cannabis

There is no specific treatment for those who abuse or are dependent on LSD or cannabis. Physical dependence, if it occurs, is only slight and the abstinence syndrome, if it develops, is correspondingly mild and does not cause significant distress. There is therefore no need to prescribe alternative psychoactive medication, and this should be avoided so that the patient learns how to cope without resorting to pharmacological solutions.

Cocaine and amphetamine

Until recently, no specific treatment was recommended for stimulant abuse on the grounds that the abstinence syndrome, if it developed, was self-limiting and not dangerous. Now, however, due to the easy availability of very pure cocaine in the form of 'crack', there are many more cases of very severe dependence with a correspondingly very distressing abstinence syndrome. It has thus become apparent that a more active approach to treatment may be necessary to help severely dependent individuals through their detoxification, otherwise the severity of their symptoms may prevent their ever becoming abstinent.

However, unlike the treatment of dependence on opiates or sedative hypnotics, there is no substitute drug to offer that will attract cocaine users into treatment and gradual detoxification by means of stepwise reduction of dosage is not recommended, because it is not successful. Drugs should therefore be stopped abruptly and treatment focuses on the relief of the psychiatric symptomatology associated with withdrawal.

1 During the initial 'crash', dysphoria with agitation can be treated with diazepam, either orally or intravenously. Neuroleptics may be used for psychotic symptoms and propranolol can be helpful in blocking effects mediated by the sympathetic nervous system (40–160 mg/day).

2 Dopaminergic drugs have proved most successful in managing the depressive symptoms and the severe craving, characteristic of the later stages of cocaine withdrawal. Daily amantadine, for example, reduces cocaine use and craving for up to 3 weeks and may be helpful early in the second phase of withdrawal. Other drugs that have been assessed include bromocriptine, laevodopa, methylphenidate and desipramine. The latter is known as an effective antidepressant and its use in cocaine withdrawal is based on its ability to increase synaptic concentra-

tion of dopamine.[31] Although some have advocated the use of methylphenidate, the introduction of another drug with potential for causing dependence to an individual known to be at risk of dependence, seems unwise. A number of other drugs have been used including low-dose flupenthixol, tryptophan, pyridoxine, L-tyrosine, and the selective serotonin reuptake inhibitors (SSRIs). To date, however, no effective pharmacological treatment has been found for cocaine dependence.[32,33]

3 Psychotic symptoms usually resolve within a few days but a phenothiazine drug or haloperidol may sometimes be necessary.

It is worth noting that some patients show considerable resistance to phenothiazines and benzodiazepines so that larger doses than usual may be necessary. Clonidine is said to be effective for the treatment of associated anxiety and tachycardia but hypotension may occur.

Those who are consuming large quantities of stimulants and who are severely dependent may require in-patient detoxification. This is indicated if there have been repeated attempts at out-patient detoxification, or if drug withdrawal leads to severe depression or prolonged psychotic symptoms. Admission enables complete dissociation from sources of drugs and from drug-using situations and also permits more attention to be paid to the patient's general health and nutritional status, which may have suffered severe neglect. However, this can only provide a temporary respite and the high relapse rate after discharge from hospital emphasizes the extreme importance of all the general measures of intervention outlined in Chapter 6.

Exciting new developments in the treatment of cocaine dependence include the development of a therapeutic cocaine vaccine, in which anticocaine antibodies block the effects of cocaine by preventing it from entering the brain. Cocaine vaccine is produced by a method similar to that used to make influenza vaccines and the ultimate aim is that patients would be immunized to prevent relapse.[34] Another approach is to increase enzymatic activity so that cocaine is removed from the body more quickly. In theory, this could be achieved by enhancing butylcholinesterase (pseudocholinesterase) activity in the body. However, both of these approaches rely on interactions outside the central nervous system and their efficacy will depend on how much contact the antibodies/enzymes have with ingested cocaine molecules; unfortunately, when cocaine is injected or smoked, it reaches the brain so quickly that duration of contact may be too short.[34]

Harm reduction

Although the overriding aim of treatment is to bring about permanent change so that those who abuse drugs and/or are dependent upon them can cope without, it is acknowledged that this may not be achieved for all those who seek help and that, even when successful, it may take a considerable period of time. A consensus therefore emerged that a more pragmatic response was indicated with greater emphasis on the need to prevent or at least to reduce the harm associated with drug abuse and dependence. This approach gained impetus because of the particular threat posed to injecting drug users and the wider community by HIV infection, and harm reduction (or harm minimization) became the main focus of attention of many agencies. In the midst of new enthusiasms it is worth noting that harm reduction is not a new response. For years, some professionals have advocated that opiate addicts should be prescribed injectable heroin, which they prefer, rather than theoretically safer oral methadone, to prevent them resorting to black market sources with all the attendant hazards. They pointed out that the harmful consequences of drug abuse are rarely due to the effect of the drug itself, but are more often due to the method of its administration and the presence of adulterants. However, since the late 1980s, harm reduction has been formally identified as an approach to treatment and encompasses a range of different goals including stopping (or reducing) injecting, sharing injection equipment, illicit drug use, prescribed drug use and offending behaviour. Other lifestyle goals may also be covered by the umbrella term of harm reduction, including a healthy lifestyle, getting a job, avoiding criminal activity, safe sex, etc.

Needle exchange schemes

Needle exchange schemes are probably the most visible component of harm reduction programmes and, ever since it became apparent that intravenous drug users are a high-risk group for contracting HIV and, latterly hepatitis C, there has been a body of opinion advocating the provision of sterile injection equipment to addicts who inject drugs. It is argued that this will be a genuine public health measure and good preventive medicine because, theoretically, if sufficient syringes were provided, there would be no need to share injection equipment at all, and the transmission of the HIV virus between addicts and from them to the nondrug-using population would be reduced.

The simplicity of this approach is appealing, but it has certain inbuilt disadvantages. There is a very real risk, for example, that the easy availability of sterile syringes and needles may make the transition to injecting easier and more acceptable and might encourage more young drug abusers to start injecting and to do so sooner; equally there may be less incentive for others to give up injecting. Such a policy could therefore lead to an increased number of injectors within the population and an increased number of severely dependent individuals. Furthermore, it would not completely eliminate the sharing of injection equipment, which is associated with socializing and communal feeling in the drug subculture and not just with the shortage of needles, so there are bound to be some individuals who would carry on sharing regardless of the hazards. In addition, there will always be occasions when the drug user forgets to carry his or her own syringe or has attempted to have a fix when he or she did not intend to.[35]

There are certain practical problems associated with the policy too, such as the number of syringes to be issued per day, and restrictions on those who may receive them. Should they, for example, be given to anyone who asks for them, even before they inject for the first time? Logically, to prevent AIDS and hepatitis they should be freely available, but many professionals caring for drug abusers feel very uncomfortable in a situation in which they seem to be condoning, if not positively encouraging, self-injection, which inevitably leads on to a more severe dependent state. A common policy is to provide syringes on a 'new for old' basis only. This prevents the accumulation of large stocks of injection equipment outside the 'system' and ensures the safe, ultimate disposal of potentially contaminated syringes and needles. However, it cannot control, nor even estimate, how many times or by how many people a returned syringe and needle has been used. In practice, in some areas where syringe exchange schemes have been introduced, local communities complain bitterly that used syringes and needles are left lying around and are a serious hazard to young children.

Although the provision of sterile injection equipment is less simple than it first appears, syringe exchange schemes have proliferated rapidly. Research into their effectiveness is difficult because of the long time lag between infection with HIV and seroconversion (presence of detectable antibody) and because HIV is not exclusively transmitted by sharing contaminated injection equipment. However, it appears that providing sterile injection equipment can contribute to the adoption of safer drug-use behaviour amongst injecting drug users and will therefore reduce the incidence of HIV among addicts.[36,37] However, it should be noted that even without providing free syringes, fear of HIV infection may bring about beneficial changes in techniques of drug administration, with a reduction in all complications due to injection.[38]

Perhaps the best way forward is to judge each case on its merits, rather than to adopt a stereotyped response. Where it is clear that a stable addict does inject regularly and will continue to do so, and if one can be confident that the injection equipment will not be shared, it may be sensible to provide syringes and needles. On the other hand, it is foolish to pretend that the chaotic polydrug abuser, who is frequently intoxicated and for whom sharing injection equipment is an integral part of drug-taking behaviour, is a safe person to entrust with a supply of syringes and needles. On a more positive note, the provision of a 'user-friendly' service, offering equipment that addicts want and need, is one way of attracting them into contact with health service professionals and thence, perhaps into treatment. Such programmes can offer holistic help and advice – for example on sexual risk behaviour – that also contribute to harm reduction in its widest sense.

Some countries have extended the concept of providing sterile injection equipment still further and have set up 'shooting galleries', specific facilities where drug addicts can self-inject with illicit drugs. The motivation for such developments may include a wish to remove addicts from the street and other places where self-injection offends many members of the public; concerns about the public health risks of needles and syringes that are disposed of in public places; and also a desire to minimize risk in the case of an overdose. Whatever the motivation, the provision of such 'shooting galleries' may contravene International Conventions and, by providing a formal outlet for illicit drug trafficking, seems contrary to the concept of prevention in its more general context.

The provision of syringes and needles to addicts has been discussed in some detail because it is of considerable topical interest. It is not, however, the only aspect of harm reduction. Another similarly controversial question has arisen about whether young solvent abusers, at risk of fatal accidents while intoxicated, should be instructed in safer techniques of solvent sniffing – such as not putting a plastic bag right over the head, not sniffing alone, not sniffing in dangerous places (e.g. roof tops, canal banks). Preventive education of this type, although potentially life saving, at best conveys a very ambivalent message about drug-taking and at worst seems to encourage the practice.

These examples emphasize the unpalatable fact that the laudable aim of harm reduction may sometimes conflict with the much more important aim of preventing and reducing the underlying problems of drug abuse and dependence. It is worth noting that the harmful consequences of drug abuse were largely ignored by the general population until one of these consequences, AIDS, became a serious threat to themselves as well. The vociferous support for harm reduction since then suggests that it is motivated more in unthinking self-interest than in a genuine concern for the well-being of drug abusers. For the latter group, the best approach is undoubtedly to encourage them vigorously to become abstinent from drugs. This is achieved more easily if it is attempted early in a drug-taking career, and ideally it should be attempted before self-injection becomes established and causes severe physical and psychological dependence. Easy access to treatment facilities is therefore a very important factor in harm reduction. Only if treatment and persuasion fail should measures that may reinforce dependence be considered.

Substitute prescribing

The use of methadone for the stabilization, detoxification or maintenance of opiate-dependent individuals has been described in some detail earlier in the chapter. One of the reasons for adopting this type of substitute prescribing is to attract more drug users to services, so that treatment, in its broader sense, can be initiated as soon as possible. It may have very positive benefits in terms of harm reduction, in that the patient may cease to use illicit drugs, may stop injecting, or at least use a sterile injection technique. However, while substitute prescribing may be a helpful tool in helping the drug-dependent individual to move towards abstinence or towards intermediate goals, there is a very real risk that this progress may be unacceptably slow and that the patient may be maintained indefinitely in an opiate-dependent state, without any clear decision having been taken that this is the right course of action for this particular patient. It follows that if the potential benefits of substitute prescribing are to be fully realized, it is essential that treatment interventions should have a clearly defined aim, and that there are well-established routes into detoxification.

Outreach services

Despite general acknowledgement of the importance of easy access to treatment and the consequent growth in drug services in recent years, the majority of drug users are not in touch with these services. Indeed, there may be a period of several years between starting illicit drug use and making contact with a helping agency. Reducing this time lag early in a drug-taking career, when intervention is most likely to be successful, is essential for effective prevention. Because waiting for drug users to attend established services is clearly an inadequate response, out-reach services have been developed that are proactive in making contact with drug users to offer them short-term help and to refer them on to appropriate helping agencies.

If outreach services are to be effective, some type of needs assessment is essential. For example, the reasons why existing services are not being used will have to be established and, if necessary, these services will be reviewed and modified so that they are acceptable and attractive to those who need them. In particular, outreach can aid the development of effective liaison and referral mechanisms between a wide range of agencies, including voluntary services and statutory health and social services.

However, outreach workers will never be able to achieve contact with all drug users, nor will they be able to achieve onward referral to an appropriate agency for all those with whom they do come into contact. Therefore, an important aspect of their work is to achieve change at community level and to achieve harm reduction by a cascading educational process. Thus, when working with a certain number of individuals, they also try to ensure that their message reaches other drug users with whom their client comes into contact. Because outreach developed as an attempt to reduce the spread of HIV and AIDS, much of the work is focused in this area, with an emphasis on advice on safer sexual practices and safer injecting practices and on practical measures such as the provision of condoms and sterile injection equipment. Effective harm reduction, however, encompasses far more than this, and outreach workers should not lose opportunities to discourage regular drug use among experimental users, to discourage injection by potential injectors, to encourage established injectors to switch to safer, oral administration of drugs and to encourage drug injectors and their sexual partners to be immunized against hepatitis.

Conclusion

It appears that, for some people, harm reduction has become an ideology and an end in its own right, rather than one component of a comprehensive and holistic approach to the treatment of substance dependence. While the concept has been embraced with enthusiasm in some countries, it remains controversial in others and this is perhaps because of some of the practices now subsumed under this heading. For example those who advocate the legalization of drugs may do so, under a 'harm reduction' umbrella. Furthermore, as indicated above, many harm reduction practices were introduced only in response to the threat of HIV/AIDS. In other words, they were public health measures, intended for the good of society as a whole, rather than focusing on what was best for the individual patient. The harm reduction measure of 'shooting galleries' can similarly be categorized as a method of social control and one which reduces the social visibility and inconvenience of drug injectors in public places. Focusing on the good of the individual patient permits greater clarity about what is genuinely harm reducing for them. Specifically, the overriding aim should always be to reduce demand for drugs and to encourage abstinence. While some harm reduction practices may be expedient in particular sociocultural settings, anything that appears to encourage drug consumption should be treated with scepticism. On the other hand, harm reduction, in the sense of tertiary prevention, is a long-established and important component of medical treatment.

Finally, it is important to emphasize that the very term 'harm reduction' risks conveying the gloomy and inaccurate message that substance dependence is not susceptible to effective treatment and that all that is possible is a reduction in the harm that it causes. Substance-dependent individuals deserve a more positive and energetic response from health care professionals.

Complications of drug abuse and their treatment

Those who abuse drugs may suffer many physical and psychological problems as a consequence of their behaviour. Some problems can be directly related to the pharmacological effects of the drugs, but many are associated with the methods of drug administration and more specifically with self-injection. Some drug abusers inject subcutaneously ('skin-popping') and some do so intramuscularly, but the most favoured route is intravenous – because this delivers the whole dose, with no wastage, directly into the bloodstream, producing the maximum effect with minimum delay, although increasing the likelihood of a toxic overdose. Whatever complications ensue, their management and the ultimate prognosis is adversely affected by the poor general state of health of many of those who are severely dependent on drugs, resulting from poor social conditions, malnutrition and self-neglect.

No attempt has been made in this chapter to cover all the possible complications of drug abuse, but to address instead those situations that are most frequent and cause particular problems. The emphasis throughout is on the practical aspects of diagnosis and patient-management.

Infective complications of injection

Whatever route is chosen, injection carries a high risk of infection. Needles and syringes are often used several times and may be shared with others. Sterilization of injection equipment, if it is attempted at all, is usually inadequate and therefore ineffective, and the skin is rarely cleaned before injection takes place. Dirty injection habits cause local infection at the site where the needle penetrates the skin and the underlying vein and more generalized illnesses, which may be of life-threatening severity. Some infections, notably hepatitis and HIV, are transmitted directly from one drug abuser to another as infected blood contaminates shared syringes and needles and other injecting paraphernalia. Drugs themselves may also be contaminated by bacteria and this may lead to a sudden increase in the death rate among injecting drug users, as occurred in the UK in 2000 when, over a

3-month period, more than 30 drug users who injected heroin intramuscularly, died. This episode appeared to have been caused by the contamination of heroin with an anaerobic *Clostridium* which, by the production of a toxin, caused the sudden onset of shock, leading to death within a few hours of the onset of symptoms.

Cellulitis and abscesses

These are local infections occurring at the site(s) of injection. Cellulitis is a spreading infection of the subcutaneous tissues. The affected area is red, swollen, painful and warm, with ill-defined borders, whereas an abscess is a localized collection of pus in a cavity. They may be caused by skin-popping or mainlining, and may be complicated by local thrombophlebitis (inflammation and clotting of a vein) and by the irritant effects of injected drugs (e.g. barbiturates). The local lymph nodes, in the axilla or groin, become enlarged and the patient usually has a fever.

Cellulitis and abscesses are very common complications of self-injection, and drug abusers often seek treatment for them in A & E departments. The affected part – usually the arm or leg – should be rested and elevated whenever possible. It should be cleaned and dressed and abscesses drained, if necessary. Swabs should be taken for bacteriological culture (aerobic and anaerobic), and sensitivity and antibiotic treatment should be initiated. The majority of infections are caused by a penicillinase-resistant *Staphylococcus*, so flucloxacillin is an appropriate choice of antibiotic (or erythromycin if the patient is allergic to penicillin), while awaiting the results of bacteriological examination. The first dose should be given by intramuscular injection.

Chronic skin infection, associated with skin-popping, may be complicated by amyloidosis, which is a major cause of renal damage (nephropathy). Deep abscesses may extend to underlying joints causing a septic arthritis. Bone infection (osteomyelitis) may also occur, most often in the vertebrae, and is usually due to septic emboli from a distant abscess.

Admission to hospital is indicated if the infection is severe or if the patient has toxic symptoms. The decision to admit the patient is often influenced by the knowledge that some drug abusers may not return regularly for further dressings and may be unreliable about taking a full course of antibiotics. It is often safer to admit the patient to hospital (if he or she consents to this), so that treatment can be properly supervised and further complications prevented.[1]

Endocarditis

Endocarditis is one of the most severe forms of infection in humans, in which the smooth lining of the heart valves, the endocardium, is infected and destroyed by bacteria. In those who do not inject drugs this process only occurs if the endocardium has been previously damaged, but in injecting drug abusers it can develop in a previously normal heart.

Infection causes the heart valves to become distorted by crumbling masses of blood clots and bacteria ('vegetations'), bits of which (emboli) break off and are borne away by the bloodstream to other organs, where they act as septic foci. At the same time, the vegetations prevent normal closure of the valves of the heart which then cannot function properly. This process is accentuated by the gradual destruction of the valve. In the majority of drug abusers with endocarditis, the infection is localized to the tricuspid valve, which is unusual in nondrug users.[2] The organism (*Streptococcus viridans*) that usually causes endocarditis is comparatively rare in drug abusers, in whom 'unusual' organisms are more likely to be responsible for the illness. For example, the majority of cases are caused by *Staphylococcus aureus*, perhaps because those who regularly inject themselves appear to have a high carriage rate of *S. aureus* in the nose, throat and the skin of the antecubital fossa. Sometimes the source of infection may be a cutaneous abscess or septic thrombophlebitis. Other organisms that are occasionally responsible include Gram-negative bacteria such as *Pseudomonas* and *Klebsiella*. The yeast fungus, *Candida,* can also cause endocarditis in drug abusers, although for this and other organisms of low virulence it may be necessary for there to have been prior valve damage before infection could occur. Such damage may develop as a result of bombardment of the endothelial surface with particulate matter present in the injected material.

Endocarditis should be suspected in any patient with a fever and a changing heart murmur, and the characteristic cutaneous manifestations (petechiae, subungual splinter haemorrhages and Osler's nodes) are present in up to 50% of patients. Staphylococcal endocarditis in particular is characterized by an acute onset and fulminant course, with many septic and embolic complications. Heart failure develops in severe, untreated cases. Diagnosis depends on positive blood cultures that should be carried out as soon as there is any suspicion of endocarditis, so a favourable outcome depends on the early initiation of appropriate antibiotic therapy. Two-dimensional echocardiography can be very useful in identifying and documenting the valve lesion and may sometimes demonstrate vegetations.

Treatment follows the same lines as for the general population and a combination of antibiotics is chosen according to the sensitivities of the bacteria identified on blood culture. Treatment should continue for a minimum of 4 weeks and, certainly at first, should be by continuous intravenous infusion, so that adequate blood levels of antibiotic are maintained.

'Blind' prescribing, before the results of blood culture and sensitivity tests are available, is very difficult because of the wide range of possible organisms. If it is absolutely essential because of the patient's clinical condition, an aminoglycoside (e.g. gentamicin) in combination with a penicillin, or a cephalosporin alone should be used, but specialist (bacteriological) advice should be sought. Surgical intervention (valve excision and replacement) may sometimes be necessary for patients with progressive cardiac failure that is unresponsive to medical management, and when it proves impossible to eradicate the infection from the valves with antimicrobial agents.

Septicaemia

Almost any organ can become infected during drug abuse by injection so that arthritis, osteomyelitis, nephritis and bacterial pneumonia may all occur in those who use contaminated syringes and needles. Any of these localized bacterial infections may, in turn, give rise to septicaemia, in which actively multiplying bacteria are no longer confined to the affected organ, but are present in the bloodstream too.

The most common cause of septicaemia in drug abusers is *S. aureus*, but *Streptococcus, Pneumococcus, Salmonella* or *Candida* – or indeed almost any microorganism – may, on occasion, be responsible for this very serious, life-threatening infection.

Septicaemia should be suspected if the patient is suffering from fever with hypotension or unexplained confusion, impairment of consciousness, renal failure or liver failure. Once suspected, the condition must be investigated by sending specimens of blood for culture (aerobic and anaerobic) to see if bacteria are present and, if they are, to establish their sensitivity to antibiotics. A successful outcome depends on the early initiation of appropriate antibiotic treatment, and while waiting for the results of sensitivity tests, it is usually necessary to start treatment 'blind' – a cephalosporin, or an aminoglycoside together with a penicillin, would be a suitable choice in this situation. Antibiotics should be given by intravenous infusion. Intensive supportive therapy is also required.[1]

Acquired immune deficiency syndrome

Acquired immune deficiency syndrome (AIDS) is caused by infection with a retrovirus, human immunodeficiency virus (HIV). Once inside the body, HIV infects cells called CD4 T-lymphocytes by first attaching to the CD4 receptors and other cell membrane molecules and then introducing its RNA into the cell. CD4 T-lymphocytes play a crucial role in mobilizing the body's immune system and, when HIV invades them and replicates within them, they are prevented from carrying out their normal functions. Thus, the infected individual's ability to fight infection is impaired and he or she becomes vulnerable to a wide range of opportunistic infections and malignancies that characterize AIDS. A few of those infected, however, appear to show resistance to disease progression (nonprogressors).[3]

The virus introduces its own RNA into the lymphocyte and then, using the viral enzyme reverse transcriptase, uses this RNA as a template to generate DNA, which is incorporated into the host cell's DNA by the viral enzyme integrase. The viral DNA then uses the cell's manufacturing processes to produce more viral RNA and proteins and more virus particles are produced. As these mature, viral protease cleaves precursor polyproteins to generate essential viral structural proteins and enzymes. New virus particles bud from the host cell and infect other cells, replicating quickly and continuously.

Tests for HIV

Infection with HIV stimulates the body to produce antibodies that appear to have little or no ability to neutralize HIV. The detection of this antibody forms the basis of the HIV antibody test. If positive, it denotes prior infection with HIV, but does not necessarily mean that the patient has AIDS or will contract it. It does imply, however, that the patient is carrying the virus and can transmit it to others. A negative HIV antibody test probably means that the patient has not been infected with HIV, but the latent period between infection and the development of a positive antibody test can be as long as 3 months, so a single, negative test may lead to a false sense of security. There are at least two types of HIV, HIV-1 and HIV-2; most laboratories test simultaneously for both. Detection of viral nucleic acid using the polymerase chain reaction (PCR) test can also be used in cases where there is a high index of suspicion but the anti-HIV antibody test is negative.

In an infected individual with AIDS, HIV antibody can be detected in high concentration in the blood and, in males, in semen. It has also been detected in low concentration in other body fluids, such as saliva, tears, urine, spinal fluid, cervical secretions and breast milk.

The CD4 T-cell count in the blood correlates with the progression of infection and can be used as a surrogate marker for the stage of HIV infection. The normal count is around 600–1500 cells/mm^3, with different values in different laboratories. In patients with symptomatic advanced HIV disease, counts below 200 cells/mm^3 are typical.

The concentration of HIV RNA in the patient's plasma is a measure of ongoing viral replication (viral load). Patients with the highest viral load are at greatest risk of rapid disease progression.

Routes of transmission of HIV

Unlike many other viruses, HIV is fragile and survives poorly outside the body, so that transmission is only by three routes and requires close contact:

Transfusion or inoculation of infected blood

The risk of infection from the transfusion of blood and blood products is now small in countries with high standards of screening donor blood. Drug abusers who share injection equipment are, however, a very high risk group. The World Health Organization's Multi-City study investigated the presence of HIV antibodies in blood or saliva of injecting drug users. This varied from below 5% to more than 50% for different cities at different points in time and also demonstrated that the situation could change very rapidly from one year to the next. Thus in New York, HIV seroprevalence in injecting drug users increased from under 10% in 1978 to approximately 50% in 1983.[4] Concern about HIV/AIDS usually leads to changes in behaviour with a move towards safer injection practices (but much less towards safer sex).[5] Stabilization of seroprevalence then occurs. However, there is no doubt that injecting drug users form a significant proportion of the HIV/AIDS population and play a significant part in its transmission.

In the UK, the 1999 Department of Health Unlinked Anonymous Prevalence Monitoring Programme found the prevalence of HIV amongst injecting drug users attending services in London to be 1 in 35.[6] Prevalence is substantially lower in other parts of the country and UK prevalence is lower than for other Western European countries. Since 1995, the rate has not changed but there continues to be a low rate of new cases through injecting drug use.

Sexual contact

Transmission of HIV can occur through both hetero- and homosexual genital contact. This is an important route of transmission from drug abusers to the general population, particularly because some drug abusers may turn to prostitution to finance their habit. Furthermore, although HIV risk among injecting drug users seems to be declining as a result of changes in their injecting behaviour, changes in sexual behaviour towards safer sex are not apparent.[7]

Materno-fetal spread

HIV may be transmitted from an infected, pregnant addict to the unborn child and, in the UK, by the end of April 1999, 39% of babies born to mothers infected with HIV were known to be infected by vertical transmission.[8] Transmission may be transplacental, usually in the third trimester, during the birth or through breast-feeding.

Clinical features of HIV and AIDS

The disease generally progresses through different stages.

Primary infection is often asymptomatic but in about 50% of cases, nonspecific symptoms occur up to 6–12 weeks after infection. These include fever and fatigue as well as rashes and swollen lymph nodes. Additional manifestations include aseptic meningitis, peripheral neuropathy and encephalopathy due to the virus entering the nervous system.

Following the acute HIV syndrome, most patients enter a prolonged asymptomatic or latent phase, during which there is a low level of viral replication. In adults this latent phase, during which the patient is infectious, may last for an average of 10 years. However, within months of infection there will be a gradual reduction in the CD4 T-lymphocyte cell count and opportunistic infections and malignancies are more likely to occur when this eventually falls below $200/mm^3$. Although asymptomatic, many patients are noted to have persistent generalized lymphadenopathy for which no other cause can be found. Some may also suffer from night sweats.

The alternative course of HIV disease occurs in 'fast progressors' who tend to have high viral loads and who move more swiftly to advanced HIV disease. Full-blown AIDS, is characterized by immunosuppression with low CD4 counts (below 200 cells/mm^3) and high viral loads. Opportunistic infections are common and they tend to recur; when there is deep organ involvement with fungi or parasites, this is difficult to eradicate. Examples of common infections in those with HIV include infection with a yeast-like organism, *Candida albicans*, that may cause persistent thrush in the mouth and throat; a serious pneumonia caused by *Pneumocystis carinii*; and an otherwise rare skin tumour, Kaposi's sarcoma, that develops in 25% of people with AIDS. Specific malignancies associated with AIDS (e.g. Kaposi's sarcoma, primary cerebral lymphoma, non-Hodgkin's lymphoma) are also common at this stage. Chronic active viral infection may also manifest itself by symptoms such as weight loss, diarrhoea, etc., lasting for more than 1 month. There may be neurological disease, due to the direct effect of HIV on the brain and spinal cord, e.g. dementia.[3]

HIV testing of drug abusers

HIV testing is available at most DDTUs.[9] Although testing is not a compulsory condition of treatment, patients at high risk (e.g. those who inject their drugs and those at risk because of their sexual behaviour) should be encouraged to have the test particularly because advances in treatment now offer the opportunity for effective intervention.

Pretest counselling

The aim of pretest counselling is to ensure that the individual is fully informed and prepared for the implications of either a positive or negative result; and to provide the individual with the necessary harm reduction advice, regardless of the result of the test. It therefore includes the following.

1 Education on viral transmission, the manifestations of HIV infection and the nature of the test. If the patient decides to be tested, it should be emphasized beforehand that two blood samples may be required both for verification of a positive result and to ensure the reliability of a negative test result if the patient had been at risk in the recent past.

2 Education on ways of reducing the risk of infection, such as 'safer sex' and of giving up injecting or, failing that, of never sharing injection equipment, including filters, spoons and water used for preparing heroin or other substances for injection.

3 Education on the implications of positive and negative results:

(a) Positive result. This means that the patient has been infected with HIV and can transmit it to others. No further test is available to predict the future course of events, so the patient found to be HIV-positive has to live with that knowledge, but in ignorance and in fear of the eventual outcome. The ability of the patient to cope with this degree of uncertainty and with the knowledge that they have been in contact with a life-threatening virus should be explored before the test is done. If the patient is pregnant, the risks to her and to the fetus should be explained.

(b) Negative result. This does not exclude the possibility of prior infection because seroconversion (presence of detectable antibodies) may take 3–6 months. Therefore, to be absolutely sure of freedom from HIV, a second test has to be carried out a few months later. A negative result is in itself no safeguard against infection in the future; just because a drug abuser has been 'lucky' up until the time of the test and has not been infected with HIV, it does not mean that the same risky practices can be continued.

4 Discussion of confidentiality. DDTUs need to have established policies regarding the disclosure of HIV test results, for example within the multidisciplinary team and to the GP, and the patient should be fully informed of this before testing. If the patient does not wish the result of his or her test to be disclosed to the GP, for example, although it might be the unit's policy to do so, he or she should be advised of alternative venues for testing, such as the genitourinary medical clinic.

5 The possible social and financial implications of the test – whatever its result – should be fully explained to the patient, who should understand that in some situations (life insurance, mortgage applications, employment) merely having had the test (even if the result is negative) may be disadvantageous, because of the implication of an 'at-risk' lifestyle. There should also be some discussion about the implications a test result may have for their relationship with their partner(s), and the patient should be encouraged to talk to their partner(s) about this in advance. At the same time patients should be warned to be

cautious about telling friends and acquaintances the result of the test because they may later regret the lack of confidentiality.

After discussion of all these points, patients should be allowed and encouraged to take enough time to think about testing and to come to a final decision. In the past, some felt that, whatever the result, their future behaviour would be the same: if HIV-negative, certain measures would be adopted to prevent their becoming infected; if HIV-positive, the same measures would be adopted to prevent them transmitting infection. They concluded, therefore, that there was no point in having the test, given that this in itself might jeopardize their future in an unpredictable way. Now, however, the advent of specific antiretroviral treatment offers real hope to those infected with HIV, particularly those in the early stages of the disease. Early diagnosis of infection is therefore very important and patients should be encouraged to have the test. This is especially important for drug abusers who are unwell, to enable a diagnosis to be made, and is vital for women who are thinking of becoming pregnant or who are pregnant.

The fact that HIV counselling has been given and the patient's decision about testing should be clearly recorded in the case notes.

It should be noted that, in certain circumstances, doctors may disclose information about a patient (e.g. their HIV status) without consent in order to protect another from risk of death or serious harm (e.g. a sexual contact of a patient infected with HIV). In such circumstances, the patient should be told before the doctor makes the disclosure and the doctor must be prepared to justify the decision to disclose information. Before disclosing against the patient's wish to maintain confidentiality, it is wise to seek advice first from an experienced colleague.[10]

Post-test counselling

The result of HIV testing should be given to the patient face to face, preferably by the pretest counsellor. Informing the patient by telephone or in writing is not appropriate.

1 Negative HIV-test result. The pretest education and counselling about risk reduction should be re-emphasized and a further test should be offered for about 6 months later.

2 Positive HIV-test result. The psychological impact of a positive result should not be underestimated and the patient must be allowed time to express their initial reactions. Education on reducing the risk of transmission of HIV should be repeated. Patients may welcome an offer of assistance in informing their partner(s) of the test result and they should be informed of support groups such as the Terrence Higgins Trust and Body Positive. A referral should be made to the appropriate local clinic dealing with HIV-positive patients.

Much of the information covered during post-test counselling will be forgotten in the shock of discovering that the test was positive. The patient should be offered another appointment within a week or so, to provide an opportunity to repeat the information and to talk more calmly about the implications of the test result. The patient should have ready access to a key worker or doctor for support.

Preventive measures: advice to patients

The risk of sharing injection equipment should be explained to all drug abusers. Those who are HIV-positive should understand their responsibility not to infect others, and should also be aware that their own risk of developing AIDS will be reduced if they stop exposing themselves to the infections carried by contaminated equipment and illicit drugs. Those currently HIV-negative put themselves at the risk of AIDS every time they share injection equipment. Indeed, it should be pointed out to all drug abusers that stopping injecting completely is the only safe behaviour, because drug abusers who inject are always at the risk of wanting a fix on impulse and of deciding to share someone else's equipment.

It should not be forgotten that drug abusers, although a high-risk group for AIDS because of their injection practices, can transmit HIV and be infected by it by other routes too. They should be advised about how to change their sexual behaviour to minimize the risk of transmission of the infection into the nondrug-abusing population. They should also be warned of the risk of sharing razors and toothbrushes which often come into contact with blood. Drug abusers who are HIV-positive should be taught how to clean up spillages of blood or urine.

Treatment of HIV and AIDS

A large number of antiviral drugs have been tried in the treatment of AIDS and there has been some relaxation of the otherwise extremely lengthy testing process for new drugs so that AIDS sufferers can have the benefit of new developments as soon as possible. The current approach utilizes combination therapy of at least three antiretroviral drugs that act in different ways on the intracellular, viral multiplication processes aiming to achieve a sustained reduction of viral load. It is important for treatment to be initiated before the immune system is irreversibly damaged.

Because of the complexities of the different treatment regimens, the management of patients with HIV disease should always be under the supervision of specialists in the field and only a brief outline of treatment is provided here. There are three major groups of antiretroviral drugs:

1 Nucleoside reverse transcriptase inhibitors (e.g. zidovudine) are incorporated into nucleic acids and inhibit the action of the enzyme that reverse transcribes DNA in the host cell from the viral RNA template.

2 Nonnucleoside reverse transcriptases (e.g. nevirapine) act in the same way but are not incorporated into nucleic acids.

3 Protease inhibitors (e.g. ritonavir) block an enzyme that is essential for intra-viral replication.

Integrase inhibitors are under development. They will halt the incorporation of the viral genetic material into the T-cell's DNA.

These drugs have a range of serious adverse side effects and also interact with each other and the choice of drug regimen depends on a variety of factors including viral load, CD4 count, previous history of treatment and patient preference. The latter is important because the drug regimes are complex and strict compliance is essential to prevent the development of drug resistance. Although drug toxicity is more likely as the disease advances, drug treatment can reduce viral replication, delay disease progression and prolong survival and, when they are used in combination, the development of viral resistance is impeded. Since anti-HIV drugs became widely available, median survival in those with HIV infection but initially free from AIDS rose by 8–14 months, depending on the patient's initial disease state.[3]

Efforts to improve the general health of the individual by a holistic approach to lifestyle are also of great importance. In addition, opportunistic infections should be diagnosed and treated promptly as primary prophylaxis has been shown to be effective. It is also essential that the need for psychosocial counselling for patients, families and friends is recognized.

Treatment of HIV infection in pregnancy

Because of the high level of risk of transmitting HIV to the fetus, active intervention is indicated for pregnant women who are infected with HIV. This takes the form of specific antiretroviral therapy, such as zidovudine, taken orally during the second and third trimesters and administered intravenously during labour and delivery. The baby is also treated for the first few weeks of life. Triple combination therapy is indicated for women with more advanced disease (AIDS) who become pregnant and this should be based on the same criteria as those used for women who are not pregnant. However, the mother should be fully involved in discussions about the potential risks and benefits of treatment.

Treatment with zidovudine can reduce vertical transmission rates by two thirds, from 25% to 8% with mild, self-limiting anaemia as the only side effect observed in neonates.

Mode of delivery

Caesarean section is recommended for HIV-positive women because this mode of delivery reduces the risk of spread of HIV from mother to baby, probably because the baby is much less exposed to maternal blood and secretions.

Breast-feeding

Breast-feeding is contraindicated for HIV-positive mothers because it significantly increases the risk of transmission of infection by at least 14%, with the risk increasing the longer that breast-feeding continues. Clearly this advice should be reviewed in countries where bottle feeding does not provide a safe alternative to breast-feeding.

Summary

With appropriate management, the risk of an HIV-positive pregnant woman transmitting infection to her child can be significantly reduced. This makes it all the more important for HIV infection to be detected early in pregnancy and injecting drug abusers, who are a high-risk group for infection, should be encouraged to be tested for HIV.[11]

Hepatitis

Most cases of viral hepatitis are due to hepatitis A virus (HAV) which is transmitted by the faeco-oral route, and which usually causes only mild disease without progression to chronic liver function impairment. However, hepatitis B (HBV) and hepatitis C (HCV) cause much more serious disease and both infections are common among drug abusers who inject themselves, because they often share injection equipment and thus transmit infection from one to another. It does not matter whether injection is intravenous, intramuscular or subcutaneous; once the skin has been breached by a contaminated needle, the infection can be introduced.

Hepatitis B

In addition to transmission via shared injection equipment, hepatitis B can also be transmitted by saliva, sexual contact and vertically from mother to child. Potential vehicles of transmission include ear-piercing, tattooing and sharing of razors and toothbrushes. High-risk groups include male homosexuals and patients who have previously had sexually transmitted diseases (i.e. populations with high promiscuity) and those from areas of the world where HBV is endemic (e.g. China, Africa). Health care workers have an increased risk of occupational exposure but do not have a higher incidence of disease.

Clinical course

Following infection there is a long incubation period of up to 6 months and during this time the patient is asymptomatic, although capable of infecting others. The virus replicates itself inside the cells of the liver and this may or may not result in acute hepatitis. The illness begins insidiously, usually with loss of appetite, nausea, tiredness and general malaise. There may be vomiting and abdominal distension and discomfort; a loss of desire for cigarettes by smokers is said to be a classic symptom; and skin rashes, joint pain and severe headaches may also occur. There may or may not be a fever which subsides when jaundice becomes apparent. The liver enlarges and becomes tender and there are abnormalities of liver function (bilirubin and transaminases). In 90% of HBV patients, liver function tests return to normal within 6 months, but clinical and biochemical relapses may occur during the recovery phase.

However, persistent HBV infection may occur, resulting in chronic hepatitis which is defined as liver inflammation (recognized by elevation of transaminase enzymes) persisting for more than 6 months. Two types of chronic hepatitis have been described: chronic persistent hepatitis, which is relatively benign, and chronic active hepatitis, which is progressive. This in turn may lead to cirrhosis, in which the liver becomes irreversibly damaged. Many drug abusers, already vulnerable to liver damage from viral hepatitis, also damage their livers by excessive consumption of alcohol. It should be noted that chronic hepatitis is now the most common cause of primary hepatocellular carcinoma – cancer of the liver. The risk of developing this cancer is estimated to be 250 times greater for chronic carriers of HBV than for those who are uninfected. Furthermore, in a minority, very serious complications may occur including hepatic necrosis, hepatic failure, cirrhosis and primary liver cancer.[12] The development of some of these conditions can be tracked via various serological tests for HBV infection.

Serological tests

Hepatitis B surface antigen (HBsAg) in the blood indicates a history of infection with hepatitis B. It stimulates the production of immunoglobulin M hepatitis B antibody (IgM anti-HBc), which is the initial antibody response to acute infection. This antibody continues to be detected in high titre in chronic carriers with liver disease whereas the presence of other hepatitis B surface antibodies (anti-HBs) usually indicates protective immunity to HBV. Chronic hepatitis is therefore related to an altered immune response to infection with HBV in which the virus is inadequately eliminated by antibodies. The persistence of immune complexes leads to a spectrum of associated extrahepatic manifestations of related immune complex disorders (e.g. rheumatoid-like arthritis, polyarteritis nodosa). The risk of carriers transmitting disease to others is assessed by more precise blood tests for other specific antigens and antibodies.

Hepatitis C

The occurrence of multiple episodes of hepatitis in drug abusers used to be attributed to infection with hepatitis A virus (HAV) or to exacerbations in a chronic carrier. However, specific antigens and antibodies have now been identified, indicating that other viruses are involved. These were previously known as non-A, non-B hepatitis agents (NANB), but hepatitis C virus (HCV) has now been separately identified as being responsible for many episodes, not only in drug abusers, but also in haemophiliacs and other recipients of blood transfusions and blood products. Indeed, although hepatitis B used to be considered as an indirect marker for the incidence of injecting drug use, hepatitis C is now considered a more reliable indicator.[13]

Sharing of injection equipment and associated paraphernalia is the most common route for transmission of infection. Other causes include body piercing, tattooing, electrolysis, and acupuncture, if equipment becomes contaminated. Needle-stick injury is a risk for health care professionals and others, if contaminated syringes are left lying around in public places; the risk of infection in this way from a hepatitis C-positive source is estimated to be between 3% and 10%. Vertical transmission, from mother to child during pregnancy or birth, can occur but is comparatively unusual with estimates of 5% or less. Breast-feeding also appears to be low risk.[14]

There is now considerable concern about HCV, which many perceive as one of the major health challenges of the millennium, because of the serious consequences of infection and the high prevalence rates now being found in many countries.[15] There is an estimated average global prevalence rate of 3%, suggesting that there are 150 million chronic carriers world-wide. In the USA for example it is estimated that there are at least 2.7 million people chronically infected with HCV, making it the most common blood-borne infection in the USA. Indeed, in industrialized countries, HCV infection now accounts for 20% of acute hepatitis, 40% of cases of end-stage cirrhosis, 60% of cases of hepatocellular carcinoma and 30% of liver transplants.[16] However, it has been found in many countries that HCV infection is not evenly distributed among the whole population and that it is much more common among injecting drug users with prevalence rates in this group of 60–80%. For example, antibodies to hepatitis C (seropositivity) have been found in 86% of drug misusers in London[17] and in 75% of UK addicts in methadone maintenance treatment. [18] This is particularly worrying because it shows that HCV is a serious threat to health to a very large group of predominantly young people.

Moreover, given the increasing number of drug abusers, there would appear to be a real risk of infection spreading from this very large pool to the general population although transmission by infected blood products has been reduced to near zero in most blood transfusion programmes and sexual transmission is much less common than for HIV, although more common amongst those with multiple partners. Prison appears to be a particularly high-risk setting with a high incidence of HCV in injecting drug users who have been imprisoned, although it is not clear whether this reflects risk behaviour in prison or the lifestyle of those who are subsequently imprisoned.[19]

Clinical course

The initial infection may be unrecognized as there are usually no symptoms or only mild and transient ones, resembling a flu-like illness. Occasionally, full-blown hepatitis occurs with jaundice at the onset. The infection clears completely only in about 15–20% of patients, leaving the remainder as potential transmitters of the disease to others. Although about 40% of those who are infected have a benign outcome – either recovering completely or having asymptomatic lesions in the liver – a significant proportion develop chronic hepatitis and become chronic carriers of the virus. Of this latter group, about 20% develop cirrhosis over a time period of 10–20 years, from which they may die and, as with hepatitis B, there is an increased risk of hepatocellular carcinoma.[12,14]

The clinical course of the disease, and specifically the rate of development of cirrhosis, is adversely affected by the use of alcohol (even in small quantities), coinfection with HIV or hepatitis B and the age of infection, with the disease progressing more slowly in those who acquire it younger.

Serological markers

As with HBV, infection with HCV is diagnosed by the presence of specific antibodies. The majority of those who have been infected have antihepatitis C antibodies within 3 months of infection, although this test may not become positive for up to 6 months. Therefore, there is a long period when the diagnosis is not confirmed and when the risk of transmission is high. It is customary to confirm a positive test with a second test. If antibodies are found, the presence of HCV RNA indicates active viraemia. Pre- and post-test counselling should be offered, similar to that described for HIV test counselling.

Delta virus

During the last decade another hepatitis virus, the δ virus, has been the subject of considerable investigation and research. It is now known that it is a unique but defective transmissible virus and that infection with it can only occur if the individual is simultaneously infected with HBV, or is a chronic carrier. Two basic categories of δ infection have therefore been identified. 'Coinfection' occurs when there is simultaneous infection with both HBV and δ virus. Most of such cases run a fairly benign course, similar to that caused by HBV alone, with progression to chronic hepatitis D occurring in only 2% of cases. 'Superinfection' with δ virus occurs when the patient first became infected with HBV some months earlier, or if he or she is already a chronic carrier. In these situations, HBV is already replicating vigorously and the δ virus can begin to replicate immediately, resulting in a very severe infection. δ superinfection is therefore associated with fulminant hepatitis and a high rate of progression to chronic active hepatitis. It is not associated with a greater risk of liver cancer, perhaps because of the high early mortality rate.[12]

Treatment

There is no specific treatment for hepatitis B in the acute stage. Bed rest, according to how the patient feels, a well-balanced, normal diet with an adequate intake of calories and abstinence from alcohol are probably the most important points. Admission to hospital for a few days may be necessary if the patient is ill and/or domestic circumstances do not permit adequate care at home. Fulminant hepatitis and death occur in less than 1% of cases at the acute stage. In severe cases, opiate withdrawal itself may be hazardous and can precipitate hepatic failure. Detoxification must therefore be very gradual and must be closely supervised. Prothrombin time should be measured three times a week, any prolongation suggesting that hepatic failure may be imminent. Disease progression will be managed according to the problems that arise.

Treatment of hepatitis C

In addition to the general supportive measures in the acute stage, treatment is now available for persistent hepatitis C infection. Combination therapy with alpha interferon and ribavirin is indicated for moderate to severe infection for previously untreated patients and for those who have responded to monotherapy but have since relapsed. Treatment continues thrice weekly for six months. It is associated with unpleasant side effects and patients need considerable support to continue treatment reliably for this length of time. However, combination therapy significantly improves the success rate of treatment in appropriately selected patients. Substance misusers are not excluded from treatment although continued self-injection with the consequent risk of reinfection is a contraindication, as is a high alcohol intake. Combination therapy is not advised for women who are pregnant.

The availability of treatment should be seen as offering new opportunities for health care professionals to work positively with substance users and to encourage them to adopt a healthier life style and to stop self-injecting.[14,20]

Preventive measures

Prevention of transmission

Because of the limitations of treatment, primary preventive measures are a high priority and, among these, a reduction in the rate of drug injection is particularly important because the risk of infection with hepatitis starts with the first injection and continues for as long as injecting does. In this context it is relevant that, even when there is a low incidence of HIV infection among injecting drug users, because of the availability of syringe and needle exchange programmes there may be a continuing high incidence of hepatitis C infection. This suggests that there may be a much larger pool of infection for hepatitis C and/or that the virus is more infective than HIV. Specifically, HCV may survive longer and be spread more successfully via the communal use of spoons, filters and other injection paraphernalia. Secondary preventive measures focus on the reduction of drinking because alcohol consumption appears to enhance the replication of HCV and produce more severe liver injury than that caused by alcohol alone.

The measures for preventing the transmission of hepatitis B and C are identical to those recommended for HIV: there should be no sharing of injection equipment and 'safer' sexual practices should be adopted. Clinical and laboratory staff are at risk of contracting hepatitis from drug abusers in the same ways that they are at risk from HIV infection. Indeed, at present there is a greater risk of hepatitis, both because more drug abusers are infected with HBV and HCV than with HIV, and because the hepatitis viruses are more resilient to destruction outside the body. The stringent procedures which have been adopted since the threat of AIDS was identified will also prevent the transmission of hepatitis. They should be routine when handling any specimen from any drug abuser who injects drugs.

Screening
In the UK and other countries where the prevalence of hepatitis is comparatively low, population screening for hepatitis is not cost-effective. However, high-risk populations, such as drug abusers who self-inject, should be screened, and, if negative for hepatitis B, they should be offered immunization. Antibody to hepatitis core antigen (anti-HBc) is the best prevaccination screening test.

Active immunization against hepatitis
The development of a vaccine for hepatitis proved difficult because of repeated failure to grow the virus in tissue culture. A vaccine of alum-absorbed, inactivated HBsAg was eventually prepared from the serum of chronic, symptomless carriers. The vaccine is safe and effective, although expensive, but is unacceptable to many people because of a perceived (but unproven) risk of transmission of AIDS and/or other infections. A more recent development has been to apply genetic engineering techniques. Genetic material (DNA) from HBV is introduced into yeast cells so that they possess some of the antigenicity of HBV and can stimulate antibody production. Any possibility of disease transmission is ruled out because only part of the genetic material from HBV is used.

The availability of an absolutely safe vaccine means that a policy of active immunization for those at risk from infection with HBV can be implemented.

Immunization should be offered to drug abusers who inject, to the staff at DDTUs and to others who are in regular contact with, and give treatment to, drug abusers who self-inject. Sexual contacts and family members in close contact with patients infected with HBV should also be immunized.[21]

Vaccination involves a course of three injections, with the second dose being given 1 month after the first and the third 5 months later. Booster doses are recommended every 5 years, but should be repeated earlier if antibody levels are low following immunization, because this indicates continued susceptibility to hepatitis.

As yet there is no vaccine for hepatitis C or δ virus. However, as the clinical course of HBV infection is much more severe if the patient also has HCV, vaccination against HBV is especially recommended for those with HCV antibodies but no evidence of immunity to HBV. Immunization against hepatitis also protects against δ virus because this virus only replicates in the presence of hepatitis infection.

Passive immunization against hepatitis

A single, acute exposure to HBV may occur if someone is accidentally pricked with a needle used by or for a patient with hepatitis, and this is an indication for passive immunization. Hepatitis immunoglobulin should be given as quickly as possible, and preferably within the first 48 hours after exposure. A dose of 3 ml (200 IU of anti-HB/ml) is usually administered and repeated 30 days later. Alternatively, active immunization with vaccine can be combined with simultaneous administration of hepatitis immunoglobulin, given at a different site.

Health care workers with hepatitis or HIV

Rarely, in the course of treating health care workers with a substance abuse problem, the diagnosis may be made of a serious communicable disease, such as HIV or hepatitis. If the health care worker is practising or has practised in a way that places patients at risk, an appropriate person in the employing authority (e.g. occupational health physician) or the relevant regulatory authority must be informed.[10]

Pulmonary complications

Pulmonary complications are common among drug abusers who inject their drugs because of the introduction into the venous system of particulate matter – either from crushed tablets or the insoluble adulterants of illicit drugs. These particles (microemboli) become trapped in the tiny arteries of the lungs, which they obstruct, causing those areas of the lung that are deprived of their blood supply to die (pulmonary infarction). Areas of inflammation – granulomas – may surround these microemboli, and the occlusion of the pulmonary arterioles may sometimes be so severe and widespread that there is an increase in pulmonary artery pressure (pulmonary hypertension). This should be suspected in a patient who complains of fatigue, breathlessness or angina. Later, there may be oedema and the patient may cough up blood. Little can be done to improve the situation and the prognosis is poor.[1]

Psychiatric complications

The abuse of potent psychoactive drugs does not always produce the desired and sought-after psychic effect but may, on occasion, lead to an abnormal and unwanted mental state. Sometimes the drug-abusing individual becomes unconscious (or drowsy), and sometimes he or she becomes very disturbed and may suffer from hallucinations or delusions. These conditions may arise because a single, very large dose of the drug was taken (overdose), or because of excessive consumption over a long period (chronic intoxication), or because the drug-abusing individual is unusually sensitive to the effect of a particular drug and develops an idiosyncratic response. Sometimes the abnormal mental state may be due to a 'flashback' – a recurrence of a hallucinogenic drug experience after the effect of the drug has worn off – and sometimes it may be due to drug withdrawal.

The patient's mental state depends on which drug has been taken and its dose, and on the individual's previous experience with drugs and dependence status. Often, none of these variables is known, so that the doctor or other health care worker is confronted with a patient in an abnormal mental state, suspected of being due to drug abuse, and has to proceed in ignorance of the underlying cause. Patient care and management is therefore based on sound general principles and there is little treatment that is drug-specific. Certain symptoms and signs are suggestive of particular drugs and sometimes there is a clear history of what has been taken. However, even apparently sound information may be misleading or may only tell part of the story: illicitly obtained drugs are often contaminated with unknown adulterants, some of which are pharmacologically active. Street heroin, for example, is often adulterated with a barbiturate and/or other sedative hypnotics, so that measures to treat a heroin overdose may be only partially effective and recovery may be complicated by an unanticipated withdrawal syndrome. In addition, deliberate polydrug abuse, overdose and dependence is common and may present difficult problems of management.

The acutely disturbed patient

Several drugs of abuse can cause disturbances of behaviour, depending on the dose that is consumed and the sensitivity and dependence status of the individual concerned. Unfortunately, there are no clear-cut psychiatric 'syndromes' to provide an instant diagnosis of the drug of abuse, and the clinical picture may be complicated by polydrug abuse. Some information may be available from the patient, or others, and this may be helpful in diagnostic and treatment decisions.

A rapid assessment of the patient's mental state should be made in all cases, to provide a record of baseline observations, before medication (if any) is started, and to describe precisely the nature of the behavioural disturbance so that emergency treatment is appropriate to the condition. A systematic approach to the description and assessment of the acutely disturbed patient is essential and a suggested format for these assessments is provided below.

1 General behaviour. What is the patient doing? How is the patient behaving? Is he or she restless, agitated, tense? Is he or she making gestures or grimaces? Is the patient showing any repetitive behaviour? Is he or she hostile or aggressive?

2 Talk. Is the patient talking much or little? Is this spontaneously or only in answer to questions? Is he or she coherent or incoherent? Does he or she use strange words? Is there flight of ideas?

3 Mood. Does the patient have a constant or labile mood? Is he or she cheerful, depressed, frightened, suspicious, anxious, perplexed?

4 Abnormal belief. Ideas of reference? Paranoid delusions? Delusions of bodily change? Delusions of passivity? Thought reading or intrusion?

5 Abnormal experiences. Hallucinations or illusions – auditory, visual, tactile? Depersonalization, derealization?

6 Cognitive state. Attitude to present condition? Aware of possible cause?

On the basis of these observations it should be possible to decide whether the patient is suffering from:

1 A psychotic illness, characterized by hallucinations and delusions in a setting of clear consciousness – often manifesting in thought disorder and lacking insight into the nature of the condition; or

2 A panic reaction, with fear as the overwhelming symptom; or

3 An organic mental state: characterized by confusion (disorientation in time and space, impaired mental functioning), and often accompanied by disorders of perception (hallucinations, illusions). The patient is often perplexed and frightened by these experiences.

Any of these three types of reaction can occur with any drug and it may not be possible to decide on clinical grounds which drug(s) caused the abnormal mental state. A physical examination should be carried out whenever possible, but this may be difficult or impossible if the patient is very disturbed and/or hostile. Pulse rate, blood pressure and body temperature should be recorded and a sample of urine sent for toxicological analysis. The vital signs should be monitored regularly until the patient's mental state is normal. Any evidence of self-injection should be noted and the size of the liver recorded.

Management

The patient should be cared for in a quiet environment with no unnecessary stimulation. Lighting should be moderate and there should be no shadowy areas that might be worrying for a delirious or paranoid patient. Above all, the room should be as safe as possible for the patient and the staff, especially if the patient becomes violent.

The staff should be adequately trained so that they can cope confidently with disturbed patients and remain calm. They should avoid moving too close to the patient, and they should not walk behind the patient, because this may seem very threatening to a paranoid individual. Talking should be quiet, but not whispered so that paranoid and delirious patients do not misinterpret what is being said.

Patients should be reassured about the nature of their experiences. It should be explained that their distressing symptoms are drug-induced and will wear off gradually, as the drug is eliminated from the body. Reorientation – telling the patient where he or she is and what time it is – and offering positive explanations may all help to calm an acutely disturbed patient. In particular, all procedures such as examining the patient and obtaining blood samples, etc. must be explained before they are undertaken.

Acutely disturbed patients are in a state of high sympathetic arousal. They may have a raised body temperature and may sweat profusely. It is easy for them to become exhausted and dehydrated, which in turn may exacerbate the underlying condition. It is important therefore that they are cared for in a quiet room where it is easier for them to rest, and that they are given plenty of fluids and actively encouraged to drink enough.

Gastric ravage and forced diuresis to increase drug excretion are rarely appropriate or possible in acutely disturbed patients. Their use in specific clinical situations is described below. It may be difficult to achieve satisfactory environmental conditions for a disturbed patient in, for example, a busy A & E department. Nevertheless, attention to the measures outlined above is positively therapeutic, reduces the risk of outbursts of violent behaviour and may obviate the need for sedative medication. In general, the best approach is to wait for the effect of the drug(s) that have caused the disturbed behaviour to wear off, rather than to intervene with more and different psychoactive drugs to counteract their effects. The latter approach often complicates the clinical picture, making diagnosis more difficult, and carries a risk of harmful drug interactions.

Drug treatment

Some patients may be so disturbed, however, that general supportive measures are inadequate and treatment with drugs is then necessary. If it has not been possible to make a definite diagnosis about the cause of the patient's mental state, an empirical approach to treatment must be adopted.

In general, chlorpromazine is used when psychotic symptoms are the most prominent feature of the patient's condition. It may be administered orally (100 mg) or intramuscularly (50–100 mg). Chlorpromazine should not be given if intoxication with phencyclidine is suspected.

Diazepam is used for panic states and severe agitation. The dose is 10 mg orally or by slow intravenous injection. The intramuscular route should be used only if oral or intravenous administration is not possible.

If an organic mental state is diagnosed, it is best, if possible, to avoid all psychoactive medication.

Differential diagnosis and specific treatments

Cannabis

When taken in sufficient dosage, cannabis typically causes a toxic psychosis with confusion, disorientation, paranoid symptoms (suspicion, delusions) and hallucinations. The combination of organic features (confusion, impaired concentration and memory) with psychotic symptoms is very suggestive of cannabis abuse. In some individuals this develops when only a small quantity of cannabis has been used, but usually it is a dose-related effect. The patient's eyes are often red, due to injected conjunctivae, and although there may be tachycardia, blood pressure is usually normal.[22]

Sometimes these symptoms are nothing more than a 'bad trip' and subside spontaneously. 'Talking down' by peers who are familiar with such adverse responses may be all that is required while the effects of the drug wear off.

Those suffering from prolonged (more than 5–8 hours) and more severe symptoms are more likely to seek professional help. If their behaviour is very disturbed and they do not respond to simple reassurance, chlorpromazine 25–50 mg intramuscularly acts as a sedative and as an antipsychotic drug.

Flashbacks may occur after cannabis use and should be treated if necessary, according to the patient's mental state, with chlorpromazine.

LSD and other hallucinogens

Although hallucinations and other abnormal perceptual experiences are the sought-after effects of hallucinogens, they are not always pleasurable, and according to the user's mental state and the setting in which drug use occurred, they may sometimes be so terrifying that they overwhelm the drug taker. Thus the typical adverse reaction to hallucinogen abuse is a state of severe panic caused by uncontrolled hallucinations.

At times the patient may be mute and withdrawn, apparently preoccupied by inner experiences, but mood is characteristically very labile and may swing suddenly to severe anxiety. Depersonalization, confusion and suspicion also occur.

LSD has sympathomimetic effects and somatic signs of its use include pupillary dilation, tachycardia, raised blood pressure and increased body temperature.

The adverse reaction to LSD usually lasts for 8–24 hours and during this time, trained and experienced staff may be able to 'talk down' a panic-stricken patient. This is achieved by helping the patient to regain contact with reality and to relax and to understand the nature of his or her experiences without being overwhelmed by them. However, if the patient is excessively agitated, medication will be necessary. Diazepam 10–30 mg orally is usually effective and can be repeated every few hours, if necessary. Chlorpromazine (50–100 mg) is sometimes used, but only if it can be established with reasonable certainty that anticholinergic drugs have not been taken (chlorpromazine potentiates the effects of anticholinergic drugs and may precipitate hypotension).

Flashbacks, if they occur, are usually self-limiting and short-lived and rarely require treatment. Occasionally they occur frequently and become distressing, in which case treatment is the same as for an acute panic attack. Patients should be warned not to take hallucinogens or cannabis again because this may precipitate further flashbacks. If flashbacks persist and become increasingly troublesome, the patient should be assessed more thoroughly for underlying psychiatric illness.

Stimulants (amphetamine and cocaine)

Chronic abuse of central nervous system stimulants causes a psychotic illness characterized by delusions of persecution, ideas of reference (e.g. believing that others are talking about, slandering or spying on him or her) and hallucinations (auditory and visual). The patient is likely to be restless, talkative and irritable and may exhibit a repetitive, stereotyped behaviour.

The highly characteristic, almost diagnostic feature, is the absence of any confusion or disorientation so that the psychotic symptoms all occur in a setting of clear consciousness and it may be difficult to distinguish this drug-induced illness from schizophrenia.

The sympathomimetic effects of stimulant drugs may produce characteristic physical signs – tachycardia, hypertension, sweating, raised body temperature and dilated pupils – but these are very variable because of the development of tolerance in the chronic abuser. There may, however, be evidence of weight loss or of self-injection.

Stimulant psychosis usually arises in the course of chronic abuse, but sometimes occurs after a single (usually large) dose. Cases that present for treatment are more likely to be due to amphetamine use than cocaine because the effects of the latter wear off quickly, before they cause excessive concern. After amphetamine, hallucinations disappear over 24–48 hours, but delusions may persist with reducing intensity for a week to 10 days or longer.

An acutely agitated and psychotic patient should be given chlorpromazine 25–50 mg intramuscularly or 50–100 mg orally and this is repeated as necessary. Haloperidol is also effective. Antipsychotic medication may only be necessary for the first 24 hours, occasionally for a few days. If agitation and anxiety are the most prominent symptoms, diazepam may be used instead.

The excretion of amphetamine can be increased and the duration of the adverse reaction reduced by keeping the patient well hydrated and by acidification of the urine by intravenous administration of ammonium chloride. Urinary catheterization is then essential and serum electrolytes must be measured frequently.

Hyperthermia (raised body temperature) is a potentially serious side effect of amphetamine overdose. It is more likely to occur in an inexperienced abuser after a large dose of amphetamine than in a chronic abuser who has become tolerant to the effects of the drug, but body temperature should be monitored in all cases. If it rises rapidly or if it rises above 102°F (39°C), it should be treated promptly by sponging with cold water, ice-packs and fanning. Chlorpromazine (25–50 mg intramuscularly) can be given, but blood pressure should then be monitored closely in case hypotension occurs. It is important to recognize and to treat hyperthermia vigorously because it may be the forerunner of convulsions. Severe hypertension is another serious complication of amphetamine toxicity, because of the risk of cerebral haemorrhage and of cardiovascular collapse. It should be treated with phentolamine 5 mg intravenously, repeated if necessary, or with diazoxide 100–150 mg intravenously repeated after 10–15 minutes if necessary.

It is important that patients recovering from stimulant intoxication should be kept in a peaceful environment, away from unnecessary stimulation. They may sleep for many hours as the effects of the drugs wear off and may later become apathetic and depressed, sometimes suicidally. Antidepressant medication may then be necessary.

Phencyclidine

Phencyclidine consumption leads to bizarre clinical states that pose particular problems of management. In doses such as those that are often obtained at street level (5–10 mg) it produces an acute confusional state with disorientation in time and place. Characteristically, the patient is very agitated and often in a state of severe panic. There may be sudden outbursts of very violent behaviour, when the drug abuser seems to have superhuman strength, alternating with periods of mutism when the individual may respond only by nodding or eye movements. The eyes are often held wide open, giving a staring appearance and nystagmus may be present. There may be severe muscle rigidity and a grossly ataxic gait. Episodes of nausea and vomiting may occur. Pulse, blood pressure, temperature and respiration rate are usually increased.

It is generally agreed that patients intoxicated with phencyclidine should be subjected to as little verbal and physical stimulation as possible, to minimize the risk of provoking violent outbursts. Ideally, they should be cared for in isolation on a cushioned floor in a quiet room. The patient should be constantly observed in case convulsions or unconsciousness occur and pulse, blood pressure and respiration should be monitored. It is best not to give any psychoactive drugs at all, but to wait for the effect of phencyclidine to wear off. Most patients can communicate normally within 2 hours and are apparently fully recovered within 4 hours. Monitoring should, however, continue for a further 2 hours. If necessary, diazepam 10–20 mg can be given orally to control violent behaviour that threatens the safety of the staff and/or patient. Haloperidol may also be used, but phenothiazines are contraindicated because they are believed to potentiate the anticholinergic actions of phencyclidine and may produce severe and prolonged hypotension. It may be necessary to restrain the patient physically to protect both patient and staff and this is achieved more safely by using people rather than mechanical restraints.

Sedatives

The chronic abuse of sedative drugs may cause acute behavioural disturbances in two quite distinct ways.

Chronic intoxication. Patients who take sedatives regularly become tolerant to their effects and tend to increase the dose. When the limit of tolerance is reached, further increases lead to a state of chronic intoxication in which the patient has slurred speech, staggering gait and nystagmus and is mentally confused. Such patients (particularly those taking barbiturates) are characteristically hostile, aggressive and uncooperative, and are often brought to medical attention because of dangerous, socially unacceptable behaviour. Physical examination often reveals characteristic signs of barbiturate self-injection: thrombophlebitis, ulcers, brawny oedema, etc.

Unfortunately, little can be done except to wait for the effect of the drug to wear off, and although during this time the patient may be extremely disruptive and difficult to manage, he or she cannot be discharged because he or she is in a state of intoxication. Pulse, blood pressure, respiration and temperature should be monitored regularly and the patient's level of consciousness recorded. If the patient falls asleep, he or she should be placed in a semiprone position and observations should continue without fail; an intoxicated, conscious patient may lapse into unconsciousness as more of the drug is absorbed into the bloodstream.

After recovery, patients should be admitted to hospital for supervised sedative withdrawal. Many refuse this option and discharge themselves, against medical advice, to resume their drug abuse. They present to A & E departments with monotonous regularity in an intoxicated condition, and it requires a high degree of professionalism to maintain impeccable medical care in the face of such recidivism. Occasionally patients are receptive to crisis intervention and agree to referral to a specialist unit.

Withdrawal. Acutely disturbed behaviour may also arise in the course of the sedative abstinence syndrome. Some patients develop a psychotic illness, similar to the delirium tremens caused by alcohol withdrawal, and characterized by disorientation, hallucinations and delusions. The timing of these symptoms depends on the duration of action of the particular sedative, so that they may arise on the second or third day after the last dose was taken, or at any time in the following 2–3 weeks. The physical signs of sedative abstinence include tachycardia, with an increase in heart rate of more than 15/minute, and orthostatic hypotension (fall in blood pressure) on standing. Patients are usually tremulous and severely agitated and may make determined efforts to obtain their drug. There may be evidence of barbiturate injection.

Once the diagnosis has been made, treatment must be prompt to prevent the onset of withdrawal convulsions. Pentobarbitone 120 mg or diazepam 20 mg should be given and the patient admitted to hospital for stabilization on sedatives and supervised detoxification.

Solvents

The clinical picture varies according to the severity of intoxication and the drug of abuse. At first, the patient appears as if drunk and may be exhilarated in mood and impulsive in activity. More severe intoxication results in an organic mental state with confusion, slurred speech and staggering gait. Hallucinations and delusions may also occur and the diagnosis is confirmed by the smell of volatile inhalants on the breath and clothes.

Patients with acute disturbance of behaviour due to solvent abuse present for treatment only rarely because the reactions are short-lived and resolve spontaneously, as the effect of the drug wears off. There is no specific treatment, but the patient should be carefully observed during the recovery period.

Compulsory treatment

Although drug abuse and drug dependence *per se* do not constitute grounds for compulsory admission to hospital, a patient may sometimes become so severely disturbed as a result of taking drugs that treatment is essential either to protect the patient, or to protect others from the patient's actions. For example, a patient may be so violent and aggressive that he or she has to be physically restrained from attacking anyone nearby. Under the influence of LSD, patients have been convinced of their ability to fly and have attempted to prove it by leaping from a window. These patients lack insight into their condition and are unlikely to consent to treatment. In such situations compulsory treatment is justified for any patient who is a danger to him or herself and/or anyone else, and is permitted under the 1983 Mental Health Act according to the following sections.

Section 2

Section 2 is relevant if the patient is seen at home or in the A & E department of the hospital. An application for admission is made based on the written recommendations of two registered medical practitioners who have examined the patient and have then completed the prescribed form. If possible, one doctor should have previous acquaintance with the patient (usually the patient's GP), while the other should be a doctor approved by the Secretary of State as having special experience in the diagnosis and treatment of mental disorder.

A patient who is admitted to hospital under Section 2 may be detained in hospital for up to 28 days, but no longer. Usually, however, the acute effects of the drug abuse have worn off long before the 28 days have elapsed, so that if a longer period of treatment is considered necessary the patient will probably by then be able to decide whether to agree to the treatment.

Section 4

If the patient is acutely and severely disturbed and in need of urgent treatment, it may not be possible to get hold of two doctors quickly enough. In this case an emergency application may be made under Section 4 of the Mental Health Act, either by a close relative of the patient or by an approved social worker. The emergency application must also be signed by one of the doctors described above (either the GP or the specialist). It lasts, as an interim measure, for only 72 hours, and during this time the second medical recommendation for hospital treatment is sought. If it is obtained, the patient can be detained in hospital for 28 days, if necessary.

Section 5

If a patient who is already in hospital becomes acutely disturbed and refuses treatment and/or tries to leave hospital when it is clear that he or she is a danger to him or herself and/or others, the patient may be detained and treated under Section 5 of the Mental Health Act. The registered medical practitioner in charge of the patient makes the formal application which can be enforced for only 72 hours. If it is not possible for a doctor to come immediately to sign the requisite form, a nurse may detain the patient until the doctor arrives, for up to 6 hours.

The drowsy or unconscious patient

Unconsciousness in the course of drug abuse and dependence is usually due to an overdose of an opiate drug or of a sedative hypnotic drug such as a barbiturate, benzodiazepine or methaqualone. Sometimes drugs of both types are taken together causing a potentiation of their effects; alcohol consumption may also contribute to the clinical picture. Prolonged solvent sniffing can also cause unconsciousness. Indeed, coma may be the consequence of an overdose of almost any drug; if it occurs after drugs such as amphetamine, LSD, cannabis, phencyclidine, etc. it is evidence of a very severe degree of poisoning.

Whatever the cause, the priorities of treatment are the same as for any unconscious patient: to establish an adequate airway and to support the circulation, if necessary. The first step, therefore, is to assess the vital signs. If there is no pulse, cardiopulmonary resuscitation should be started immediately. If the heart is beating, the patient's breathing should be assessed. Central nervous system depressants cause respiratory depression so that slow, shallow breathing is common and there may even be apnoea (breathing stops). If respiration is absent or inadequate, assisted ventilation by mouth-to-mouth resuscitation or Ambu-bag inflation should be started. In hospital, endotracheal intubation can be performed and the patient established on a ventilator. If intubation and ventilation are not needed, an oropharyngeal airway will prevent the tongue from falling back and obstructing the airway. Oxygen may be administered because these patients are usually hypoxic, but this should be done carefully in case the relief of hypoxia precipitates apnoea. The patient should be nursed semiprone to keep the airway clear and to prevent the aspiration of vomit.

Once urgent first-aid measures have been carried out, a rapid physical examination should be made. The following points should be noted to aid diagnosis and so that appropriate action can be initiated.

1 *Blood pressure.* Low blood pressure (hypotension) is common after barbiturate overdose. Because a systolic blood pressure of less than 80 mmHg may cause brain and kidney damage, it should be treated promptly: intravenous fluids should be administered, preferably with central venous pressure monitoring to prevent fluid overload. High blood pressure may occur in amphetamine intoxication and can be treated with a beta-adrenoreceptor-blocking drug (e.g. propranolol).

2 *Pulse.* If arrhythmias occur, ECG (electrocardiograph) monitoring should be initiated so that appropriate treatment can be started.

3 *Chest sounds.* Severe pulmonary oedema is a life-threatening complication of opiate overdose. It should be treated with positive pressure ventilation. Aspiration pneumonia is common after opiate overdose because of depressed reflexes and opiate-induced vomiting.

4 *Pupil-size.* Pin-point pupils are (almost) diagnostic of opiate use, but pilocar-pine, used in the treatment of glaucoma, also causes miosis. Pupillary constriction may be absent after opiate use if large amounts of amphetamine or cocaine were taken at the same time. Prolonged hypoxia, caused by respiratory depression and leading to cerebral (brain stem) anoxia, produces fixed, dilated pupils. In other words, the absence of pin-point pupils does not rule out the possibility of opiate overdose.

5 *Breath odour.* This may indicate consumption of alcohol or solvent sniffing.

6 *Evidence of trauma.* Note especially any head injury that may be contributing to unconscious state.

7 *Evidence of injection.* Needle marks, abscesses, fibrosed veins, etc. suggest long-term drug abuse and probable dependence. The possibility of the emergence of an abstinence syndrome should be borne in mind.

8 *Liver size.* Enlarged liver and/or presence of jaundice suggests impaired liver function. All resuscitative measures should be planned to minimize the risk of precipitating hepatic failure.

9 *Body temperature.* Hypothermia is common in patients who have been unconscious for a long time, and particularly after barbiturate (or phenothiazine) overdose. It is easily missed unless the temperature is taken (rectally) using a low-reading thermometer. The patient should be wrapped in blankets to conserve heat and not exposed unnecessarily for examination and investigation. Hyperthermia (after stimulant overdose) should be treated promptly with sponging, ice-packs and fanning.

10 *Investigations.* Blood should be taken for toxicological analysis, for blood sugar, urea and electrolyte estimation, and for a blood count. Emergency management cannot wait for the results of these tests, but they establish a baseline which may be helpful for future decisions about treatment.

11 *Additional measures.* If hypoglycaemia is suspected, administer 50 ml of 50% glucose solution. According to the general condition of the patient (level of consciousness, pulse, blood pressure, respiration) the following measures may be necessary:

(a) an intravenous line can be established to provide rapid access to the circulation, if this proves necessary;

(b) an indwelling urinary catheter may be inserted to monitor urinary output and 50 ml of urine sent for toxicological analysis as soon as possible. Because drugs are concentrated in the urine, they are more likely to be detected there than in the blood sample;

(c) cardiac monitoring can be initiated;

(d) gastric lavage may be appropriate if the drug is known to have been taken orally within the previous 4 hours. It should only be done if the heart rate and circulation are stable and should only be attempted in an unconscious patient if there is a cuffed endotracheal tube in place to prevent the aspiration of stomach contents.

Specific measures

Opiate overdose

If unconsciousness is thought to be due to an overdose of an opiate drug, the opiate antagonist, naloxone, can be given. It should be administered intravenously in a dose of 0.4 mg (1 ml), and this can be repeated at intervals of 2–3 minutes until sufficient naloxone has been given to reverse the effect of the opiate overdose: respiration (rate and volume) increases, systolic blood pressure increases, the pupils dilate and the level of consciousness improves. The total dose of naloxone that is required to achieve this improvement varies, according to the dose of opiate that was taken and on pre-existing physical dependence on opiates. There is usually some response after two or three doses, but more may be needed for the full effect.

The duration of action of naloxone is shorter than that of many opiates, so that there is a risk that the patient may slip back into unconsciousness as the effect of naloxone wears off. It is essential, therefore, that the patient should remain under observation after he or she regains consciousness, so that repeated doses of naloxone can be given if necessary. This is especially important if the overdose is of methadone or of the even longer-acting L-alpha-acetylmethadol (LAAM), when monitoring should continue for at least 72 hours. In such cases, continuous intravenous infusion (2 mg naloxone diluted in 500 ml saline) obviates the need for repeated injections and the rate of infusion can be adjusted to maintain consciousness, respiration and blood pressure at satisfactory levels.[23]

The response to naloxone in cases of opiate overdose is so reliable that a lack of response implies that opiates have not been taken, or are not the cause of the patient's present state. Up to 10 mg naloxone (in divided doses) can be given to establish this point, and as naloxone has virtually no effect when administered alone, this therapeutic trial has no adverse effect if the patient's condition is not due to opiate overdose (but see below).

Naloxone should be administered cautiously to those who are (or are suspected of being) physically dependent on opiates. Once the respiratory depression has been counteracted, 'surplus' naloxone precipitates the opiate abstinence syndrome. This is short-lived (because of the short duration of action of naloxone) and although not hazardous for the patient, is uncomfortable and distressing. If it occurs, the patient should be reassured that it will not last long, but no attempt should be made to overcome it by giving opiates.

Later, when the effects of the overdose have completely worn off, an opiate-dependent individual will manifest signs of opiate withdrawal. This should be managed by restabilizing the patient on methadone, using the procedure described in Chapter 7.

Naloxone is generally considered to be a pure opiate antagonist, devoid of pharmacological activity except for its reversal of opiate effects. It may, very rarely, cause hypertension, pulmonary oedema and cardiac arrhythmias (usually only in those with an underlying cardiac abnormality). The risk of these serious adverse effects is so small that naloxone continues to be recommended for the treatment of opiate overdose.

Benzodiazepine overdose

Flumazenil is a specific benzodiazepine antagonist with high affinity for benzodiazepine receptors, where it competitively binds and displaces benzodiazepines. It is therefore very useful in the management of benzodiazepine overdose but only by intravenous administration. Although it is rapidly absorbed following oral administration, little of the drug reaches the systemic circulation because of immediate metabolism in the liver and effective oral doses are accompanied by side effects. Intravenous administration of 1 mg flumazenil over a period of 1–3 minutes is usually sufficient to abolish the effects of therapeutic doses of benzodiazepines. Patients with suspected benzodiazepine overdose should respond to a cumulative dose of 1–5 mg, given over 2–10 minutes. Indeed, a failure to respond to 5 mg of flumazenil makes the diagnosis of benzodiazepine overdose unlikely – or at least suggests that this is not the primary cause of the sedation. Because the half-life of intravenous flumazenil is about 1 hour, the duration of its clinical effectiveness is limited and additional courses of treatment may therefore be necessary if sedation recurs.[24] Careful observation of the patient is therefore essential, so that a lapse into unconsciousness does not go unnoticed or untreated.

Other sedative hypnotics

There are no other antagonists for the treatment of sedative overdose so that the keynote of treatment is good supportive care (which should also be provided to patients with benzodiazepine overdose). Forced alkaline diuresis used to be advocated for patients in deep coma, but this procedure is not without risk and it is now recognized that it is useful only for severe phenobarbitone poisoning. Charcoal haemoperfusion is used for patients with severe barbiturate poisoning whose condition fails to improve or who deteriorate despite good care.

Particular problems may occur when those who are dependent on sedative hypnotic drugs take a larger than usual dose and become unconscious. Their initial management is the same as for any patient with a sedative overdose, but when the effect of the drug wears off, the abstinence syndrome will become manifest. If it does, it must be treated promptly so that serious complications (e.g. fits) are prevented. Thus the possibility that the patient is dependent on sedatives must be borne in mind so that he or she can be questioned about drug-taking habits when consciousness is regained. In addition, patients should be monitored carefully after recovery, so that the important, early signs of the abstinence syndrome are not missed. If these signs are present, a suitable sedative drug should be given, e.g. phenobarbitone 120 mg or diazepam 20 mg, and the procedure for stabilization and gradual detoxification described in Chapter 7 should be adopted. Drugs should not be prescribed in the absence of objective signs of withdrawal, even if the patient claims to be suffering from this and asks for drugs.

Another problem, seen most often in those who are dependent on barbiturates and/or methaqualone, is that the patient becomes very restless on recovery from a period of unconsciousness. Such patients may be hostile and aggressive and refuse to stay in bed, staggering around and generally being very difficult to manage. As they are still in an intoxicated condition it is undesirable to prescribe a sedative drug which may precipitate a further episode of unconsciousness. If absolutely necessary, a small dose of chlorpromazine can be administered.

Phencyclidine overdose

Large doses of phencyclidine cause stupor or coma, in which the eyes usually remain open, although the patient only responds to deep pain. The pupils are constricted and there may be roving eye movements, dysconjugate gaze and nystagmus. There is often severe muscle rigidity and episodes of jerky, tonic-clonic movements and facial grimacing. Repeated episodes of vomiting can occur and hypersalivation is common. Life-threatening complications include convulsions, severe hypertension and cardiac arrhythmias (cardiac arrest). Respiratory depression is more likely to develop if opiates, sedatives or alcohol have been taken too.

Gastric lavage can remove large quantities of phencyclidine from the stomach and should be attempted. However, endotracheal intubation is often very difficult because of intense laryngeal spasm and, if intubation is essential for the purpose of ventilation, large (anaesthetic) doses of muscle relaxant may be required.

Severe hypertension should be treated promptly to prevent cerebral haemorrhage. Diazoxide 100–150 mg should be administered as an intravenous bolus and repeated after 10–15 minutes if necessary. Convulsions should be treated with diazepam which is administered slowly and intravenously. The usual dose is 5–10 mg, repeated if required at 10- to 15-minute intervals.

Convulsions

Convulsions arising in the course of drug abuse and/or dependence usually occur in one of two situations.

1 During withdrawal from a high dose of sedatives in a dependent individual.

2 During severe intoxication with certain drugs: usually stimulants (such as amphetamine or cocaine) or phencyclidine or, more rarely, after very high doses of opiate drugs (such as morphine, pethidine or dextropropoxyphene), or LSD or methaqualone. Convulsions may also develop if prolonged hypotension has led to cerebral anoxia, or if the drug abuser has a low 'epileptic threshold' so that fits are precipitated by any one of a number of reasons.

Single, short-lived convulsions do not necessarily require treatment. If they occur repeatedly or are prolonged, they should be treated with intravenous diazepam (preferably in emulsion form) injected at the rate of 5 mg/min until the fits are controlled. A dose of 10–20 mg is usually sufficient and can be repeated, if necessary, after 30–60 minutes. If convulsions recur, diazepam can be administered by slow intravenous infusion. Because of the risk of respiratory depression when diazepam is given intravenously, equipment should be available for intubation and ventilation if necessary.

Once the emergency treatment of convulsions has been carried out, their cause should be assessed. Patients suffering from the sedative abstinence syndrome should be stabilized on an appropriate drug (diazepam or phenobarbitone) and should undergo supervised detoxification.

Special problems

The pregnant addict

Pregnancy

The antenatal care of the pregnant drug addict or drug abuser has exactly the same aims as for the nondrug-abuser – to keep the woman in good health for her own sake, and to give her the best chance of delivering a healthy child. Achieving these aims is often complicated not only by the pharmacological effects of the drugs the mother uses but also by her lifestyle.

To start with, the diagnosis of pregnancy and hence the initiation of antenatal care may be delayed because there is a high incidence of abnormal menstrual cycles and amenorrhoea during opiate administration, which often resolves when drug use is interrupted. Thus, it may happen that a woman who has become pregnant while temporarily abstinent assumes that her subsequent amenorrhoea is due to a resumption of drug-taking, and does not present to an antenatal clinic until well into her pregnancy, when her increasing weight and enlarging abdomen become apparent. This late presentation may be particularly disadvantageous for those living in poor environmental conditions and with poor nutrition who need the vitamin and mineral supplementation routinely provided during pregnancy. Others may attend antenatal clinics, but are frightened to admit their dependence and conceal it from obstetricians and others.[1,2]

However, once aware of their pregnant condition, many drug addicts do approach their GP or another agency for advice. Their motivation to come off drugs may be high at this time because they are afraid that their new-born child will be taken from them, or at least placed on the Child Protection Register, if they are still taking drugs at the time of birth. It is very important that these women, with all the normal emotional sensitivity and vulnerability of pregnancy, plus their additional anxieties and feelings of guilt, should be handled with tact and sensitivity, so that they are attracted into and are retained in treatment and that nothing deters them from seeking further help.

The majority of pregnant drug addicts are dependent on opiates that cross the placenta and affect the fetus directly. Constantly exposed to these drugs, the fetus also becomes dependent on them and suffers from withdrawal if the mother is deprived of her drugs. This may precipitate fetal distress or death or induce premature labour.[3] On the other hand, an opiate overdose may also affect the fetus adversely. A similar situation arises with those dependent on sedative hypnotics, but this type of drug dependence may be particularly hazardous for the fetus because it is often associated with a chaotic lifestyle, alternating episodes of intoxication and withdrawal, with rapidly fluctuating blood levels of the drug. Obviously, if the mother injects drugs, the fetus is constantly exposed to the risk of infection and the effects of unidentified adulterants.

Whenever possible, pregnant women should be encouraged to come into hospital at least for the initial assessment period and, in an effort to engage all patients in treatment, clinic and in-patient units should be more flexible than usual and ready to make exceptions to their usual policies. The ideal management is to assist the pregnant woman to come off drugs as comfortably and as early in pregnancy as possible. Ideally, the patient should be drug free for at least 2 months before the expected date of delivery as this will ensure a nonaddicted infant, even if there is some uncertainty about dates.

For opiate-dependent patients, methadone withdrawal should be achieved gradually, to avoid precipitating fetal distress or premature labour, and the withdrawal programme should be individually tailored according to the severity of dependence, the stage of pregnancy and the general level of cooperation and motivation. When a pregnant patient is unable to cope with being drug free or has presented too late in pregnancy for complete withdrawal to be feasible, then maintenance on the lowest possible dose of oral methadone is an acceptable alternative to the ideal. Generally, and empirically, a dose of 25–30 mg or less of methadone daily is acceptable. It is essential that pregnant barbiturate addicts should be weaned off their drugs and should adopt a more stable lifestyle.

Liaison with the obstetrician and with local social services is essential during the treatment of pregnant patients. In many cases it can be anticipated that a case conference will be arranged after the birth to consider the degree of risk to which the baby is exposed and to plan appropriate action. This should be explained to the mother who should be reassured that each situation is assessed individually. It may then be a powerful inducement to her to cooperate fully with the treatment regime and to withdraw from drugs, if she knows that being drug free at delivery and achieving stability substantially improves her chances of keeping her child. On the other hand, if she believes that the child will automatically be removed or placed on the Child Protection Register, she may retreat from any source of professional help only to reappear near term, or even in labour. By this time the baby is genuinely at risk and the opportunity for positive action has been lost.

Antenatal screening

All pregnant addicts (and those planning to have a child) should be encouraged to be tested for HIV antibodies and for hepatitis. The woman will then be able to make an informed choice about whether or not she wishes to continue with the pregnancy (or whether or not she wishes to become pregnant). Secondly, if she is found to be positive for HIV or hepatitis, she can be offered appropriate medical treatment, as can the baby, if she continues with the pregnancy. The management of HIV in pregnancy is discussed in Chapter 8.

Labour

Pain relief in labour

The management of pain relief in labour for women who have been using opiates during pregnancy can be more difficult than usual because the dose of opiate required to achieve adequate analgesia for the mother may be too high as far as the baby is concerned. An epidural anaesthetic may therefore be indicated and this, as well as other approaches to pain control, should be discussed with the mother beforehand so that her anxieties can be acknowledged and discussed and so that her wishes can be taken into account.

Infection control in the labour room

Although drug abusers who self-inject are more likely to be HIV-positive and more likely to be carriers of hepatitis virus, no special precautions need be taken for them in the labour room over and above those taken for any other woman. This of course assumes that all delivery units maintain a high standard of care, with adequate precautions being taken for every delivery, so that there is then no reason to single out and stigmatize women who are positive for these infections, and staff are not at risk when dealing with undiagnosed cases.

The neonate

Congenital abnormalities

A major concern for the pregnant drug abuser is the fear that her baby will have a congenital abnormality attributable to drug-taking in pregnancy. In fact, there is little evidence that any of the common drugs of abuse are teratogenic. Although LSD produces chromosomal damage in human leucocytes in culture, and can cause congenital malformations in rats and mice, there is no firm evidence of its teratogenicity in humans. Similarly, although cannabis has been suspected of causing limb deformities, this is a fairly common abnormality, so that anecdotal accounts of such abnormalities in babies born to cannabis abusers do not prove causality. There have been similar stories about the effects of cocaine abuse on the fetus, but again little in the way of proof of teratogenicity.

When interpreting reports of teratogenicity, it should be remembered that the majority of drug abusers are polydrug abusers and may not remember which drugs they took during the critical period of teratogen sensitivity in the early weeks of pregnancy. Furthermore, even if they do remember, illicit drugs are usually impure and may be contaminated with unknown adulterants that may, themselves, be teratogenic. This serves to emphasize the point that, although none of the common drugs of abuse have definitely been implicated as teratogens, their consumption along with unknown contaminants is a violation of the general principle that no unnecessary drugs should be taken during pregnancy.[3]

Low birthweight

Numerically, a far greater problem than the potential risk of teratogenicity is that of low birthweight, which has frequently been reported in babies born to mothers dependent on opiates.[4] Indeed, in one study, 31% of such babies were light for gestational age. The significance of low birthweight is its association with increased infant morbidity and mortality, but it is not clear to what extent these adverse effects are attributable directly to the drug of abuse or to the pregnant addict's lifestyle. There may, for example, have been repeated episodes of drug withdrawal during pregnancy, affecting blood flow to the placenta and impairing fetal growth. Repeated episodes of infection and maternal undernutrition may also have undesirable effects. It has been suggested that cannabis and cocaine, by impairing fetal oxygenation, may contribute to poor growth. Both drugs increase maternal blood pressure and heart rate, and cocaine causes uterine vasoconstriction; cannabis, like cigarette smoking, impairs oxygenation by substantially increasing blood carboxyhaemoglobin levels.

A final point worth noting in relation to low birthweight is that the majority of drug abusers smoke and drink alcohol too. Both of these drugs are known to be associated with low birthweight, so that identifying the additional effects of specific drugs of abuse is very difficult.

Neonatal abstinence syndrome

There have been many reports of a neonatal abstinence syndrome developing in babies born to opiate-dependent mothers. It arises because the blood-borne supply of opiates on which the baby has become dependent during its intrauterine life is abruptly cut off. The infants are described as hyperactive, irritable and restless, with tremors and sometimes convulsions; some may have gastrointestinal disturbance with vomiting.[3] The onset of the neonatal abstinence syndrome depends very much on the duration of action of the opiate on which the mother is dependent. In an infant born to a heroin-dependent mother, signs are usually apparent within 24 hours, but may be delayed to the second or third day, whereas in infants born to methadone-dependent mothers the withdrawal syndrome does not usually start until 48–72 hours after birth and may be delayed even later.[1,3,5]

It should be emphasized that the neonatal abstinence syndrome does not always occur, but depends on the dose of opiate taken by the mother, the duration of her dependence and the timing of the last dose in relation to the time of delivery. When illicit opiates continue to be abused during pregnancy, the adulterants may also affect the manifestations of the abstinence syndrome.[6]

Treatment should be initiated if withdrawal signs are observed. A number of treatments have been tried over the years, including the inhalation of opium smoke and a variety of sedatives, such as paregoric (camphorated tincture of opium), barbiturates and chlorpromazine. Breast-feeding has been advocated if the mother continues to take opiates on the grounds that they are believed to be secreted into breast milk and can thus ameliorate the abstinence syndrome. On theoretical grounds, however, the administration of opiates to the infant after delivery is contraindicated, as any metabolic changes induced by exposure to them in utero are likely to be accentuated by their continued use. Chlorpromazine is generally recommended as the drug of choice, but it should be started only if there is evidence of progression in the number or severity of the signs of withdrawal. The dose should subsequently be reduced in a stepwise fashion every 2 or 3 days. Prophylactic treatment, with chlorpromazine or any other drug, is not recommended, because it is unjustifiable to expose those who are not going to manifest the withdrawal syndrome, or those who will do so only mildly, to yet more unnecessary drugs. Instead, an alert watch should be kept so that signs can be treated promptly, if and when necessary. Problems may arise when the mother's drug use is neither known nor suspected, so that diagnosis of the infant's physical condition is delayed.

With the increasing use of psychotropic drugs, many of which have a dependence-producing capacity, other withdrawal syndromes have been described in neonates. The signs of barbiturate withdrawal in the new-born are similar to those of opiate withdrawal although their onset is often delayed, sometimes for up to 4–7 days after birth. This delay can itself be hazardous as mother and baby may be discharged before the withdrawal syndrome manifests itself. Cases of benzodiazepine withdrawal (similar to barbiturate withdrawal) in infants have also been described. Experience in managing neonatal sedative hypnotic withdrawal is limited, but phenobarbitone is a logical choice of drug treatment to minimize the risk of convulsions.

The effects of maternal amphetamine abuse on the neonate are not clear. Although withdrawal signs have been described occasionally, it is not apparent whether these are really due to amphetamine or to concomitant use of opiates.

HIV and the neonate

It is very important that babies born to HIV-positive mothers should be tested for the presence of antibodies and maternal consent for this should be sought. Ideally, this will have been discussed with the mother at some time during her pregnancy, rather than being left until after delivery, when the new mother is likely to be emotionally labile.

Risk of transmission is increased by higher viral load (see Chapter 8), more advanced clinical HIV disease or lower CD4 cell count, and with prolonged rupture of membranes, premature birth, or low birthweight, or events risking fetal exposure to maternal blood.[7,8]

It should be noted that a positive HIV test at birth does not necessarily mean that the baby has been infected, because babies are born with the mother's antibodies, which persist for up to 18 months. An antibody test at this later date will give more reliable information, but as this is a long time to wait, other blood tests may be carried out in the interim that may help to determine whether or not the child has been infected.

Hepatitis and the neonate

Babies born to mothers who are hepatitis carriers should be immunized as soon as possible after birth, or at least within 12 hours of birth, because this significantly reduces the chance of the baby developing the persistent carrier state. Infants of mothers who are HBV-DNA-positive (indicating active viral replication) are most at risk and active immunization with the vaccine should be combined with simultaneous passive immunization (administration of hepatitis immuno-globulin) at a different site. This has been shown to have a success rate of over 80% in keeping infants HBsAg-negative at 1-year follow-up. Infants born to mothers who are HBsAg-positive, but HBV-DNA-negative have a low risk of becoming HBsAg-positive and immunization may not be necessary for these children.

Breast-feeding

Although breast milk is acknowledged to be the best food for the new-born baby, other factors must be taken into account when advising drug abusers about breast-feeding. Firstly, the mother's HIV status is an important consideration. HIV has been found in breast milk and it is thought that transmission to the baby via breast-feeding can occur. For this reason, HIV-positive women in the UK have been advised not to breast-feed. However, in countries where adequate substitutes are not available, the advantages of breast-feeding may outweigh the potential risk. There appears to be a low risk of transmission of hepatitis C virus in breast milk.[9]

It must also be remembered that many drugs that may cause toxicity in the infant enter breast milk in pharmacologically significant quantities. Barbiturates and benzodiazepines, for example, do enter breast milk and can cause lethargy and drowsiness in the infant. Therefore, if the mother is still receiving these drugs because detoxification before delivery was not possible, it is not advisable for her to breast-feed her baby. The same advice applies to those maintained on opiates (heroin or methadone) and to those who are likely to abuse illicit drugs after discharge from hospital. As a general principle, breast-feeding is no longer considered the best method of alleviating the neonatal abstinence syndrome (from any drug) and the mother should be advised to bottle-feed.

The child at risk

Once the hazards of the neonatal period have passed, the question remains of whether there is any longer-term effect of the baby's prolonged exposure to drugs in utero. Various studies of children born to opiate-dependent mothers have reported abnormal behaviour patterns in these children as they grow older, and developmental delays are said to occur.[10] Later, impaired concentration, hyperactivity and aggression have also been noted. It is, however, impossible to know if these patterns of behaviour and development are more likely to occur in children born to opiate-dependent mothers than to nondrug-dependent mothers and, if they do, whether they are due to intrauterine exposure to opiates or to their childhood environment, particularly if parental drug abuse continues.

Drug use by parents does not always indicate that they are bad parents. Nevertheless, there is a natural and often severe anxiety about the well-being of children in such a family. This is partly because the harsh facts of child abuse have become apparent to all, through wide exposure in the media, so that the prevention of any more horrifying instances is now of overriding importance. This has led to some local authorities automatically putting the children of addicts on the Child Protection Register, sometimes at birth. Indeed, in some countries it is routine for a baby born to a drug-addicted parent to be removed from the mother at birth, on the grounds that the child is perceived to be at risk of abuse or neglect by reason of their parents' drug-taking. The opposite point of view is that children of drug abusers are no more or no less at risk than children born to any other group of parents, but undoubtedly the reality lies somewhere between these two opinions – some children are at risk and some are not. Preliminary research suggests that abuse is no more common by drug-using parents than by the rest of the population, but that there is an increased incidence of injury as a result of accidents associated with drug use.

It is clearly of the utmost importance, whenever a drug abuser who is also a parent approaches a treatment agency for help, that the child is not overlooked and that the child's welfare receives specific and deliberate attention during the assessment procedure. It is essential to identify their physical and emotional needs and to make an accurate assessment of the risks to which they are exposed because of parental drug abuse. This assessment must be made in a systematic fashion so that a complete picture is built up of that child's lifestyle. Then, and only then, should a decision be made about his or her future care. The specific questions to be answered by the assessment procedure are shown below.

1 Provision of basic necessities.
   (a) Is the accommodation adequate for children and are rent and bills being paid? (How much do drugs cost and how is the money raised?)
   (b) Does the family remain in one area or do they move frequently? If so, why?
   (c) Is there adequate food, clothing and heating?
   (d) Does the child attend school regularly and how is he or she achieving at school?
   (e) Are the child's emotional needs being met adequately?
   (f) Has the quality of child care changed since drug abuse began? Does it improve during periods of abstinence?

2 Home environment.
   (a) Do other drug abusers share the accommodation; is the family living in a drug-using community?
   (b) Is the accommodation used for selling drugs?
   (c) Is the child left alone while parents are procuring drugs?
   (d) Does the child have to assume parental responsibilities?
   (e) Is the child taken by the parents to places where they may be at risk?
   (f) Is the child engaged in age-appropriate activities?

3 Pattern of parental drug use.
   (a) Type, quantity and method of administration of drug?
   (b) Are drugs used in the child's presence?
   (c) Is drug use stable or chaotic?
   (d) Is there polydrug abuse?
   (e) Is alcohol abused?
   (f) Does the drug-abusing parent swing between periods of intoxication and periods of withdrawal?
   (g) How does this affect child care?

4 Health risks to child.
   (a) Where are drugs kept?
   (b) Can the child gain access to them?
   (c) If drugs are used by injection, where are syringes and needles kept?
   (d) Are they shared?
   (e) How are syringes and needles disposed of?

5 Family's support and social network.

    (a) Is there a drug-free parent (or supportive partner)?

    (b) Do parents and children associate primarily with drug abusers, nonabusers or both?

    (c) Are relatives aware of drug use? Are they supportive?

    (d) Will parents accept help from relatives or friends and/or other agencies?

6 Parents' perception of the situation.

    (a) Do parents see their drug use as harmful (or potentially harmful) to themselves or their children? Are they aware of the health risks of their drug-taking practices to the children?

    (b) Do parents place their own needs before those of their children?

    (c) Are parents willing to cooperate with monitoring of the situation by nurseries, schools, health visitor, social worker, etc?

When all this information is elicited, it gives a very good idea of what life is like for the child in that household and, in particular, of the degree to which the child's life is affected by parental drug use, or indeed revolves around that drug use. It will be established, for example, whether there are times when the parent is unconscious from a drug overdose when an unsupervised child might play with a dirty syringe, or take tablets that have been left lying around. If the quality of parenting changes little during episodes of abstinence, there may be scant grounds for optimism that things will improve after detoxification. Many such factors must be taken into account, but from the point of view of the child, the single most important factor that may make home life possible is the presence of a nondrug-using, supportive parent or their partner.

This type of assessment procedure should be carried out regardless of whether it is the father or mother who is abusing drugs. It is of course more important if it is the main care provider (or the only care provider in a single-parent family), usually the mother, who is dependent on drugs, but clearly many of the risk factors are independent of which parent is involved; bottles of tablets or dirty syringes left lying around where an unsupervised toddler can reach them are always dangerous. In some families, both parents abuse drugs and this exposes the child to even greater risk. The age(s) of the child(ren) concerned is also relevant. Younger children are at greater physical risk of neglect and accidental injury and there may be clear evidence of failure to thrive. Older children, although better able to fend for themselves physically, are more likely to recognize drug-taking and to understand its significance and so may be more emotionally vulnerable.

When all the information about the child and his or her lifestyle has been gathered, a management plan must be formulated. Where a team approach is adopted for the care of drug abusers, it is essential that a keyworker should be nominated who will maintain contact with the family and who will assume special responsibility for the welfare of the child. It is all too easy, in the midst of dealing with the multidimensional problems of drug abuse, to forget, or at least to overlook, the most vulnerable and least articulate members of the family. It is crucial to have one member of the team whose responsibility it is to remind others of the existence of the children and to safeguard their interests.

The management plan should then identify the existing and potential risks to the children and define the particular circumstances that would, if they arose, give rise to special concern. The name and telephone number of the responsible social worker to be contacted on such an occasion should be recorded and accessible. The way in which the family's situation will be monitored and the children will be visited must be decided, and a date set when the child care aspects of the case will be reviewed. The particular needs and difficulties of the children should be discussed and the ways of dealing with them decided. Many families with a drug-abusing parent are already known to other agencies (social services, probation service, GP) and it is essential that close liaison is maintained with them. They may be able to play a valuable role in monitoring the situation, but feel unable to complete the total assessment without specialized aid. Again, it is the responsibility of the keyworker from the drug-dependence treatment team to liaise with other involved professionals, so that the situation does not arise in which a child's problems are known to many agencies, but appear to be the responsibility of none. Where there are preschool-age children, the family's health visitor will usually be contacted as he or she is in an excellent position to observe the children for any evidence of failure to thrive, neglect or physical abuse. For older children it may be appropriate to contact the school, where teachers who see the children every day are well placed to monitor their well-being. Parental consent must, of course, be obtained before schools or other agencies are contacted and confidential information disclosed, but in some situations concern about the child may make it necessary to override the wishes of the family. Satisfactory resolution of a conflict between the needs of the child and the rights of the parent requires good judgement and a high degree of professionalism. In rare cases, under the Children's Act of 1989, if the parents refuse to cooperate in a full assessment of the child's situation, even though the professionals involved believe that there is a risk of significant harm to the child, a Child Assessment Order can be made. This allows a full enquiry to be made into the state of the child's health and development and the way in which he or she has been treated, to decide what further action, if any, is required.

If it appears that there is immediate risk to the child – for example, if drug abuse is chaotic with periods of intoxication, when the parent becomes aggressive, or if a young baby is suffering physical neglect – clearly the child must be removed promptly from the family home. This may be done by means of an Emergency Protection Order, followed by a court case, which may lead to permanent removal of the child or plans for the parent's/parents' rehabilitation; sometimes wardship proceedings are initiated in the High Court. Such actions are fortunately uncommon. It is more likely that although there is no immediate risk to the child, there is some concern and anxiety about his or her welfare that cannot be adequately monitored and protected. In this situation, a case conference should be called to which all the involved and relevant professionals are invited, as well as the family. The outcome will depend on the individual circumstances, but it is likely that either the child will be removed from the family (by one of the proceedings outlined above), or that the child's name will be placed on the Child Protection Register. This means that there will be active involvement of a social worker with the family and further case conferences to monitor the progress of the child will be held. Liaison and communication between the different professions are formalized and every possible supportive service for parents and child is utilized.

It must be emphasized, however, that it is the exception rather than the rule for a formal case conference to be necessary. While recognizing the potential hazards for children growing up in a drug-abusing household, there is no need to exaggerate their problems, that can usually be adequately managed in a less formal manner by the team of professionals caring for the family. A policy of automatically putting all these children on the Child Protection Register may not substantially improve their management, and risks alienating their parents from all professional help. The rehabilitation of the drug abuser and the family, on which the child's welfare ultimately depends, may thus be adversely affected. A far better approach is to assess each family separately, in the way suggested here, and to respond to the children's needs in an individually appropriate manner.

The drug-abusing doctor: the 'professional' addict

The problems of doctors who abuse drugs have long been recognized and there has always been a tacit understanding that they are a 'special' case. In part, this is one consequence of a medical rather than a criminal approach to addiction, with the medical profession responding with empathy to the problems of one of their own kind, but in some ways the 'professional' addicts (doctors, dentists, veterinary surgeons, pharmacists and nurses), are genuinely different from street addicts. They have access to, and usually take, pharmaceutical preparations of drugs which they obtain by a variety of deceptions. The most commonly abused drugs (after alcohol) are the manufactured opiates, particularly pethidine, but also dextromoramide and dipipanone, morphine and sedative hypnotics such as the benzodiazepines. Self-medication for pain and occupational stress are often cited as reasons for the initiation of drug abuse. Professional addicts suffer fewer complications of drug abuse because they use pure, unadulterated drugs and, if they inject, because they have sterile injection equipment and employ sterile techniques. However, the purity of their drugs means that they can have high levels of intake more easily than street addicts and many may become severely dependent. Their drug-taking is nearly always a solitary activity: doctors, unlike those with no profession, or with a job they do not value, have invested a lot in their career and have much to lose financially and in status and self-respect if their drug-taking is discovered. Many doctors successfully conceal their drug dependence for long periods of time and carry on working with apparently little, if any, impairment of their clinical activities. It has even been reported that doctors on high doses of opiates have been able to become suddenly abstinent with no evidence of the withdrawal syndrome, and it was suggested that it was the overwhelming fear of detection that effectively suppressed the expected manifestations.[11]

Eventually, of course, drug abuse and dependence is likely to come to light because of problems with family, personal health or work. There may be a deterioration in personal appearance, frequent emotional crises, admissions to hospital for illness or as a result of accidents, and so on. Abnormal behaviour with staff or patients may be noticed and there may be inappropriate clinical responses. The 'locked door' syndrome has been described – when the doctor has a drink or takes drugs in privacy. There may also be frequent job changes, with many drug-abusing doctors ending up in temporary positions as locums or in deputizing services.[12]

The identification of doctors with drug problems is usually difficult because they commonly deny that any problem exists – they may deny any use of drugs at all, or if they do admit taking drugs, rationalize this as a consequence of certain recent problems (rather than their cause). They usually minimize the dose of drug taken, the frequency of administration and the duration of this practice. Their denial and rationalization is compounded by the behaviour of friends, colleagues and family, who often have a shrewd suspicion of what is happening, but who are usually reluctant to discuss it openly. Eventually, their conspiracy of silence becomes a covert collusion, so that they cover up deficiencies and avoid any action that might publicly expose the drug-taking behaviour. This protective behaviour enables the continuation of the drug abuse and helps the doctor to avoid or minimize its consequences. In the long term such protection, however well intended, is unhelpful. It delays the initiation of treatment because affected doctors are unlikely to seek help on their own initiative, and it completely ignores the well-being of their patients and the hazards that this drug abuse exposes them to. It should be clearly understood, therefore, that doctors and other health professionals have an ethical responsibility to take action if they feel that a colleague has a drug problem that impairs (however slightly) his or her ability to practise medicine.

In the UK, this is spelled out by the General Medical Council who state 'You must protect patients when you believe that a doctor's or other colleague's health, conduct or performance is a threat to them'. And also 'Before taking action, you should do your best to find out the facts. Then, if necessary, you must follow your employer's procedures or tell an appropriate person from the employing authority. . . . The safety of patients must come first at all times'.[13]

The best approach, in this situation, is to discuss the problem with other senior colleagues who are in close working relationship with the affected doctor, so that they can exert their influence in a positive and beneficial way, encouraging him or her to admit to the problem and to seek help for it. This confrontation, clearly not a comfortable situation for anyone, must be carefully planned so that it achieves the desired response. It is often better if two doctors approach their drug-abusing colleague together, one perhaps from the same specialty to offer support and friendship, the other a specialist in drug abuse, or perhaps a doctor recovering from drug abuse, to give expert practical advice on treatment. The affected doctor must not be allowed to rationalize the drug-taking and deny the problem, but must face up to the fact that he or she has a problem of which others are also aware. It should be understood that the intervention, which is probably resented as an intrusion into private affairs, is prompted by a genuine concern for the health and well-being of the doctor and that the colleagues, far from trying to stop him or her practising, are looking for a way towards recovery so that medical practice can be continued. At the same time, there should be no doubt that a refusal to seek help will have very serious implications for his or her future career. The doctors confronting the drug abuser should have a plan of action ready, so that they can offer positive suggestions about where and how to seek help. This will reduce the sense of despair that may ensue when the problem, with all its implications, has to be faced for the first time. The intensity of this despair should not be underestimated: it may, in some doctors, lead to attempted suicide. Prompt access to treatment facilities is therefore essential and it may be helpful to emphasize that this can be arranged outside the immediate sphere of work and contacts so that confidentiality is, as far as possible, maintained and damage to self-respect minimized.

Once this hurdle – of confronting the doctor and of forcing him or her to confront the problem and do something about it – has been overcome, the outlook improves considerably. Doctors who have been persuaded by a sympathetic, nonjudgmental approach to enter a treatment programme are likely to complete it, and probably have a better than average chance of making a complete recovery. Some, however, having taken very high doses of pure drugs for many years, have a severe degree of dependence and their prognosis is poorer – itself a very good reason for colleagues to practise early rather than late intervention. For all, detoxification is just the first stage of treatment and, like all other addicts, they require long-term help and support during their rehabilitation. Regular attendance at a doctors' self-help group may be of value and long-term treatment with the opiate antagonist naltrexone has been reported to be particularly effective in preventing relapse amongst highly motivated, abstinent 'doctor addicts'. Those who do become abstinent should be given every opportunity to resume medical practice, although continued supervision, including urine tests, will be necessary for some time. They may need to retrain to enter a field of medical practice that gives less easy access to drugs, and it may be necessary, with their consent, to inform a senior colleague of their previous history so that effective monitoring in the workplace is possible should a relapse occur.

It must be acknowledged that some doctors enter treatment, not after friendly persuasion by their colleagues, but by routes in which coercion is more overt. For those doctors who come to the attention of their professional disciplinary organization because of their drug abuse, resumption of medical practice will only be permitted when there is clear evidence of successful treatment and subsequent supervision. In the UK, for example, the General Medical Council (GMC) may receive information about a doctor's drug-taking from members of the public or the profession, from health authorities or the police. They advise that doctors should always be referred to the GMC if local action would not be practical, or if it has been tried but has failed; if the problem is very serious, or if the doctor has been convicted of a criminal offence, and they note that abuse of drugs or alcohol are common examples of serious problems in doctors and their practices that are referred to the GMC.[14]

Rather than initiating disciplinary procedures, this information is referred to the Preliminary Screener who decides whether action by the GMC under its health procedures is required. If it is decided that a doctor's fitness to practise does require investigation, the doctor is invited to undergo medical examination. After this, and if the doctor agrees to abide by the recommendations made about his or her treatment, supervision and professional practice, no further proceedings are taken, except to continue to monitor the case. If, however, the doctor refuses the medical examination or refuses to undergo treatment and continues to abuse drugs, then the case will be referred to the Health Committee, which may suspend the doctor's registration or impose conditions upon it.

Comorbidity

Concurrent substance misuse and psychiatric disorder is often described by the term 'dual diagnosis' or 'psychiatric comorbidity'. However, the simplicity of this terminology is misleading because relationships between the two components may be difficult to disentangle. For example, moderate substance use can affect the brain's neurochemistry and lead to psychiatric symptoms or syndromes, while intoxication, dependence and even withdrawal have their own specific effects. Furthermore, substance use may exacerbate or alter the course of a pre-existing mental disorder, or may mask it. Alternatively, a primary mental disorder may precipitate a substance use disorder, which in turn can lead to psychiatric syndromes.

Classification

Five main categories of comorbidity can be identified, although in some chronically ill patients it may be impossible to identify into which category they fall.[15,16]

1. Primary diagnosis of a major mental illness with a subsequent (secondary) diagnosis of substance misuse which adversely affects mental health. This may arise, for example, if there is self-medication with drugs or the use of alcohol to relieve psychiatric symptoms.
2. A primary diagnosis of drug dependence with psychiatric complications leading to mental illness. For example, depression (which may be suicidal) may occur in the course of substance misuse.
3. A concurrent substance misuse and psychiatric disorder, with the former exacerbating or altering the course of the latter.
4. The psychiatric disorder exacerbates or alters the course of substance misuse.
5. An underlying traumatic experience resulting in both substance misuse and psychiatric disorders, for example in post-traumatic stress disorder.

DSM-IV, with its multiaxial diagnosis, can be very useful in understanding the classification of comorbidity.

Prevalence

It is perhaps not surprising that, with increasing substance misuse over recent decades, there has been a growing awareness of, and interest in, dual diagnosis, and a number of studies have been carried out to ascertain its prevalence and to explore the links between specific morbidities and particular drugs. In the USA, for example, one study found that 41–66% of those with an addictive disorder also had at least one mental disorder, and that 51% of those with a mental disorder had at least one addictive disorder.[17,18] Similarly, in the UK, 10% of psychiatric in-patients were found to have an alcohol problem, while 40% of those with an alcohol problem had a dual diagnosis.[19]

These findings highlight a key issue in prevalence studies based on clinical samples because people with two or more conditions are more likely to seek professional help and enter treatment than those with just a single problem.[20,21] The results of a national household survey carried out in the UK are therefore of particular interest. This demonstrated a clear relationship between dependence on nicotine, alcohol and drugs and psychological morbidity, with 12% of the non-dependent population assessed as having any disorder compared with 22% of the nicotine-dependent, 30% of the alcohol-dependent and 45% of the drug-dependent individuals. Furthermore, 12% of drug-dependent individuals were assessed as having two or more disorders compared with only 1% of the nondependent population. This very marked association persisted even after various social and demographic variables were controlled for, so that it was possible to conclude that a drug-dependent subject was about three times more likely to have a disorder compared with a nondependent subject; alcohol- and nicotine-dependent individuals were about twice as likely to have a disorder than a nondependent subject. When the nature of the psychiatric disorder was explored in more detail, it was found that this relationship persisted across a range of psychiatric diagnoses with anxiety, depressive, phobic and panic disorders all occurring more frequently in the drug-dependent subjects.[22]

A study on the general population was also carried out in Australia, in the National Survey of Mental Health and Well-Being (NSMHWB), involving a sample of 10 641 adults and exploring the relationship between alcohol, cannabis and tobacco use and mental health. This, too, found an association between substance use and different patterns of comorbidity in the general population, with alcohol demonstrating a 'J-shaped' relationship with affective and anxiety disorders: alcohol users had lower rates of these problems than nonusers, while alcohol-dependent individuals had the highest rates. Tobacco and cannabis use (as in the UK) were both associated with increased rates of all mental health problems although, when factors such as demographics, neuroticism and other drug use were controlled for, cannabis use was not associated with anxiety or affective disorders. However, in common with tobacco use, cannabis dependence was correlated with screening positively for psychosis.[23]

The Australian study also investigated the prevalence of 'homotypic' comorbidity – the cooccurrence of two different substance use disorders – and found that separately, alcohol, cannabis and tobacco use were each associated with an increased likelihood of using the other drugs being studied and also that they were associated with the problematic use of other drug types, with the use of cannabis being the strongest marker for other types of drug abuse or dependence. Such findings must of course be taken into account when exploring 'heterotypic' comorbidity – dual diagnosis with disorders from two separate diagnostic groups. It is self-evident that some comorbid diagnoses are inevitably related to the same substance; for example, the psychiatric syndromes associated with alcohol withdrawal (e.g. delirium tremens) can only occur if there is alcohol dependence, which is likely to be associated with episodes of intoxication.

Aetiology

Identifying an association between psychiatric disorders and substance dependence does not, however, throw any light on the causal relationship between them and various theories have been put forward.[24] The common factor model proposes that there are underlying factor(s) contributing to the development of both the substance misuse disorder and the psychiatric diagnosis. Intuitively, this seems particularly likely in relation to antisocial personality disorder (ASPD), which is the most common psychiatric disorder amongst injecting drug users (although the diagnostic criteria for the former include some that are secondary to drug misuse).[25] In contrast, the hypersensitivity model postulates a biological vulnerability to psychiatric disorder resulting in sensitivity to small amounts of alcohol or drugs. Alternatively, there might be a premorbid psychiatric vulnerability that leads to early involvement in the use of nicotine, alcohol and other substances as a form of self-medication for unpleasant symptoms. Prospective studies that could resolve some of these issues would require a large number of young people followed up into adulthood, with monitoring of their consumption of nicotine, alcohol and other substances, both prescribed and nonprescribed. In the absence of such studies, a bidirectional model is perhaps the most useful and highlights the importance of screening those with substance use disorders for psychiatric morbidities.

Management

There is only limited information available on the outcome of different interventions for patients with dual diagnosis, but existing evidence suggests that there are increased levels of suicide, disengagement from, or noncontact with, services and poor compliance with medication and treatment regimes. Service provision therefore needs to be able to address these problems. In the absence of a universally accepted model of service provision, three different approaches have been described:

- Consecutive treatment, with programmes provided consecutively by the mental health and substance misuse services depending on the presenting problem;
- Parallel treatment, with the care of the patient provided by both services concurrently, facilitated by communication between the two services;
- Integrated treatment, with a single treatment system (a dual diagnosis team) in which the individual's substance misuse and psychiatric disorder are treated by the same clinician.

Consecutive treatment and parallel treatment both suffer from the disadvantage that each health problem is treated as a separate entity and the patient is seen by two different teams; unless communication between the teams is good, medical responsibility may not be defined sufficiently clearly. Integrated treatment is therefore considered by some to be the optimum approach and might involve a number of different treatment approaches such as an integrated out-patient service, an integrated community service, a specialized in-patient facility and an assertive outreach service. However, the evidence base for this expensive model of service provision is inconclusive, and it results in an isolation of dual diagnosis from mainstream service provision, with the added disadvantage that staff in mainstream services become progressively deskilled in managing patients with dual diagnosis.

Given the high prevalence of dual diagnosis and the lack of integrated teams to care for these patients, a pragmatic approach that makes best use of existing resources must be adopted and a Care Programme Approach (CPA) that coordinates community mental health teams and substance misuse teams probably represents the best way forward. The essential elements of the CPA are a systematic assessment of health and social care needs; an agreed care plan; allocation of a key worker/care coordinator; and regular review of the patient's progress. Although this appears straightforward and simple, many mental health professionals remain anxious about their ability to manage dual diagnosis patients with complex needs and this highlights the need for this issue to be included in all undergraduate and postgraduate training programmes for mental health professionals.

Admission to hospital

Although most patients with dual diagnosis can be managed in an out-patient or community setting, some severe cases require admission to hospital for assessment, diagnosis, treatment and planning of future care. A particular focus of concern amongst general psychiatrists is that patients who misuse drugs may have a detrimental effect on the ward regime, particularly if psychiatric symptoms are worsened by illicit drug use, leading to a potential risk to the safety of other patients, staff and others. It is therefore necessary to consider preventative strategies, such as a treatment contract for all patients, agreed on admission, that they will not use/misuse or hold in their possession, any other drugs (licit or illicit) unless prescribed as part of the treatment programme. While such arrangements rely on patient cooperation and are not legally enforceable, they do provide a framework for the management of problems that may arise in the course of the admission.

At this point it is also worth noting that a search of a patient or his or her possessions (including urine toxicology), without consent and without lawful authority, constitutes a trespass to the patient. A search would be lawful if there were reasonable grounds for suspecting that the patient is in possession of substances or articles that could be used to harm him or herself or others or was in possession of a controlled drug in contravention of the Misuse of Drugs Act

(1971). If it is suspected that a patient may be under the influence of illicit drugs, the obvious dangers of such substances reacting with prescribed medication or other consequences of drug use, would justify the responsible medical office in carrying out some investigation, such as urine toxicology, under the common law duty of care to the patient.

Drug-dependent patients on general medical and surgical wards

Drug-dependent patients may also require admission to hospital for the treatment of a problem unrelated to their drug dependence, or for one of its many complications. Their admission to a general ward, where the staff are unused to drug-dependent patients, may induce considerable anxiety, because they are often perceived as a potential source of unspecified 'trouble'. It may be helpful in this situation to regard drug-dependent patients, like diabetic patients, as having an underlying condition that requires careful, ongoing management, while they simultaneously receive specific treatment for a superimposed problem. Specialist help and advice can be obtained about the underlying drug dependence, and the admission to hospital may thus prove to be a valuable opportunity to engage the patient in long-term treatment for the drug dependence.

The question of prescribing maintenance doses of the drugs of dependence only arises for those who are dependent on opiates and/or sedative hypnotic drugs who will become physically distressed if their drugs are suddenly withdrawn. Patients admitted urgently for the treatment of acute medical or surgical conditions can rarely tolerate the additional physical and mental stress of drug withdrawal, so that this is not an appropriate time to consider detoxification programmes. If the patient is receiving a regular prescription for opiates from a clinic or elsewhere, statements about the daily dosage requirement can and should be checked with the prescribing doctor, and the maintenance prescription can then be continued in hospital.[26]

If no such information is available because the patient uses illicit drugs, it is wiser not to accept his or her demands unquestioningly, but to give nothing at first, observe the patient carefully, and prescribe only if and when the manifestations of the opiate abstinence syndrome begin. Some patients may have only a slight degree of physical dependence and minimal tolerance, and if their uncorroborated claims about the necessary dose are met in full, the greater purity of the pharmaceutical preparation may result in unexpectedly large doses being given, with the risk of ensuing intoxication. It may also cause more severe physical dependence, so that by the time of discharge the patient is taking higher doses than on admission. On the other hand, patients who are given insufficient drugs to control the abstinence syndrome are more likely to discharge themselves prematurely or to persuade friends to bring extra drugs in for them. It is therefore necessary to titrate the dose of prescribed opiate according to the individual's need, using the method of stabilization outlined on p. 257. Methadone, which can be prescribed to addicts by any doctor, without the requirement of a licence, is a suitable choice of opiate.

The same principles of management apply to those who are dependent on sedative hypnotic drugs. They should be stabilized on a sedative drug of the same class as that on which they are dependent as soon as they show any signs of the potentially dangerous abstinence syndrome.

Because drug-dependent individuals often abuse a range of different drugs, they may unwittingly become physically dependent on more than one. Medical staff should be aware of the possibility that someone diagnosed and treated as opiate dependent may also be at risk of developing the sedative abstinence syndrome and should be alert to the need to treat it promptly with the appropriate drug, should it arise unexpectedly. Because long-term maintenance on sedative drugs is not a feasible treatment option, a decision must be made according to the individual needs of the patient about when drug withdrawal should be initiated and how it should be coordinated with other aspects of treatment.

Although it is common for drug-dependent patients to inject their drugs, this should not be permitted in hospital. Their admission can thus be used to show them that drugs taken orally can adequately control and prevent the abstinence syndrome, and to encourage them to adopt this much safer method of drug administration. If medical reasons preclude oral administration, the drugs should be administered intramuscularly.

Opiate-dependent individuals who require analgesics preoperatively or for severe pain can be given opiates if these are indicated, but they will require higher than usual doses because of acquired tolerance. As a rough guide, they will need the usual analgesic dose in addition to their usual maintenance dose. If heroin is required for the relief of pain due to organic disease or injury, it can be prescribed for an addict by any doctor, without the need for a special licence. In practice, this situation arises only rarely, as there is a natural reluctance to prescribe heroin to those who are dependent on opiates.

Staff should be aware of the possibility of the problem of visitors bringing in illicit drugs and may, on occasion, have to refuse admission to undesirable visitors. Similarly, routine procedures for the security of drugs on the ward must be strictly implemented, so that no opportunities for abusing drugs are offered to individuals who, because of the severity of their dependence, may not be able to resist them. Patients' freedom to wander about should, where possible, be curtailed and they should be informed at the outset that regular urine samples will be taken and screened for psychoactive drugs. In summary, a caring but firm approach should be adopted, with certain 'ground rules' established at the outset. This should be coupled with an assurance that withdrawal symptoms will be adequately control-led and that they will receive adequate analgesia.[26]

Drug-dependent patients in accident and emergency departments

Drug-dependent individuals present frequently to accident and emergency (A & E) departments, either following an overdose or with some other drug-related problem. It is rare for them to attend for a medical problem that is not directly or indirectly caused by their drug-taking. Some patients of no fixed abode, or with no general practitioner (GP), use one or more A & E departments as their source of primary health care and attend frequently for one thing or another, becoming well known to all the staff. Others are brought in unconscious, with depressing regularity, following repeated overdoses.

Such recidivism is one reason why drug-dependent individuals are unpopular in A & E departments, where nonspecialist doctors can feel unskilled and ill-equipped to deal with them. However, the basic tools of history-taking, observa-tion, physical and mental state examination and investigation are all that is required. The doctor needs to be informed of the statutory aspects of addiction and to be aware of local specialist services that are available for onward referral. A written, departmental policy or guidelines for the management of intoxication and drug prescribing for drug abusers is helpful.[27]

Drug withdrawal and drug-seeking attendance

Some drug-dependent individuals attend A & E departments asking for and sometimes demanding drugs, on the basis that their prescribed supplies have been lost or stolen. Commonly, elaborate stories are told to account for this, or they may present themselves as temporary residents who are unexpectedly 'stranded' and unable to return to their treatment unit for their routine prescription. Attendance at night, when verification is impossible, is common. Others may complain of severe symptoms of withdrawal. In these situations, the golden rule must always be that nothing should be prescribed unless there are clear physical signs of the appropriate abstinence syndrome, which should be carefully documented. In particular, it may be necessary to resist manipulative statements, such as that the refusal to prescribe will force the individual to resort to illegal activity. Any deviation from this principle may mean that nondependent, casual users are provided with pharmaceutically pure preparations of dependence-producing drugs, or that the hospital is used deliberately by drug-dependent individuals as a supplementary source of supply; this will increase the severity of their dependence and may contribute to a drug overdose. It is imperative, therefore, that a careful history should be taken to corroborate the account of dependence, and that a thorough physical examination is carried out to establish the nature and severity of the claimed abstinence syndrome.

Of course, if there is any evidence of the sedative abstinence syndrome, treatment should be prompt to prevent the onset of withdrawal fits. Nowadays, barbiturate withdrawal is rare, but can be managed initially by giving phenobarbitone 120 mg orally. It has largely been replaced by benzodiazepine dependence, often as one component of polydrug abuse. Those dependent on benzodiazepines and/or alcohol should be given diazepam 20 mg orally. Their condition should be reviewed after 1 hour, when the intense agitation and distress associated with sedative withdrawal should be at least partially relieved. At this stage, when patients are calmer and more receptive to advice, every effort should be made to encourage them to be admitted to hospital for stabilization and detoxification. The risks of unsupervised sedative withdrawal should be fully explained, and patients should understand that if they come into hospital, they will be given medication to prevent the recurrence of the previous distressing symptoms. Some patients consistently refuse to be admitted to hospital; unless their mental state warrants compulsory admission to hospital under the 1983 Mental Health Act, they cannot be detained, and should be allowed to leave. In other cases, there may be a lack of availability of beds. In such cases, urgent referral should be made to psychiatric or drug-treatment services, or patients should be strongly advised to consult their GP as soon as possible. In the meantime, they can be provided with an adequate dose of their sedative drug to prevent the onset of the abstinence syndrome before they contact their GP. For example, they may need 20 mg diazepam 6-hourly, as takeaway medication for a minimum period, i.e. overnight. They should not be given supplies for a longer period because of the likelihood that they will take an overdose, inject it or supply it to someone else.

The clinical situation of opiate-dependent individuals experiencing the abstinence syndrome, although equally distressing, represents no serious danger, although pregnant women need special consideration. (It is not unusual for female addicts to claim falsely to be pregnant and onsite pregnancy testing is useful if the pregnancy is not obvious on physical examination.) If symptoms are mild, consideration should be given to prescribing for symptomatic relief only, perhaps using a combination of a low dose of a phenothiazine (e.g. chlorpromazine or haloperidol) and an antispasmodic, antidiarrhoeal drug (e.g. co-phenotrope, one to two tablets qds). More severe cases may be given methadone mixture 20 mg orally and should then be observed for 1 hour, by which time they should be feeling much better. They should be advised to seek treatment for their opiate dependence and, if possible, referred for specialist advice. A urine specimen taken before methadone administration may be helpful in any future assessment. The opiate abstinence syndrome is not, on its own, an indication for urgent admission to hospital, nor is there any need to prescribe methadone for the patient to take home.

Milder analgesic drugs, i.e. codeine, dihydrocodeine and dextropropoxyphene preparations are dependence forming. Although the patient may, originally, have been prescribed them during treatment for a genuinely painful condition, those who then become dependent on them often obtain supplies by attending several GPs and A & E departments with plausible symptoms such as back pain. Physical examination and investigations may be unhelpful in distinguishing between simulated and actual pain and the doctor should be particularly cautious if the patient requests an opiate painkiller or has attended previously in similar circumstances. Prescribing a nonsteroidal anti-inflammatory drug would be preferable. Patients who present with more extravagant simulations of very painful conditions such as renal colic may suggest Munchausen's syndrome, in which dependence on opiates is only one component of the disorder. Buprenorphine and pentazocine are also abused and may be sought by attenders at A & E departments claiming to have chronic, painful conditions. In assessing these patients, the doctor needs to achieve a balance between prescribing to relieve suffering and withholding addictive medication from those who are using it inappropriately. The general principle remains that, if in doubt, only small quantities should be prescribed and the patient referred to their GP, who should be informed of their attendance at hospital.

Drug overdose

It is also common for drug-dependent patients to attend the A & E department after a drug overdose and the management of such cases is described in Chapter 8. Many of these patients are likely to be unconscious and, unless there is evidence of self-injection, or they are known to the staff of the department, their dependent status may not be suspected. Those who are dependent on sedative hypnotic drugs are likely to present in a state of chronic intoxication when they may be verbally and sometimes physically aggressive towards staff and other patients. Although in this condition they may be extremely disruptive to the functioning of a busy department, so that most staff would prefer them to leave, they should not be discharged in this abnormal mental state. Specifically, they should not be removed by the police to be held in police cells. There is always a risk that these patients may lapse into unconsciousness and that skilled medical care may be urgently required. Hospitals that have to cope regularly with these patients sometimes designate a special area of the A & E department where they can be contained and subsequently sleep off their overdose under medical supervision. When they have recovered a more normal mental state, they should be persuaded to seek help for their underlying dependence.

It is worth emphasizing that A & E staff have a key role to play in the diagnosis of drug dependence, and particularly in identifying drug-dependent individuals among the vast numbers involved in incidents of deliberate self-poisoning. There is clear evidence that many of those who take a drug overdose apparently accidentally, or in a suicidal attempt or gesture, are in fact dependent on these drugs. This may be established if a careful and detailed history is taken with attention paid to points such as the past history of drug overdose, the number of drugs taken, the duration of drug-taking and so on, rather than concentrating only on the management of the presenting incident of overdose. Awareness of the possibility of drug dependence will lead to earlier diagnosis and earlier intervention and probably to a better prognosis.

Engagement in treatment

Drug-dependent patients present to A & E departments with a whole range of other problems, of course. The management of many problems has been described elsewhere in this book but in some ways the treatment of the immediate complications of drug dependence is only a minor component of the total management of these patients in A & E departments. What is far more important is that these departments are often the only point of contact between drug-dependent individuals and health care professionals, and are therefore their only route into treatment for their drug dependence. It is therefore essential that the staff who treat them for the complications of their dependence try wholeheartedly to engage them in long-term treatment, rather than adopting the 'sticking-plaster' approach of dealing with the immediate problem and sending the patient away as quickly as possible. It is, of course, completely understandable if they feel like doing just that. As a group, these patients are demanding, difficult and unpopular. Staff who are unaware of the nature of drug dependence do not fully understand the overwhelming compulsion to take drugs and perceive the attendant complications as self-induced and unworthy of much sympathy. In addition, many drug-dependent patients are very uncooperative, particularly when intoxicated, and they rarely express any appreciation for what has been done for them. In other words, they are ungratifying patients to whom the staff are likely to have hostile attitudes.

It requires a high degree of training and professionalism for staff to overcome these attitudes and to respond to drug-dependent patients in a more constructive way. For example, the continual reattendance of a patient can be used to establish a relationship that may eventually be instrumental in persuading that patient to accept a referral to a drug-dependence treatment unit (DDTU). Such help should be offered whenever a drug-dependent patient attends for treatment because there is evidence that at a time of crisis – when recovering from an overdose, or after experiencing the effects of drug withdrawal – the patient may be particularly receptive to intervention, and this opportunity to engage the patient should not be lost.

To facilitate the referral process, staff need to have ready access to and knowledge of local advice and treatment agencies, preferably in the form of a comprehensive directory of local services. If the A & E department is in a hospital with a drug unit on site, it is mutually beneficial to establish liaison and referral procedures. A Drug and Alcohol Liaison Service that can be 'on-call' to deal with problems as they arise can offer very valuable support that enables staff to feel more confident about dealing with these problems.

Data collection and statutory requirements

The strategic response to drug-abuse problems depends on information and knowledge of their scale and nature. In the UK, all Regional Health Authorities have now established Drug Misuse Databases (see Chapter 2), which, at St George's, includes information on the use of alcohol. For these, information is collected on anonymized forms, covering any drug abuse problem. Clearly, this database offers the potential for comprehensive monitoring of drug-abuse problems, provided that all agencies involved with drug abusers participate by completing the forms and A & E departments should do this routinely for any attendance by a substance abuser.

With the enlarging scope of recreational and experimental drug use, and the development of designer drugs, the A & E department is in the frontline of coping with the adverse effects, and there may be few sources of detailed knowledge of the pharmacological and physiological actions of these new drugs. Good record keeping will assist in increasing knowledge and, at all times, a urine sample should be collected for toxicological analysis of any attender who is suspected of having a drug-abuse problem. Although the result of analysis is unlikely to be immediately available to influence the management of the patient at that time, it can prove extremely useful in the follow-up and continuing care of the patient.

Drug-dependent patients in the general practitioner's surgery

With the growing number of drug abusers and drug-dependent individuals in the population, GPs are likely to see them more often and have an important role to play in their treatment and management. Although some individuals with drug-related problems recognize that they have a problem and seek help for it, others may approach their GP about an apparently unrelated complaint. An alert doctor, aware of the dependence-producing liability of many of the newer psychoactive drugs, may be able to recognize drug dependence in its early stages and to intervene before it becomes severe and difficult to treat. In particular, it is now recognized that although symptoms such as anxiety, tremor, insomnia and depression, as well as many somatic symptoms, may indicate underlying psychiatric illness or other personal problems, they may also be the early manifestations of the benzodiazepine withdrawal syndrome, and a clear indication of physical dependence upon these drugs. Sometimes the drugs may have been prescribed by the GP, but such is their widespread availability nowadays that the patient may have 'borrowed' them and/or have used up an old supply, and the doctor may well be unaware of this self-medication with prescription-only drugs.[28,29]

Another common way for GPs to come into contact with a drug-dependent individual is to be approached by someone seeking treatment as a temporary or private patient for a chronic, painful condition requiring potent analgesics, or for insomnia, requiring a prescription for hypnotics. The history is often very plausible, but it transpires later that it is a total fabrication and that the patient has approached a number of doctors, sometimes under an assumed name, in a deliberate attempt to obtain a prescription for drugs on which he or she is dependent. It is, of course, an offence for a patient who is already receiving controlled drugs on prescription from one doctor not to disclose this fact to another doctor who is also going to prescribe them. However, there are many who are not deterred by this and who have a 'collecting round' of several doctors. This is particularly likely to occur with those who are dependent on opiates, and is an excellent reason for the GP approached to communicate with local substance misuse services. If the patient is found to be dependent on opiates (or sedatives), drugs should only be prescribed if there is clear objective evidence of the appropriate withdrawal syndrome, and then only as a single dose, preferably to be consumed on the premises. Doctors who prescribe more liberally are likely to find that, as word gets round, they are visited by many more such patients, eager to benefit from a 'soft touch'. Because these patients may be quite prepared to break the law in order to obtain their drugs, it is essential that drugs, syringes, needles and prescription forms are not left unattended.[30]

If it becomes apparent that a patient is abusing drugs or is dependent upon them, or if the GP suspects that this may be the case, the first step must be a thorough assessment of the patient's drug problem. This should include a full drug history and examination of the patient's physical and mental state. It is essential to establish whether or not the patient is physically dependent on any drug. If the doctor has had long contact with the patient (and often the family), he or she is likely to be familiar with the patient's social situation, but if not, this is an area that requires clarification. Observed specimens of urine should be taken for drug screening as the findings may provide helpful corroboration of the patient's history.

The problems of drug abuse and drug dependence are now so great that it is not possible for every case to be referred for specialist treatment, nor is it desirable that this should be done. Indeed, many patients, and particularly those who have become dependent on sedative hypnotic drugs, in the course of medical treatment, may deeply resent referral to a special clinic that they perceive to be the last resort of treatment for 'junkies' and the like. For others in an early stage of a drug-taking career and with only a mild degree of dependence, it may be positively disadvantageous to introduce them to a clinic where they are likely to meet more experienced drug takers and be introduced to the drug subculture. Finally, and perhaps most important of all, the GP is likely to have a longstanding acquaintance with the patient that can be used to enhance psychotherapeutic counselling. Management of substance dependency in the primary care setting can be facilitated by 'Addiction Prevention Counsellors' or by 'Primary Care Addiction Liaison' or indeed any service that encourages the development of shared care between the GP and the local, specialist DDTU.[31]

However, some patients have such severe and complex problems that they need all the multidisciplinary resources and expertise of a specialist drug-treatment clinic. Opiate abusers, for example, using other drugs as well; sedative abusers taking large doses of these drugs and who are therefore at risk of withdrawal convulsions; and those chaotic drug abusers whose life has become wholly centred on drugs and drug-taking, cannot be satisfactorily treated in a general practice setting, and should be referred to a specialist treatment facility.

When the GP decides to treat the patient him or herself, the goal of treatment is always to help the patient come off drugs, rather than to offer any maintenance treatment. If the patient is physically dependent on opiates or sedatives, a contract should be agreed between doctor and patient specifying the drug to be prescribed, the total duration of treatment and the rate of dose-reduction. If methadone is indicated, prescription must be on a daily basis and six hand-written prescriptions will be required each week. Pharmacological treatment is only appropriate for those who are dependent on opiates or sedative hypnotics (e.g. benzodiazepines, barbiturates). No drugs should be prescribed for those who are dependent on stimulants such as amphetamine. During detoxification it is best to avoid prescribing any other psychoactive substances. Apart from the obvious risk of causing dependence on yet another type of drug, it is very important that the patient should learn nonpharmacological responses to symptoms and problematical situations. Counselling, psychotherapy and instruction in simple techniques of relaxation may all be helpful and will also convey this important message. However, if symptoms of insomnia, anxiety and craving are severe and distressing in a patient who is otherwise doing well, a neuroleptic such as chlorpromazine or haloperidol can be prescribed. These have few or no addictive properties and the patient is very unlikely to escalate the dose. Drug-dependent patients should be seen at least weekly and there should be frequent, preferably random, urine tests. Every effort should be made to involve the patient (and their family) in local self-help groups and other activities conducive to a drug-free lifestyle.[31,32]

Patients who have been referred to a specialist DDTU may continue to consult their GP for other apparently unrelated conditions. On no account should any psychoactive drugs be prescribed for these patients without prior consultation with the responsible doctor at the DDTU. For example, if the patient is complaining of severe symptoms of drug withdrawal it is very important that the clinic doctor should be aware of this, so that treatment can be adjusted accordingly rather than the picture being clouded by the patient obtaining drugs from another source. In addition, there is also the risk that some patients may try, quite deliberately, to obtain extra drugs from their GP, and the clinic should be informed of this drug-seeking behaviour.

Substance abusers detained in police custody

Substance abusers are frequently detained in police custody and the advice of forensic physicians (police surgeons) is often requested in these circumstances. These doctors are experienced in dealing with issues such as the individual's fitness to be detained, the need for treatment and fitness for interview. However, if the detainee needs to be transferred to hospital, other doctors and health care professionals become involved in their care too, and it is important that they also are aware of particular issues that are relevant to detainees.

The rights and clinical safety of the detainee

Individuals detained in police custody are entitled to the same standard of clinical care as any other member of the public and the overriding responsibility of the forensic physician is the clinical safety and well-being of the detainee.[33] Fitness for detention must therefore be assessed first and transfer to hospital may be indicated if, for example, there is an allegation that the detainee has taken drugs prior to their arrest and there is concern about the level of consciousness. It must also be remembered that signs of intoxication may not be immediately apparent but may develop later, particularly if long-acting drugs have been swallowed immediately before arrest. Although a limited period of observation may be possible in the police station, it is inappropriate for nonmedical personnel, such as custody officers, to observe a detainee for prolonged periods.

Consent should be sought for any examination that is undertaken on a detainee, who also has the right to have prescribed treatment continued while they are in custody, as long as it is clinically safe to do so. Thus, if the detainee has medication prescribed for him or her in his or her possession, its continued use can be authorized. Sometimes it may be necessary and possible to contact the pharmacist or prescribing doctor to verify details of the prescribed drug. However, on occasion, and particularly if the detainee claims to be suffering from withdrawal symptoms from drugs obtained illegally, treatment will be prescribed at the discretion of the forensic physician. In this situation, a careful and well-documented history and examination is essential; it should be remembered that substance abusers may not be frank and that inconsistent information may be given for some perceived secondary gain. However, an honest history is more likely if the detainee has confidence in the forensic physician and in his or her independence of the police.

The history should include details of current and past substance use including alcohol, as well as previous experience of withdrawal symptoms and the physical and psychological consequences. Physical examination should include seeking signs of withdrawal or intoxication and signs of physical illness or injury that may be consequent on substance misuse. The possibility of head injury should not be overlooked, particularly in a patient who may appear intoxicated or who is behaving strangely. Mental state examination should establish whether there is any mental disorder, which may be drug-related or coincident; this may have legal implications for the offence or affect the assessment of fitness for interview. Risk assessment (of both self-harm and risk to others) should be covered.

Detainees who are intoxicated need to be closely monitored and transfer to hospital is essential if there is concern about the level of consciousness. Onsite urine testing may be available at the police station and may give valuable additional qualitative (rather than quantitative) information about whether a drug has been consumed.

Prescribing and drug administration

If a decision is taken that medication is necessary to alleviate symptoms and signs of opiate withdrawal, for example, the doctor may prescribe a drug, such as codeine, that he or she carries with him or her. National Health Service prescriptions must not be issued for persons detained in custody, for whom drugs should be prescribed on a private prescription, to be paid for by the police. Although all medication in the police station is usually held by the custody officer, on behalf of the detainee, no police officer may administer controlled drugs nor measure out doses of methadone or other medicines. The doctor should therefore ensure that prescriptions are dispensed by the pharmacist in single doses and, if a detainee requires drugs, he or she administers them to him or herself under the supervision of the forensic physician. This does not necessarily require the forensic physician to be present at the time, only that he or she has authorized this treatment. Good practice guidelines suggest that the physician would not authorize treatment without having previously examined the patient. Injectable preparations are utilized only in exceptional circumstances, and in such cases the forensic physician would administer or personally supervise drug administration.

In the case of female detainees who are pregnant, it is important that the consequences of substance use or withdrawal on the fetus are not overlooked (e.g. the potential effect of opiate withdrawal on precipitating fetal distress, miscarriage or premature labour).

Discharge from hospital

An individual who is well enough to be discharged from hospital may not be fit enough for detention in a police cell. The hospital doctor should take this into account before discharge and, if necessary, recommend reassessment by the forensic physician when the detainee returns to the police station, because this does not happen automatically.

Intimate searches

The authorization of a police officer of the rank of Superintendent or above is required before an intimate search can be carried out. It must be carried out at a hospital or other medical premises (not a police station) by a registered medical practitioner or registered nurse, and the responsibility for performing the examination lies with the forensic physician and not the hospital doctor. The forensic physician must have obtained informed consent from the detainee and permission from senior medical or nursing staff at the hospital or other medical premises concerned. It can only be carried out if there are reasonable grounds for believing that the person has concealed a class A drug intended for supply to another or to export and that an intimate search is the only practicable way of removing it.

Fitness for interview

Forensic physicians and other doctors may be asked for their opinion about a detainee's fitness for interview. Before offering this opinion they should be aware of the proposed time and likely duration of the interview. They will then need to establish whether there is evidence of substance abuse; if the patient is currently under the influence of drugs and/or alcohol; whether there is evidence of the abstinence syndrome; and whether the detainee is fully aware of his or her surroundings, is well enough to cope with a stressful interview, can understand the questions put to him or her and can instruct solicitors.

Particular problems arise if the individual concerned is suffering from drug withdrawal because of the risk of giving a false confession, which is later retracted. This may occur because detainees believe that compliance will result in early release with charges being dropped or altered, while stubborn denial leads to further detention and difficulty in obtaining necessary drugs. In particular, the physical and mental distress caused by drug withdrawal may make it difficult for the individual concerned to retain coherence of his or her story and to maintain his or her defence, when questioning is carried out by skilled interrogators. If drugs are prescribed to alleviate the abstinence syndrome, it may later be argued that the treatment itself impaired the individual's fitness for interview and this may affect the admissibility of any confession.

False confessions can be categorized as voluntary, coerced-compliant, coerced-internalized and accommodating-compliant. Drug addicts wanting early release to enable them to secure their next 'fix' are clearly at risk of making a coerced-compliant false confession. Coerced-internalized confessions may happen if detainees believe that they may have committed a crime even if they have no recollection of this because of an awareness that their memory is impaired by drug consumption and/or because they have come to distrust their own memory.

In general, although mild opiate withdrawal may not impede interviewing, severe withdrawal may result in the detainee being unfit for interview until symptoms subside (2–3 days) or are treated with an opioid substitute. Similarly, the withdrawal of sedative hypnotics from a severely dependent individual may severely impair fitness for interview until the patient has been stabilized on a long-acting sedative drug.

Where a detainee is obviously intoxicated, it is customary to wait until the effects of the drug(s) wear off before the interview begins. However, when hallucinogenic drugs have been taken, the mental state may fluctuate markedly in the recovery stages and it may not be apparent that the detainee is not fit to be interviewed immediately.

Young people in custody

The increasing prevalence of substance misuse by young people has resulted in more finding their way into police custody. They frequently have co-morbid psychiatric disorders and there may be a history of deliberate self-harm. Assessment must include an exploration of these issues, including enquiry about drinking patterns. Children and young people should be kept informed about what is happening to them in terms of their clinical treatment. Although it is normal practice to obtain the consent of the parent or other person with parental responsibility before carrying out an examination or initiating treatment, it is recognized that, in some cases, children are competent to make a decision for themselves.

Arrest referral schemes

Access to arrest referral schemes is increasingly being emphasized and forensic physicians are well placed to encourage detainees to make use of this facility, to provide a referral and to provide information to the arrest referral worker (with the consent of the detainee).

Driving licences

In the UK, holders of driving licences or those applying for a licence are obliged by law to notify the Driver and Vehicle Licensing Agency (DVLA) as soon as they become aware that they are suffering from a 'prescribed disability' (as set out in the regulations of the Road Traffic Act) or any other condition likely to make the driving of a vehicle a likely source of danger for the general public. Drug and alcohol misuse and dependence are prescribed disabilities and patients should be told of their legal duty to inform the DVLA. If they fail to do so, their driving licence and insurance may be considered invalid.

The current UK regulations are in line with the requirements for medical standards of driver licensing set out in the 2nd EC directive. If there is evidence of persistent use of cannabis, Ecstasy and other 'recreational' drugs including amphetamines, LSD and hallucinogens, the consequence is a 6-month driving ban; this period is doubled for other drugs (amphetamines, heroin, morphine, methadone, cocaine, LSD/hallucinogens, including the abuse of Ecstasy and other psychoactive substances that are currently fashionable) if dependence is confirmed. Urine screening may be required. A 'Till 70' licence will be restored only after satisfactory independent medical examination, and urine tests negative for drug abuse. The patient is recommended to seek help from medical or other agencies during the period off driving. It should be noted that patients on consultant-supervised oral methadone, buprenorphine or other substitution therapy can normally have a driving licence, subject to annual review; however, if patients are receiving methadone-maintenance treatment intravenously, it is recommended that their driving licence should be refused or revoked.[34]

The above rules apply to those with an 'ordinary', Group 1 licence for cars and motorbikes. Those holding vocational, Group 2, licences for vehicles such as lorries and buses, can expect to have their licence refused or revoked for 1 year for persistent use of cannabis, Ecstasy, etc. or for 3 years for dependency on amphetamines, heroin, morphine, methadone, cocaine or benzodiazepines, during which time there should be no evidence of dependency or continuing misuse. On application for a licence, a specialist medical examination is required with a negative urine screen for drugs of abuse.

Persistent solvent abuse also requires driving to cease and the DVLA to be informed. The licence would be restored after medical enquiries confirm no continuing abuse.

Epileptic fits or seizures may occur in conjunction with drug abuse, and there is an obligation to notify the DVLA of this. In this situation, the ordinary licence (Group 1) would be revoked for 1 year after a single or multiple seizure(s). Group 2 (vocational LGV/PCV) licences would be revoked for 5 years following a single drug-related seizure or for 10 years where multiple seizures have occurred.

The non-prescribed use of benzodiazepines and/or the use of 'supratherapeutic' dosage, whether in a substance withdrawal/maintenance programme or otherwise, constitutes misuse/dependency for licensing purposes. Persistent misuse of, or dependence on, benzodiazepines confirmed by medical enquiry will lead to licence refusal or revocation until a minimum 1-year period free of such use has been attained (Group 1). For Group 2, a minimum 3-year period free of use must be attained.

Some patients continue to drive and fail to notify the DVLA despite advice to do so. Under these circumstances the GMC advise that the doctor should make every effort to persuade the patient to stop driving, if necessary informing the next of kin. If a doctor believes that a particular patient, when driving, is a grave risk to the public at large (perhaps because of a chronic state of intoxication due to sedative hypnotic dependence), he or she may consider overriding normal standards of medical confidentiality and informing the DVLA. This is a matter for the clinical judgement of the individual doctor, who should be prepared to justify the decision if it is questioned. Relevant clinical information should be disclosed in confidence to the medical advisor at the DVLA but, before doing so, the doctor should inform the patient of the intention to contact the DVLA. Once the DVLA has been notified, the doctor should inform the patient of this in writing.[34]

Persistent alcohol misuse confirmed by medical enquiry and/or by evidence of otherwise unexplained abnormal blood markers requires license revocation or refusal until a minimum 6-month period of controlled drinking or abstinence has been attained with normalization of blood parameters. For Group 2, the minimum period is 1 year. When there is alcohol dependence, a 1-year period free from alcohol is required, and in Group 2, this is extended to 3 years.

Travelling abroad

Drugs such as amphetamines, barbiturates and the opiates in Schedules 1–3 of the Misuse of Drugs Regulations (Chapter 12) are subject to legal restrictions on their import and exportation. However, ordinary travellers are allowed to import or export and possess limited quantities of medically necessary controlled drugs, by virtue of an 'open general licence' held at the Home Office. This is intended to cover an average prescription for 15 days, and up to 500 mg methadone would be reasonable. Larger quantities, even if the drugs have been legally prescribed, require an individual export licence which is issued by the Home Office (drugs branch). This facilitates passage through British customs but, like the 'open general licence', has no legal status outside the UK. Details of the import licence required by the country of destination (if importation is permitted at all), can be obtained from that country's embassy.

The question of an addict taking drugs abroad is most likely to arise for stable opiate addicts on methadone maintenance who want to go abroad on holiday. If the doctor in charge of the patient's treatment has personal contact with colleagues in DDTUs in other countries, it may occasionally be possible to arrange for methadone to be prescribed by them for the period of the holiday. Generally, however, it must be accepted that opiate dependence significantly curtails an individual's freedom to travel – and this may be used as an additional incentive for coming off drugs.

Follow-up and treatment outcome

Introduction

Those who have read the earlier chapters of this book will appreciate that there is no quick solution, no 'cure' for drug abuse, and anyone who has come into contact with drug abusers will know, from personal experience, that they can be one of the most difficult groups of patients to treat.

So what does happen to them? What is the outcome for drug abusers and drug-dependent individuals? Do they get off drugs or are they always addicted? Do they carry on taking drugs until they kill themselves or are they likely to die from an unrelated illness? If they become abstinent, what brings about this fundamental change, and when is it likely to occur? Does treatment 'work'? If so, which treatment is 'best'?

There are no simple answers to any of these questions. Drug abusers are a heterogeneous population, and the individuals who make up that population have different personality attributes and exist in different life situations. They suffer from one or more of a range of drug-related problems, of variable severity, and the eventual outcome of their drug abuse, like its initiation, depends on the unique interaction between drug, individual and society. To this already complex formula must be added yet another variable – the effect (if any) of treatment intervention. Thus, while one heroin-dependent individual may successfully achieve and maintain abstinence, another attending the same clinic may die from an overdose, while a third may attain stability when provided with a regular prescription for methadone. Similarly, among a group of adolescents experimenting with glue sniffing, most will 'grow out of it', but an occasional youngster will persist in abusing solvent for many years and may, in the process, seriously damage his or her liver and kidneys.

Endless anecdotal examples could be given of patterns of drug abuse and of the different outcomes that ensue. Most research, however, has concentrated on what happens to those who abuse opiates, sometimes with a tacit assumption that all opiate abusers are necessarily dependent on their drug and are therefore 'addicts'. In contrast, there is a striking paucity of information about what happens to those who abuse other drugs and/or are dependent upon them, and this yawning gap in our knowledge base is usually papered over by extrapolations from studies of opiate 'addicts'.

Definition of 'treatment'

Before trying to evaluate the effect, if any, of treatment, it is helpful to be clear about what is encompassed by this term. An expert group convened by the World Health Organization defined treatment as: 'The process that begins when psychoactive substance users come into contact with a health provider or other community service, and may continue through a succession of specific interventions until the highest attainable level of health and well-being is reached'.[1]

They suggested that treatment should have three main objectives:
- Reduce dependence on psychoactive substances;
- Reduce morbidity and mortality caused by or associated with the use of psychoactive substances; and
- Ensure that users are able to maximize their physical, mental and social abilities and their access to services and opportunities and to achieve full social integration.

Defining 'outcome'

In addition, there is often a lack of clarity and little agreement about what exactly is meant by 'outcome'. Drug-taking status is an obvious component of any assessment procedure, but it must be precisely defined. For example, an individual who has successfully become abstinent from opiates may then abuse a whole range of other drugs such as cannabis, alcohol and sedatives, and may become dependent upon one or more of them. How should this person be described as far as outcome is concerned? In a multidimensional approach to drug abuse, detoxification and abstinence are rarely the only goals of treatment. Elimination or reduction of criminal activity, cessation of all illicit drug use and the establishment of socially acceptable behaviour, such as obtaining employment, maintaining a basic standard of living by legitimate means and maintaining stable relations with family and friends, are all considered important and may be included as outcome criteria in the evaluation of treatment.[1] In a methadone maintenance treatment programme, they are of course the most important indicators of the success of the treatment.

Time scale for assessment

Another question that needs to be addressed is the timing of assessment procedures. Exactly when should 'outcome' of treatment be assessed? For those undergoing detoxification, completion of the detoxification programme is a major landmark of their treatment, and the proportion who manage to reach it is an indication of the acceptability of the treatment programme to patients – an important factor when patient motivation is crucial to recovery. However, in a chronic and relapsing illness, evaluation at a single point in time is not enough; to be meaningful it must extend over months and years and this in itself raises further problems, particularly when different treatment modalities are being compared and different goals of treatment are included. For example, those individuals who are imprisoned, or go into hospital, or decide to enter a therapeutic community, have limited opportunity to use illegal drugs, commit crimes or become employed, and this may affect the result of outcome assessment. Sophisticated analysis of data can control for time at risk in outcome studies, but the important point to be grasped here is that bland statements of success of different treatment strategies should never be taken at face value. Claims of '75% cure rates' for drug dependence require further clarification. When are 75% of patients considered 'cured'? At the end of a course of treatment? If so, what has happened after 6 months, or 1 year? If 75% of patients are abstinent from their original drug of abuse, how many are taking a substitute drug from the same class; how many are using alcohol or other drugs? When these points are clarified and taken into account, the figures for 'successful' treatment are usually much lower – and more meaningful. On the other hand, beneficial consequences of intervention and treatment may not be manifest immediately, and may not therefore be recognized as a consequence of treatment. For example, even if relapse to drug-taking occurs within days of completion of a detoxification programme, the experience of abstinence, albeit temporary, may be instrumental in a later decision to enter a therapeutic community or to engage in other long-term treatment programmes.

The difficulties of assessing the outcome of treatment for drug abuse are compounded by a basic ignorance of what might be termed the 'natural history' of the condition, making it difficult to know whether any changes following an intervention are causally related to the treatment intervention or might have occurred anyway. Many studies evaluating treatment compare illicit drug-taking, employment status, etc. in the year following the treatment intervention with what was happening the year before. Any differences are attributed to the effectiveness or ineffectiveness of the treatment process.

It is important to remember, however, that professional intervention is only one factor in a complex and ever-changing situation and it is arrogant to assume that it lies at the root of all subsequent change. For example, an opiate addict undergoes detoxification in an in-patient unit and, after being discharged, continues to attend a nonuser's group regularly; after vocational rehabilitation he is able to gain regular employment and never abuses opiates, or indeed any illicit drug, again. Is this happy ending due to the effectiveness of in-patient detoxification, or could the fact that his wife is pregnant and has said that she will leave with the baby unless he comes off drugs and gets a job, explain why treatment on this occasion was successful? Or could it be that he has attained sufficient maturation of personality that he can now cope without drugs? Undoubtedly, all of these may be important factors independently and their interaction may account for the patient eventually achieving abstinence. Statistical evaluation of outcome is necessarily complex but it is now apparent from studies of 'self recovery' that access to social services support combined with active support by family, friends, etc. can be influential in assisting recovery.[2]

Natural history of drug dependence

One of the reasons why it is impossible to be definite about the outcome of drug dependence and to evaluate accurately the effect of treatment intervention is because of our ignorance of the natural history of the condition. Indeed, the very term 'natural history' is somewhat misleading because it assumes the existence of a predictable pathological process with an inevitable course, whereas in any discussion of drug abuse and dependence there is constant awareness of the way in which external factors interact to affect the course of events.[3] In the absence of a 'typical' natural history, it may be more helpful to consider drug dependence in terms of different drug-taking 'careers'. Examination of a large number of these careers may permit the extraction of certain commonalities that tell us something about the nature of drug dependence and its eventual outcome.

Relapse and remission

First and foremost, it is clear that although there are many routes into drug abuse and thence to drug dependence, once the dependent state has been reached it is generally a chronic condition lasting for years rather than months, and one that is difficult, but not impossible, to overcome. Within this long-term perspective, it is also clear that it is a condition of relapse and remission. Very few drug-dependent individuals achieve permanent abstinence the first time that they try, and of those who eventually achieve it, the majority have had several, often numerous, attempts. They may have tried to become abstinent, but only managed a temporary reduction in dose, or they may have become abstinent but resumed drug-taking within days, weeks or months. It is sometimes assumed that this cycle of abstinence and drug-taking is a consequence of treatment and its subsequent failure, but a similar pattern of behaviour is reported by addicts attending DDTUs for the first time. A carefully taken history usually elicits an account of at least one, and often several, episodes of abstinence achieved on the individual's personal initiative and with no professional intervention.

It is very important that all who work with or who have contact with drug-dependent individuals understand the fluctuating nature of the condition. Resumption of drug-taking after a period of abstinence is then not perceived as failure, but as an indication of the severity of the underlying addiction, and it becomes the cue not for recrimination but for a more energetic attempt to induce another remission. Furthermore, the natural cycle of relapse and remission must be borne in mind in any assessment of treatment outcome, just as it is in the evaluation of other fluctuating conditions such as multiple sclerosis.

Longitudinal studies

In the absence of information about what happens to drug-dependent individuals who remain aloof from all professional intervention, it may be possible to gain some understanding of the natural history of the condition by following the fortunes of cohorts of addicts over a number of years, accepting that any 'treatment' or contact with health care professionals is just one component of the totality of a drug-taking career. An historic study along these lines was initiated in 1969 of 128 subjects being prescribed heroin at London drug clinics. They were followed up by record searches and personal contact for 10 years by which time, 19 (15%) had died, 49 (38%) were still attending the clinic and 60 (47%) were not. Of the 49 individuals still attending the clinic in 1979, all were receiving prescriptions for opiates (methadone and/or heroin) and the majority had received prescriptions continuously for the 10-year period.[4] On the whole, other aspects of their lives were unproblematic and the majority were employed. It appears that they had settled down into a life of fairly safe but chronic addiction and it seems unlikely that this would have changed in the future. It is often assumed, when addicts stop attending the clinic and are lost to follow-up, that they have probably resumed drug-taking. This study, which made energetic and thorough attempts to trace addicts and to confirm their drug-taking status, suggests otherwise; over the years the number of people remaining addicted declined, and after 10 years 38% (estimated) had stopped using heroin and other opiates. Having become abstinent, they did not generally abuse other drugs or alcohol. By 1979 their average period of abstinence was more than 6 years and it seemed unlikely that drug-taking would be resumed thereafter.

In another study, a cohort of all 83 addicts attending a London drug clinic in July 1971 was followed up 11 years later by a search of medical notes and Home Office records.[5] At that time, 29 (24%) were known to be still using drugs, the majority receiving injectable methadone on prescription despite an 'official' clinic policy of weaning addicts off injectable drugs. Once again, as in the study described earlier, this group showed a definite move towards stability, with a marked fall in the number having complications of drug use or being involved in criminality, and a slight increase in the attainment of stable relationships and regular employment. Whether this increased stability was a result of continued and often uninterrupted prescription of opiate drugs, or the cause of their prescription is not clear. It may be argued, for example, that it was the provision of a regular supply of opiates that kept addicts out of trouble and permitted the development of a stable and uncomplicated lifestyle – but it could also be true that continued prescribing was a consequence of the addicts' underlying stability because a chaotic lifestyle (abuse of other drugs, excess side effects, etc.), would probably have led to cessation of prescription.

Whatever the reason, in two long-term studies of British opiate addicts attending drug clinics, about 30% settled down to a state of chronic but uncomplicated addiction. It is interesting that a third, somewhat different study reported a similar result: 86 injecting drug users, most of whom used opiates, attended a clinic that did not prescribe opiates at all. After a follow-up period of up to 6 years, 30% were continuing to inject regularly, many of them having subsequently attended clinics which did prescribe for them.[6]

The importance of early intervention

Another finding to emerge from many studies carried out in drug clinics is that if abstinence is going to occur, this is more likely in the early stages of a drug user's career. For example, when 40 patients who became drug free were compared with 40 patients at the same clinic who did not become drug free, the mean time between claimed first use of opiate and first attendance was 3.9 years for the group who became abstinent, but was 8.7 years for the others.[7] The message is clear from many sources that it is the less chronic addicts who are likely to become abstinent in the short term, and that short-term or early improvement is more likely to lead to long-term improvement. This phenomenon has been described as the 'rush' in the numbers becoming abstinent early in their drug-taking career, followed by a much slower 'trickle' of addicts coming off over subsequent years. The slow but steady decline over the years in the numbers continuing to be dependent may be evidence of the effect of maturation – that, eventually, many addicts will 'grow out of' drug-taking.[8]

Mortality

Mortality rates

It is widely believed that to be an 'addict' (i.e. an opiate addict) is to dice with death. Indeed, many people believe that early death is the inevitable outcome of addiction. Mortality statistics refute the latter belief while confirming the hazards of the condition. For example, an oft-quoted study of addict deaths between 1947 and 1966 estimates their mortality rate to be 28 times that expected for a population with similar demographic characteristics.[9] Since then, there have been many studies of addict deaths, but their differing research methodologies make interpretation and comparisons difficult. In general, however, most of these studies report that 2–3% of addicts are dead within 1 year of making contact with a clinic or helping agency.[10]

However, addiction is a chronic condition and it is also important to find out what happens to those who survive the first year. Do more and more addicts die as time goes by, or is mortality concentrated in the early years of an addiction career, with 'stable' addicts, who have learned to live with their addiction, surviving comfortably into old age? The answers to questions such as these are relevant to an understanding of the natural history of addiction, but they are difficult questions to resolve because of the difficulties of following cohorts of addicts over long periods and of knowing when and why they died. It may be labouring the obvious to point out that the eventual outcome for any cohort (addict or not) followed for a sufficiently long period of time will be a 100% mortality rate, but this emphasizes the statistical problems surrounding the study of chronic conditions with an increased mortality rate.

Despite these pitfalls, mortality studies are useful investigative tools. One source of information in the UK used to be the Home Office list of those addicts, previously notified, who were then removed from the index by reason of death. During the 15-year period, 1967–81, 1499 notified addicts died, and when they were divided into annual cohorts, according to the calendar year in which they were first notified, it was found that approximately 1.6% died within that calendar year and that 3.3% died by the end of the subsequent calendar year (Fig. 10.1).[10] These percentages were fairly constant over the whole of the study period, which encompassed a range of different enthusiasms and policies for treating addiction: in the early years, clinics opened and started to prescribe heroin; then injectable methadone was substituted and then oral methadone. Clinics became more reluctant to prescribe opiates and usually did so only as part of a therapeutic contract. None of these measures seem to have had any impact on early mortality and the uniformity of the results over the 15 years suggests that these death rates perhaps represent the elusive 'natural history' of addiction. When the results are corrected to reflect annual mortality, rather than death within a specific calendar year, the true death rate for the first year approaches 3%, for the second year 1.9%, and for the third 0.7%. When the older, 'therapeutic' addicts were excluded from the calculations, mortality due to recreational opiate addiction was found to be approximately 16 times that expected for a similar population of nonaddicts.

Other studies have also described this high mortality rate. For example, a Swedish study of 188 opiate users reported a mortality rate of 18.3% after 12

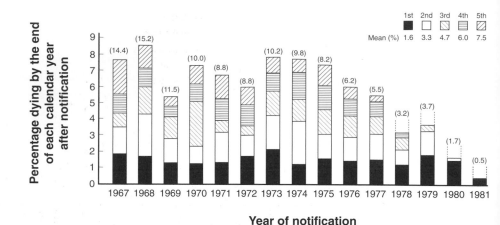

Fig. 10.1   Mortality among cohorts of addicts notified each year. Figures in parentheses are percentages of each annual cohort dead at follow-up (1982). (Source Ghodse et al.[10])

years,[11] and 11.9% mortality was reported in an English cohort of 128 heroin addicts followed up for 22 years.[12] However, with these comparatively small samples, it is difficult to understand underlying whole population trends and, for this reason, the Home Office study described above is particularly important because it describes what happens to *all* newly notified addicts. When it was updated in 1993 it covered a period of 27 years during which the cumulative newly notified study group comprised 92 802 addicts and a total of 687 673 person-years.[13] By the end of 1993, there had been 5310 deaths, giving an annual crude death rate of 7.7/1000 person-years, lower than that described in a 12-year Australian study of 307 addicts on methadone maintenance, which reported a mortality rate of 11.1/1000 per year.[14]

In the British Home Office study (Fig. 10.2), the median age at death was 30.6 years and 91% of deaths were of nontherapeutic addicts. Over the 27-year study period there was a consistent decline in overall age-adjusted death rates from 19/1000 person-years in the first decade of the study to 10.5/1000 person-years in the last decade. This occurred at a time when there was a general reduction in death rates at all ages and increased life expectancy associated with better quality health and social care provision. Simultaneously, there was much greater involvement of the primary health care sector in the care of addicts, along with improved specialist services and these changes have undoubtedly led to addicts having much better access to mainstream health services and better treatment for life-threatening conditions such as hepatitis. Furthermore, there have been general improvements in A & E departments which commonly deal with drug-related emergencies.

Within the overall improvements in death rate it is interesting to note that there

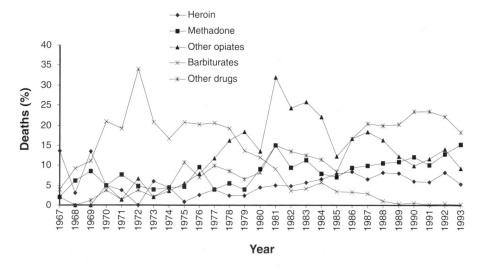

—◆— Heroin
—■— Methadone
—▲— Other opiates
—✕— Barbiturates
—✳— Other drugs

Fig. 10.2   Percentage of drug-related deaths per year, 1967–93.

are very different death rates in the different age groups. In the last decade of the study, for example, the average annual death rate per 1000 person-years was 3.2 for those aged 15–24 years, 8.3 for those aged 25–34 years, 13.9 for those aged 35–44 years and 10.7 for those aged 45–54 years. Furthermore, while the death rate declined over the 27-year period for the total population, this did not apply to all age groups, with the death rate of those aged 35–44 years increasing by about 40% in the last decade of the study in comparison with the first. Overall, the Standardized Mortality Rate for females was higher than for males throughout the study.

Cause of death

What do these young addicts die of? Even with long periods of administration, pure opiates do not cause direct tissue damage, and it is evident from this study that a substantial proportion of addicts can and do survive for a long period. However, it is perhaps not surprising that drug-related deaths do account for 64% of deaths, with heroin and barbiturates accounting for the smallest percentage during the 27-year period. Barbiturates used to be a major cause of addict deaths but have been in decline since 1972, with other opiates (morphine, dipipanone and dextromoramide) now accounting for the highest number of deaths. Deaths related to methadone were relatively stable until 1990 when an increase in trend occurred which has persisted. There has also been an increase in deaths related to other, nonopiate drugs.[13] These worrying trends may be attributable to the prescription of drugs to addicts far in excess of their therapeutic needs, with consequent 'leakage' of prescribed drugs to the illicit market. In part this may be due to doctors not adhering to good practice prescribing guidelines, but in some cases addicts may deliberately seek substitution therapy for opiate and/or ben-zodiazepine dependence from two or more sources simultaneously. Published data for methadone and morphine consumption confirms an increasing trend in the UK.[15]

These mortality findings are not confined to notified addicts. A study carried out in the coroners' courts of Greater London identified 134 deaths due to drug addiction in the period 1970–74, of which only 79 (59%) were addicts who in life had been notified to the Home Office. At that time, many (71) deaths were primarily due to barbiturate overdose, and only 44 of the addicts were known to the Home Office.[16] A more recent study in 80 coroners' jurisdictions in England and Wales of deaths due to psychoactive drugs, found that about 68% of all cases studied had a history of drug abuse.[17]

In summary, although opiate dependence is not invariably fatal, many, pre-dominantly young people, die from it. The mortality rate in the earlier years of dependence appears to have remained fairly constant over a number of years, suggesting that this is perhaps an unvarying component of the 'natural history' of the condition. Subsequent mortality may be more markedly affected by 'external' factors. In the UK, addicts' deaths are usually due to drug overdoses and pre-scribed drugs are at the core of this aspect of the problem. Far from being a new phenomenon, prescribed drugs have always played a large part in addiction in Britain and this may be the inevitable consequence of a medical, rather than a criminalizing, response to addiction. These findings emphasize how, even in death, addiction is intimately involved with and influenced by apparently periph-eral issues. Mortality rates are decided not only by the severity of the dependence syndrome, but also by the availability of drugs to the general population, which in turn is closely related to doctors' prescribing practices

Outcome of treatment

The high mortality rate of opiate dependence emphasizes the severity of the condition for some individuals and, on a wider scale, drug abuse and dependence have far-reaching implications for society as a whole. The need for effective treatment is clear and becomes daily more important as the numbers involved increase steadily. It is no longer sufficient to offer treatment on an *ad hoc* basis; its usefulness must be assessed. In this context, it is important to be precise about the goals of specific treatment modalities. For example, if treatment is aimed at reducing criminality and illicit drug abuse, it is necessary to know if it actually has this effect and for what proportion of patients. Similarly, if the purpose of a treatment programme is detoxification, it is useful to know what proportion of patients actually achieve abstinence and whether other methods of detoxification are better or worse at achieving this. If an out-patient programme is aimed at preventing relapse, how many people stay drug free and for how long?

The answers to these questions are important, primarily for the sake of the individual, but they also have important financial implications. When large numbers of patients are involved, resources (staff, time, money) should not be wasted on ineffective treatment, and if comparable treatment programmes yield similar results, it is common sense to adopt the most economical. Cost-effectiveness may be further improved if patient characteristics can be identified that permit patients to be assigned to the treatment that is most likely to help them attain achievable goals.

Despite the obvious difficulties of treatment evaluation, many research studies are addressing this problem – or at least some aspect of it. None can give a complete answer about the 'best' treatment, but separate studies, focusing on specific answerable questions, are providing worthwhile information. Gradually, a picture is emerging, as yet far from complete, that shows some of the effects and consequences of different treatment interventions.

Outcome evaluation studies

The National Treatment Outcome Research Study (NTORS)[18] has been the largest study into treatment outcomes in the UK. It is a prospective longitudinal cohort study involving the monitoring of 1075 drug misusers admitted into treatment in the 1990s, from 54 different treatment facilities including both residential and community services. Although there are some serious reservations about the methodology of this study, it demonstrated considerable improvements in substance use, health and criminality 2 years after the end of treatment. For example, regular heroin use fell by 43%, cocaine and amphetamine use fell by 60% and benzodiazepines by 70%. Acquisitive crime was reported to fall by more than 75% and drug trafficking by 80%.[18]

As always, vast studies have been carried out in the USA on a scale unknown elsewhere. The Drug Abuse Reporting Programme (DARP),[19] for example, described 44 000 patients attending 52 different agencies from 1969 to 1974. Follow-up research strategies and patient characteristics of 6402 patients were selected for follow-up. The treatment modalities studied included methadone maintenance (MM), therapeutic communities (TC), out-patient drug-free (DF) programmes (mostly nonopiate drug users) and short-term detoxification (DT). Outcome was defined as 'highly favourable' if there was no use of illicit drugs (except less than daily use of cannabis) and no arrests or imprisonment during the year, and as 'moderately favourable' if there was no daily use of illicit drugs and no major criminality (i.e. <30 days in prison; no crimes against the person or crimes of profit). Sophisticated statistical analysis, with 'time at risk' adjustments, demonstrated that the most favourable outcomes were associated with MM, TC and DF and that patients on these three programmes did about equally well. Those on short-term detoxification programmes and those who registered with one of the treatment agencies, but never actually engaged in treatment, had significantly poorer outcomes. Since then, meta-analysis of MM studies has confirmed a statistically significant relationship between treatment and the reduction of illicit opiate use, HIV risk behaviours and drug and property crimes.[20] It was also found that psychosocial counselling, as part of treatment programmes, had a positive impact on outcome.[21]

Also in the United States, the Drug Abuse Treatment Outcome Studies (DATOS), has reported on further evaluation studies, analysing the treatment results of 96 programmes (10 010 patients) 1 year after the end of treatment in the 1990s. This demonstrated a two thirds reduction in 'hard core drug use' – i.e. drug use at least weekly – for cocaine and heroin, and a reduction in involvement in illegal activities by more than one half. Both DARP and DATOS demonstrated that results were better with longer engagement in treatment with 90 days (3 months) appearing to be a critical minimum level.[19]

In this context, it would be expected that residential rehabilitation, for example in a therapeutic community, should be helpful and the Treatment Outcome Prospective Study (TOPS) confirmed this. While regular use of drugs was reported by 31% of clients in the year before admission to residential programmes, for those who received at least 23 months of treatment, this reduced to zero during the first 90 days of treatment and then stabilized at 12% at 3–5 years after treatment.[19]

Collectively, these findings are of interest and importance. Firstly, many studies confirm that treatment works. Secondly, they confirm clinical experience and commonsense expectation that in a chronic illness, change is unlikely to be effected by fleeting contact with treatment. This emphasizes the importance of retention in treatment as a phenomenon in its own right. The consequences of drop-out can be serious both for the patient and for society as a whole and if drug abusers are going to be helped, they must stay in contact with the helping agency. We need to know who the drop-outs are and why they leave treatment. Some studies have already suggested that retention in treatment (or outcome) can be predicted from psychobiological testing or from typologies derived from cluster analyses of patients' characteristics. Thus personality traits, once studied from the point of view of the aetiology of dependence, may come to be of more interest as predictors of outcome.[22,23] From such studies has come the concept of 'matching' patients to the treatment facility that is most likely to be successful and which also provides best value for money because, if some patients benefit equally from all treatment programmes, it makes financial sense to manage them in less expensive out-patient treatment programmes rather than in costly in-patient units. However, it is worth noting that in the survey of British addicts being prescribed heroin in 1969, there were very few differences between those who were going to continue taking opiates and those who were going to stop. They could not, for example, be differentiated on characteristics such as social class, sex, employment, crime, drug use or income, so that prediction about prognosis and treatment would have been very difficult. In fact, the main difference seemed to be that those who subsequently stopped taking opiates were younger, had a shorter history of addiction and were prescribed smaller doses of opiates.[8]

Retention in treatment

Of course, the prescription of opiates to addicts when they present for treatment is an important, often essential, component for retaining them in treatment. The extent to which addicts should get what they want as a way of attracting them to, and keeping them in treatment, is a difficult question to resolve. The point is elegantly illustrated by research carried out in London in the 1970s, when some patients attending a clinic were offered injectable heroin (undoubtedly the drug of choice for most opiate addicts), while the rest had oral methadone. A year later, three quarters of the heroin group were still attending the clinic compared with less than one third of the methadone group, most of whom had left treatment early in the year. However, those receiving heroin had changed very little – they continued to take their heroin and most were still involved in the drug subculture. In other words, heroin had kept them in contact with the treatment agency, had maintained the status quo of their addiction and had reduced their involvement in criminal activity. In contrast, after a year, the methadone group had polarized into two subcategories. Some had given up drug use altogether and were not involved in criminal activity, but others were injecting illicit opiates regularly and had a high conviction rate. It seemed, therefore, that the more confrontational approach of not giving the addict the preferred drug 'precipitated' abstinence for some, at the price of effectively driving others away from the treatment agency altogether.[24]

The interaction between treatment and the wider society

Public debate on this issue has became more vigorous with the advent of AIDS, because of concern about protecting the general population from this disease. A body of opinion believes that the general purpose of the treatment of addiction should change from one that emphasizes abstinence for as many addicts as possible, to one of 'harm reduction' – ostensibly the reduction of harm that addicts may do to themselves, but also with the clear purpose of reducing the harm they may do to society as a whole – for example, reducing drug-related crime and reducing the risk of transmission of AIDS. Since then, with a vociferous lobby in favour of 'decriminalisation' of drug use that is currently categorized as illicit, the arguments have changed again. These debates illustrate how the treatment of addiction and its evaluation can be radically affected by societal factors. It is this ever-shifting background that makes assessment of treatment outcome so difficult.

Discussion

Despite the very patchy nature of our knowledge, it is possible to draw together some of the information that has been gathered and to present the rudiments of an answer to the question posed at the beginning of this chapter, 'What happens to addicts?'

Firstly, it is apparent that opiate dependence is a serious condition with a high mortality rate. This is particularly worrying because of the youth of those concerned and because of the feeling that they may have stumbled into drug abuse and dependence because of a combination of circumstances, and that death is too high a price to pay for youthful error.

Nevertheless, a diagnosis of opiate dependence is not a death sentence. The majority of opiate abusers do survive – some settling into a state of chronic dependence, with areas of their life, other than drug-taking, more or less normal and involving stability of relationships, home and employment. It appears that this group can function normally only if they take an opiate regularly and that their drug is as necessary for them as insulin is for a diabetic, or vitamin B_{12} injections for someone with pernicious anaemia. Others become abstinent. Those who are young and have a shorter history of addiction are the most likely to achieve this outcome – which is undoubtedly the safest and most satisfactory.

It is therefore important to encourage everyone who seeks help to attempt abstinence while their chances of achieving it are highest, and before they become entrenched in a permanent drug-taking lifestyle. Not everyone will achieve abstinence in the early stages of their drug-taking career, and even those who do are likely to need several 'tries'. It is worth pointing out that the prognosis for 'new' addicts, presenting in the twenty-first century, may be better than that established for addicts who presented for treatment in the late 1960s and 1970s. 'Modern' drug addicts have a daily dose of opiates that is much lower than their counterparts in the 1960s, so on pharmacological grounds their dependence can be considered less severe.

At present, there is no sure way of predicting at the beginning of a dependence 'career' which route a particular individual is likely to follow. It seems as if the most stable and 'settled' are the most likely to end up as stable, chronic addicts, but in the UK this may be a reflection of a system that permits opiate maintenance. It also appears that those with the most severe psychological problems do less well, often continuing to abuse a variety of drugs in a chaotic fashion. They suffer the medical, legal and social consequences of their drug abuse until such time as they do eventually 'mature' into abstinence, settle down into a more stable pattern of drug-taking, or kill themselves. Mortality statistics suggest a hard core, apparently unhelped by treatment, who die early in their addiction career, and this bears out clinical experience of a group who do badly whatever measures are attempted.

Research over the last 20 years appears to demonstrate that treatment can and does work. Health care professionals and drug-dependent individuals themselves must therefore hang on to the fact that a good proportion can achieve abstinence and be considered 'cured'. This is rarely achieved rapidly – drug dependence is a chronic condition unlikely to be affected by brief encounters with treatment intervention – but if a prolonged period of help is accepted, this offers real hope of drug abstinence. Compulsory 'help', in terms of enforced abstinence during imprisonment, is rarely useful because relapse is more likely to occur upon release.[25]

In addition to the effects of treatment on patients, it is also worth considering the economic impact of successful treatment although cost–benefit analysis is a relatively recent development in addiction studies. One study, for example, estimated that the treatment of 6500 heavy cocaine abusers in the USA would reduce cocaine consumption by one tonne per year.[26] With nearly a quarter of a million admissions for the treatment of cocaine abuse per year in the USA, it is easy to calculate that this could significantly affect the illicit cocaine market. Reductions in the cost of crime following treatment of cocaine dependence have also been demonstrated and cost–benefit ratios suggested significant returns on investment in both long-term residential and out-patient drug-free centres; other potential areas of benefit are health, disease avoidance and employment.[27] In the UK, for example, it has been claimed that for the main specialist treatments, every £1 spent on treatment saves more than £3 in the cost of addiction to the community.[28] In the USA, it has been estimated that every $1 spent saves the community $7.[29]

In many European countries an even higher proportion of heroin abusers are in contact with treatment agencies than in the USA and, again, this has the potential for significantly reducing demand for heroin and thus making a contribution to prevention initiatives (see Chapter 11). In other words, apart from the benefits to the individual, energetic approaches to treatment are likely to have wider societal benefits too.

So far attention has focused exclusively on the outcome of dependence of those addicts who have come to 'official' attention and who have remained within its range long enough for someone to assess what happens to them. But what of the rest? Undoubtedly, 'out there', beyond any statistics or follow-up studies, are many opiate-dependent individuals who make only fleeting contact with health-care workers and many who make no contact at all during the course of their drug-taking career. Their numbers are unknown, but it is abundantly clear that they exist: drug abusers approaching a clinic for the first time characteristically report a history of many years of drug abuse and long periods of regular self-injection; some make contact only briefly and never return; they describe friends who have injected regularly for years who have never sought help. Sometimes, this is due to a reluctance to become involved with a clinic or any official body, sometimes because they fear they will be prescribed inadequate quantities of opiates. Whatever the reason, and with a covert activity such as illicit drug abuse there may be many, these addicts and their fate remain unknown.

This profound ignorance seriously affects our understanding of the outcome of opiate dependence. It is rather like trying to understand the outcome of a streptococcal infection by studying only those admitted to hospital with the more sinister consequences such as rheumatic heart disease, arthritis or Sydenham's chorea, while ignoring all those with more common manifestation such as tonsillitis and cellulitis. It is therefore worth making a guess at what happens to these unrecognized thousands.

Undoubtedly, some die with their addiction still undetected and unknown to any authority until they die as a consequence of it. Mortality statistics do not, however, suggest that the majority of young unknown addicts perish. Some probably become chronically dependent, obtaining drugs regularly from illicit sources, but it is impossible to believe that they all go on to a state of permanent, covert, chronic dependence. In the 40 years since the beginning of the drug-dependence explosion in the UK, such a large population would have developed that it is unlikely that it could remain excluded from all statistics. Presumably, therefore, many become abstinent, probably in a very similar way to those who achieve abstinence by means of professional help – with periods of voluntary abstinence, followed by relapse into drug-taking, until eventually some achieve permanent abstinence. Indeed, it may be very common for abstinence to be achieved in this way with no professional intervention, because the individuals concerned are likely to be young and at an early stage of their addiction career – just the group most likely to become successfully abstinent. Those who present for professional treatment, on the other hand, are likely to be the more severely dependent who can no longer afford to support their escalating drug habit.

This emphasizes the point that although opiate dependence is a serious and chronic condition, there is cause and room for optimism. Abstinence is an attainable outcome for many, perhaps even the majority, and treatment is a way of propelling more drug-dependent individuals towards that outcome, more rapidly than they might otherwise have reached it. However, the importance of treatment is much greater than any theoretical 'success' rate. The fact that treatment exists is a clear statement that the dependent state need not be permanent, that drug-dependent individuals can be helped and that they are worthy of help. By its very existence, treatment offers hope, sparks motivation, and improves outcome; and these benefits extend beyond those who are in formal receipt of the different treatment interventions.

Although this chapter has focused on opiate dependence and its outcome, some of the observations that have been made clearly apply to other forms of substance dependence too. The chronic nature of dependence and the pattern of relapse and remission are common to all types of drug dependence, including alcohol and tobacco, and it is possible to identify similar types of outcome. For example, people attending slimming clinics for years to obtain regular prescriptions of amphetamine, or those taking barbiturates or benzodiazepines regularly for insomnia, equate with chronic, stable opiate addicts on methadone maintenance. Similarly, there are individuals who take sedative hypnotics for many years. The plethora of self-help groups that have sprung up tell eloquently of the difficulties of achieving abstinence – whatever the underlying drug of dependence. It is these (and other) underlying commonalities that justify different types of drug dependence being treated in similar ways, despite the different pharmacological properties of the drugs involved.

Prevention of drug abuse

Introduction

In the light of our knowledge of the consequences and complications of drug abuse, of the difficulties of treatment, and of the high mortality rate, the old adage, that prevention is better than cure, is beyond dispute. For drug-related problems, the value of prevention goes way beyond the individual benefits it confers, important though these are for the people whose lives are thus preserved. Prevention is also crucial for society as a whole and this is more apparent now than ever before. Drug trafficking, associated as it is with organized crime on an enormous scale, can threaten the very fabric of society by undermining law and order and the economy. In addition, the advent of AIDS, which is probably the most serious threat to the health of the world population since the Black Death, has made the prevention of drug abuse by injection relevant to everyone. No longer can drug dependence and abuse be shrugged off and ignored by those who are not affected; it is now in the immediate interest of everyone in the community that effective preventive measures should be adopted.

Although the need for prevention is clear, the best course of action is not. Because the causes of drug abuse are multiple, interrelated and multidimensional, its prevention is similarly complex. Unlike an infectious disease, there is no single causative factor to be opposed or countered by a single preventive measure, and it has proved very difficult to identify and assess which factors among many might be susceptible to preventive intervention.

It is not surprising, therefore, that different cultures and societies choose and employ quite different preventive measures, and that these will need to vary in response to new trends in drug abuse.

Definitions of prevention

A traditional approach has been to classify preventive measures as primary, secondary or tertiary.

- *Primary prevention* aims to prevent the initiation of drug abuse. Limiting the availability of drugs is an important component of this strategy, usually combined with educational programmes for those perceived to be at risk of starting to experiment with drugs.

- *Secondary prevention* depends on the early identification of drug abusers so that they can be treated promptly, to prevent the development of a state of severe dependence and to reduce the total number of those dependent on drugs.
- *Tertiary prevention* involves the treatment of those with a severe drug abuse or dependence problem, with the aim of mitigating the effects of harmful use. On the principle that most newcomers to the scene are introduced to drugs by an experienced user, vigorous efforts at treatment should also have a preventive effect.[1]

At all levels of prevention the keystone of any approach is to reduce drug availability by statutory control. At one stage, this was the only way of tackling drug-abuse prevention, but it has gradually become apparent that, on its own, this is never sufficient. Unless total eradication of supply is achieved, which is impossible, drug abuse continues. The modern approach therefore is to couple the goal of reducing the supply of drugs with that of reducing demand for them recognizing that, while neither approach is sufficient on its own, each augments the effectiveness of the other. The importance of demand reduction received international acknowledgement in the 1988 United Nations Convention against Illicit Traffic in Narcotic Drugs and Psychotropic Substances (see Chapter 12).[2]

Reducing the availability of drugs of abuse

The basis of all strategies to control the availability of drugs of abuse and dependence is statutory control and law enforcement. In all countries, laws are passed to control the production, supply, import, export, sale, prescription and possession of these drugs. The underlying principle is that there should be sufficient drugs available for any genuine, medical need, but no surplus, and that these drugs should be 'guarded' (i.e. controlled) to ensure that none are diverted for illicit abuse.[3,4]

The measures used to control the availability of drugs vary according to the type of drug involved. Different methods of control are used for prescription drugs (e.g. methadone, barbiturates, benzodiazepines, amphetamines) and for illicit street drugs (e.g. LSD, cocaine, cannabis, heroin). In the UK, heroin occupies a unique position: it can be medically prescribed, but because most of the abused heroin is smuggled into the country, many of the measures used to control its availability are the same as those employed for illicit drugs rather than for prescription drugs. Although cocaine can still be prescribed in the UK, this rarely happens.

Illicit drugs

The illicit street drugs currently causing most concern globally are heroin, cocaine and cannabis. Large quantities are smuggled into the major consumer countries – USA, Canada, Western Europe, Australia, New Zealand – from the producing countries, which are mostly in South and Central America and Asia. The main thrust of preventive action in the consumer countries has been to try to keep the drugs out by vigorous customs control at national boundaries, coupled with equally vigorous police activity to detect and prosecute those who buy and sell the drugs. Severe penalties are usually imposed on those who buy and sell large quantities of these drugs. However, it is generally admitted that only a fraction of the total imported is ever detected, and although massive seizures are frequently made, this appears to have little effect on drug availability. Because of their own failure to keep drugs out, the consumer countries have looked further afield and have encouraged attempts to reduce availability by curtailing production abroad. Crop eradication, by burning or spraying with herbicides, financial inducements for crop substitution, destroying illicit factories where drugs are extracted and purified, and destroying airstrips to prevent drugs being moved out, have all been tried. Despite immense input in terms of time, money and effort, the plant crops from which the drugs are extracted (opium, cannabis, coca) continue to be grown, apparently in increasing acreage, because they are far more profitable than any other crop. Stopping their cultivation would adversely affect employment, income and standard of living – and not just for those immediately involved in this activity.

Income from these crops may be integral to the producer country's economy and those who control the drug trade are very wealthy and usually have considerable political power. In addition, the producer countries themselves have, so far, had comparatively little experience of serious drug problems because there the drugs are consumed in a socially controlled way, as they have been for centuries, by smoking or chewing the vegetable matter rather than in a highly purified and potent form. The drug problems of the rich, importing countries, have up to now caused little concern to producers and have seemed an inadequate reason for tackling a difficult and politically unpopular problem. Recently, however, the picture has changed and several of the producer countries have begun to experience the real impact of a serious drug problem. A more determined effort to eradicate excessive crops may thus become more acceptable to their population.

An additional impetus for action in these countries is that there is now serious concern about the environmental impact of illicit cultivation of narcotic drugs, that now accounts for an increasing proportion of tropical deforestation. Land-clearing techniques such as 'slash and burn' in the depths of the rainforest, often in steep-sloped mountain environments, lead to a high degree of soil erosion and nutrient depletion. Problems are compounded by high levels of chemical use, in the form of herbicides, fungicides and fertilizers. Furthermore, it is now common for drug extraction and purification to take place in clandestine refineries close to the site of cultivation, and toxic by-products are dumped indiscriminately, polluting water supplies that are used to irrigate food crops, causing significant public health risks.

However, the distinction between producing, transit and consuming countries has now become blurred and most countries are consumers of a wide variety of drugs. Furthermore, the production and manufacture of some substances now takes place nearer to the consumers and, as far as synthetic drugs and psychotropic substances are concerned, trafficking may take place in many different directions simultaneously. A number of developing countries now have manufacturing capacity for the licit as well as the illicit market and hydroponic cultivation of high grade cannabis is widespread in some industrialized countries. The availability of appropriate chemicals and precursors essential for manufacturing controlled drugs is another factor in the international market and drug-trafficking scene. The globalization of economies, trade and communication makes the identification of the source of production, manufacture and trading via intermediary agents, very complex. Preventive measures thus have to tackle *all* aspects of the problem, which is made more difficult by the larger number of agencies that are now involved in supply reduction and interdiction. This requires an adequate legal system to cope with highly technical legal enforcement issues as well as money laundering, confiscated assets, controlled delivery, etc., which are beyond the scope of this book. All such measures to reduce availability must be complemented by a reduction in drug demand and the importance of moving away from a dichotomous model to a continuum, in which both demand and supply reduction are fundamental to prevention, cannot be exaggerated.[5]

There is some evidence that sustainable alternative development will have an effect on the eradication of cultivation of narcotic crops, providing that there is adequate financial and technical support over a long period of time; this, of course, requires political will, international support and collaboration[1,6]

Whatever the measures taken by individual countries, there is little cause for optimism. If crops of cocaine, opium and cannabis are forced out of one geographical area, there is every likelihood that they will be grown, equally successfully, elsewhere in the world, and for the same reason. The potential profit is so enormous that even large increases in the cost of production have only minimal impact on the final profit margin. Even if there were total crop eradication world-wide, chemists, spurred on by the promise of those profits, could undoubtedly synthesize any of these drugs in illicit factories, just as LSD, amphetamines and many designer drugs are synthesized today.[1,7,8]

Prescription drugs

Because drugs such as barbiturates, benzodiazepines and amphetamines are (or should be) available only on prescription, the doctor who prescribes them, and who therefore acts as the 'barrier' between the drugs and the general population, is the key figure in any attempt to reduce their availability. Improving doctors' prescribing practices may therefore be an important preventive strategy, both in terms of reducing the likelihood of an individual becoming dependent on drugs in the course of treatment and in terms of reducing 'overspill' of prescribed drugs to the black market.[9]

In the course of their training, doctors learn about psychiatric illnesses and the psychoactive drugs available for their treatment. Once qualified, however, they see many patients with symptoms suggestive of psychiatric illness, but who are not suffering from an identifiable disease state. Patients complain, for example, of nonspecific symptoms such as depression, anxiety, sleeplessness, inability to cope and headache, that reflect life's stresses but do not necessarily indicate psychiatric illness. They are normal responses, experienced by most people at some time or another, to a difficult situation, and if the situation is very difficult, the symptoms too may be very severe. The point at which they are felt to be sufficiently severe to seek medical help varies from one individual to another, and the point at which drug treatment is judged to be necessary is similarly arbitrary. Because the symptoms are often very distressing, and because modern psychoactive drugs can provide almost immediate relief, it is a natural and humane response to offer symptomatic treatment by prescribing these drugs. The doctor is well aware that in many cases the treatment is not curative but the principle of symptomatic treatment is, after all, a well-established component of clinical care. For these patients the underlying problem, whether personal, interpersonal or social, is usually beyond the doctor's power of intervention.

Although well intentioned, the lax prescribing of psychoactive drugs often has unintended effects on the individual concerned and has become so widespread that it has far reaching consequences for society as a whole. For the individual, the rush to provide symptomatic relief may mean that the underlying condition is not investigated and is never identified. To make matters worse, the drugs themselves may further impair the patient's ability to cope with the problems. The drugs are potentially harmful, with a variety of side effects. They are liable to abuse and may be taken in overdose, giving rise to considerable problems of diagnosis, treatment and rehabilitation. There is always a risk of dependence, even when taken under controlled medical conditions. Most important of all, however, is that inappropriate prescription to individuals contributes to a vast pool of these drugs within the community as a whole. How many households, one wonders, do not have a supply of psychoactive drugs, often the remnants of earlier courses of treatment? It is these medicines, legitimately obtained on prescription and now as easily available as any 'over the counter' medication, that provide a never-ending source of drugs for abuse and dependence, just as surely as the fields of opium poppies and the plantations of coca bushes and cannabis.

The education of doctors in the rational prescription of psychoactive drugs is therefore crucial to reducing their present, very liberal availability. Doctors should learn from a very early stage of their training the full implications of their prescribing habits. Their training should prepare them adequately to cope with the many patients who will present complaining of the nonspecific symptoms outlined above. A scientific approach to the prescription of psychoactive drugs must be inculcated from the beginning, before casual and unthinking habits become entrenched. For example, the specific condition or symptom to be treated must be clearly identified, and the decision to prescribe a psychoactive drug must be made on the positive grounds of its effectiveness, rather than for negative reasons, such as the patient's expectations or the doctor's need to be seen to be responding. The drug with the least potential for abuse should be prescribed, although alleged differences between drugs of the same class should be treated with scepticism. The dose and the appropriate duration of treatment must be decided. Prescription of the optimum dosage is very important: too small a dose is pointless, exposing the patient to many of the risks of treatment for little or no therapeutic benefit; too large a dose increases the risk of toxicity and dependence and means that more of the drug is available to spill over into the communal 'pool'. Patients should understand at the outset that treatment with any of these drugs will be for a limited period, usually only for a few weeks. This period depends, in part, on the pharmacological properties of the drug and, in particular, on the time taken for tolerance to develop to the effects of the drug. Once this occurs, the prescribed dose is no longer effective and to continue the drug at that dose is of little or no use. Side effects should be monitored throughout and patients thought to be at risk of developing dependence on the drug should be identified at the start. All of these decisions and observations are usually made automatically when non-psychoactive drugs are prescribed, but the usual clinical approach is often abandoned when psychoactive drugs are involved, perhaps because it seems less appropriate if the underlying problems are social rather than medical.

Once the stage has been reached when prescribing becomes a positive, therapeutic decision rather than a semi-automatic response, there are likely to be many more occasions when the prescription of psychoactive drugs is seen to be wholly inappropriate. For example, if the real cause of the patient's anxiety is a long-standing social problem, there is little point in prescribing benzodiazepines for a month, which is the maximum advisable duration of treatment with these drugs for anxiety.

Similarly, chronic insomnia is rarely benefited in the long term by treatment with hypnotics. In these or similar situations, when a pharmacological solution is seen to be inappropriate, it may still be very difficult for the doctor to withhold symptomatic relief when confronted by a patient suffering real and distressing symptoms. It is therefore very important that doctors become familiar with practical and effective alternative treatment strategies, such as behaviour therapy, psychotherapy, counselling, etc. Some of these methods may appear technical and difficult when described in scientific jargon, but they are often no more than the application of commonsense principles to patient management.[9] In practice, most doctors employ them unconsciously as part of their total therapeutic relationship with their patients. If any attempt to reduce the availability of psychoactive drugs is to be successful, these nonpharmacological responses will have to receive far more attention in medical education than at present, so that they become a recognized and a respectable component of the therapeutic response, rather than merely second-rate 'alternatives' or 'afterthoughts' to prescribing. Behavioural approaches have the additional advantage of helping people to take responsibility for their own problems, rather than expecting a pharmacological solution, and in the long term may help to reverse the trend towards the medicalization of psychosocial problems.

Medical education, therefore, has a crucial role to play in reducing the availability of prescribed drugs for abuse. This begins with undergraduate education, where basic information about psychoactive drugs and the consequences of their abuse should be formally taught and should receive the attention merited by a condition that can cause widespread public health and social problems. Because there is a constant stream of new psychoactive drugs coming into the market all the time, it is essential that during their undergraduate education, doctors also acquire the skills necessary to evaluate information about new drugs, so that extravagant claims for effectiveness and lack of dependence liability can be assessed critically.[10] Undergraduate education, however, is only the starting point. The practising doctor, as well as keeping abreast of new drugs and treatments, is also exposed to a variety of influences. Continuing education is essential, and it is important that all the institutions and organizations that are in a position to train and influence the doctor exert their influence in the direction of the rational use of psychoactive drugs. Their involvement may take the form of seminars, conferences, articles in journals, etc., and they also play an important role in liaising with other bodies such as government and pharmaceutical industries.[4,9]

The role of pharmaceutical companies in training doctors is often ignored because it is felt that their ultimate goal, of increasing the sale of their products, opposes the aims of rational prescribing and of reducing the availability of psychoactive drugs that might be abused. However, because governments can and do impose strict control on drugs that are widely abused, the optimal prescribing of their products is ultimately in the best interest of the pharmaceutical companies too and their role in research and information dissemination is too important to be discounted.[1,11]

The risks of certain drugs, such as cocaine, heroin and other opiates, are seen to be so great that special legal restrictions are imposed upon their prescription. The degree of restriction and the drugs involved vary from country to country, but the basic principle is that clinical freedom to prescribe as the doctor wishes is sacrificed for the sake of control, because the drugs concerned are being widely abused. Such measures are usually imposed in response to an upsurge in abuse and are intended to prevent the situation worsening. Their effectiveness may be reduced by a shift in the pattern of abuse to another, less restricted and therefore more easily available preparation. In other words, the problem is not eliminated but transferred to new areas. It is for this reason that imposing restrictions, although sometimes necessary as an immediate response, is far less significant as a long-term preventive measure than genuine improvements in prescribing practices. Some countries have carried this restriction a stage further and have adopted a national drug policy with only a very limited number of drugs available for prescription. The psychoactive drugs included in this list have been well tried out in practice and the information necessary to ensure their proper use is available. New drugs are added to the list only if they have clear-cut advantages over existing drugs.[12]

Other health care professionals, apart from doctors, are also involved in controlling the availability of psychoactive drugs. In some countries, for example, many of these drugs can be obtained 'over the counter', without the need for any prescription, and the pharmacists who sell them and who have a vested financial interest in their sale must be included in any educational initiatives.[13] Even in countries where prescriptions are always required, pharmacists may be important in detecting abuse and may be able to exert a beneficial influence on patients who seek their advice about taking psychoactive drugs. In some parts of the world, community nurses too may have supplies of these drugs under their control.

Reducing the demand for drugs of abuse

The great difficulties of reducing the availability of drugs for abuse emphasize the need to reduce public demand for them: if no-one wanted heroin or cocaine, the illicit market for them would collapse; if there were no longer the expectation that the doctor can and therefore should relieve all discomfort, far fewer prescriptions for psychoactive drugs would be required. Demand reduction, however, is a preventive approach that attracts comparatively little attention because it depends heavily on worthwhile, but un-newsworthy educational campaigns to influence society's attitude towards drugs and drug-taking. Unfortunately, one need look no further than the next cigarette smoker to know that there is no straightforward relationship between education – teaching people about drugs and the dangers of drug abuse – and actually changing their drug-taking behaviour. Spelling out the risks of a particular type of drug abuse does not necessarily mean that those who indulge in it will actually stop doing so and there is evidence that ill-chosen material, intended to scare people away from drug abuse, may instead arouse an interest in the topic and stimulate some individuals, who would not otherwise have become involved, to try drug-taking for themselves.[14]

The content of any educational effort is therefore of the greatest importance. Broadly based health campaigns that encourage healthy lifestyles are generally agreed to be the best approach. Within this framework, healthy eating, participation in sport and physical activities and the appropriate use of medicines are emphasized.

In other words, the message is positive – what should be done to achieve and maintain a healthy lifestyle, rather than emphasizing what is forbidden or dangerous. The individual is encouraged to assume personal responsibility for his or her own health, which would clearly be damaged if drugs were abused. The advantage of this sort of approach is that with appropriate modification of presentation and detail, it is suitable in its broad outline for all ages and all groups. From primary school onwards, the emphasis is on a positive attitude towards health, and within this framework the safe use of medicines can be emphasized: that they should be taken only when necessary for the treatment of illness, that medicines should always be stored safely, that one person must never take another's medicine, and so on.

From this baseline position it is possible to move on quite naturally to non-pharmacological responses for coping with both physical and psychological symptoms. It is very important that people learn that there is not always a 'pill for every ill' and that for many conditions for which there is no cure, symptomatic relief, using traditional, homely remedies is appropriate. A child given lemon and honey for a sore throat, rather than a medicated lozenge, or a hot-water bottle for a stomach ache, rather than a spoonful of medicine, is being taught by practical experience that the first response to discomfort is not necessarily a pill, a medicine, or a drug, but commonsense self-help. Such lessons carried on into adulthood teach that mild psychological symptoms too may be managed by nonpharmacological methods. In this context, one can question whether it is wise for indiscriminate pill-taking of any sort to be positively promoted in any way. Should 'over the counter', nonprescription medicine be widely advertised on television, for example? Should children take daily vitamin pills, when a good diet can supply their needs? Practices such as these run contrary to the basic message of only taking medicines when absolutely necessary, to treat recognized disease states, and they invest medicine-taking with an undesirable ordinariness.

Although it is very important that the trend of recent years to medicalize social problems should be reversed, it is equally important that the proper use of medicines should not be discouraged. Amid all the concern about psychoactive drugs and the catalogue of problems consequent on their use, it should not be forgotten that it is this group of drugs that has revolutionized the care of the mentally ill during the last 40 years or so. The drugs have permitted many who would otherwise have been confined to institutions to live within the community and have removed much of the stigma of mental illness. It is essential, therefore, that efforts to limit inappropriate use of drugs in general and of psychoactive drugs in particular, do not develop into a general condemnation of all drug-taking. There are many people for whom it is absolutely essential to take drugs regularly, perhaps on a daily basis, perhaps for life, for the treatment of physical or mental illness. Those with a genuine requirement for such treatment should not be discouraged from this wholly appropriate use of drugs, nor made to feel guilty about it.

Once again, doctors have an important role to play in this long-term, public education programme. Their attitudes towards prescribing and their prescribing practices may significantly affect their patients' attitudes too. Doctors who pre-scribe rationally and who explain their decisions to their patients can make a medical consultation a genuinely educational experience and can contribute regularly to the prevention of drug abuse.

In addition to the education of the community as a whole, specific target groups can be identified for whom more specialized campaigns may be appropriate. Young people are usually perceived as a group for whom preventive education is most important, perhaps because much drug abuse starts at this age, when it is intimately related to peer-group pressure and youthful curiosity.[15,16] It is also a time for rebellious attitudes and behaviour, when campaigns against drug abuse may have exactly the opposite effect, stimulating an interest in drugs just because they are 'anti-authority'. At this time, life skills training may be particularly appropriate in helping them develop basic personal and social skills so that they can better cope with the everyday problems with which they are confronted. These programmes focus on providing young people with the information and skills needed to resist social pressures to use drugs as well as reducing the potential motivation for drug use by helping the development of greater social confidence and self-esteem.

Many other target groups can also be identified.[17] Young professionals, who may be tempted to take cocaine as a symbol of their success; old people who sleep poorly and who would like regular prescriptions for hypnotics; doctors, with their prescription pads always in front of them – all can be recognized as being at special risk, and worthy of special preventive efforts.

For these more specialized preventive campaigns it may seem appropriate to focus the anti-drug message on the particular drug that is the current cause of concern. This permits a simple and direct communication to get the immediate message across, but by stressing the hazards of a particular drug, it is out of tune with modern thinking about the much bigger problem of substance abuse as a whole. Instead, where possible, it should be integrated within existing frameworks and health care programmes, making best use of opportunistic interventions.[18,19] For example, older adolescents may be approached through programmes in youth training or work-experience schemes, while the health promotion clinics established by primary health care teams for specific patient groups can play an important preventive role in which active patient participation is encouraged. Pregnant women, for example, attending antenatal clinics and aware that the health of their unborn child is dependent on their own good health, may be particularly receptive to health education. Similarly those consulting a doctor or admitted to hospital offer a window of opportunity for brief interventions, perhaps using very brief questionnaires to establish habits of substance use and then offering information, advice and opportunities for seeking help if necessary. Another potentially fruitful population for opportunistic intervention is the prison population, particularly because substance abuse is so prevalent in this group.

Community involvement

When substance abuse becomes endemic in a particular area, it often provokes a reaction in the local community who become deeply resentful of its impact on their lives and who, with appropriate leadership, may group together to combat the problem. The community response may develop in a number of different ways. For example, some seek to enhance law enforcement, perhaps by organizing citizen patrols, working closely with the local police force and informing them of ongoing drug activities. Other approaches include civil justice efforts by taking drug dealers to court, developing local treatment and prevention programmes and also more general actions that unite local residents into vibrant communities by engaging them in action to improve their communities and the local environment by direct action (collecting litter, removing graffiti, organizing activities for children).

In the USA during the 1970s, parent movements formed a significant part of such grass-roots prevention activities. In general, they focused on the social and environmental factors that were believed to be contributing to drug escalation among young people and developed very clear goals for primary and secondary prevention. They emphasized an uncompromising 'no-use' message rather than recommending the 'responsible use' of illegal and harmful drugs and ensured that drug education materials accurately reflected the findings in medical and scientific literature about the effects of different substances. They also organized intensive campaigns in many areas to ban the sale of drug paraphernalia, even though they were opposed by powerful groups campaigning for the decriminalization of cannabis. Evaluation of such activities is not simple but their strategies appear to have contributed to the steady decline in drug use by adolescents and young adults during the late 1970s and the 1980s, which was associated with their perception that substance misuse was indeed harmful.

Unfortunately, these hopeful trends began to decline in the early 1990s at a time when there was growing pressure to decriminalize cannabis and when substance abuse was increasingly being glamorized in song, films and fashion. Of course the media have been, and indeed still are, widely used in drug abuse prevention campaigns.[20]

Role of the media

There is also an awareness that the media can influence people's attitudes to substance abuse in a more indirect way.[21] For example, millions of people regularly watch television 'soaps' and their portrayal of substance abuse has the potential to provoke widespread discussion about such issues and also to affect public perceptions and responses. It is therefore essential that such programmes adopt responsible approaches and do not seek to glamourize substance abuse. Similarly, it is important that the significant role models for young people – pop stars, actors, sportsmen and women and the like – are aware of their potential influence particularly on young people and use this to reduce demand for drugs and certainly not to promote them.

Pharmacological approaches

One approach to preventing dependence on prescribed drugs has been to try to modify the chemical structure of drugs to reduce or eliminate their dependence-producing liability. Pharmaceutical companies are constantly producing new psychoactive drugs for which they make extravagant claims in this respect. Usually, however, when more people start to use the drug, its dependence potential becomes apparent and cases of abuse and of dependence on it are reported. So far, this approach to preventing dependence has been strikingly unsuccessful, as evidenced by the barbiturates, which were replaced by non-barbiturate hypnotics such as methaqualone, which in turn gave way to benzodiazepines.[22] Now that these too have come under the cloud of dependence, a new anxiolytic has appeared opportunely on the market, and the same claims are being heard again.

Although solvents are not prescribed drugs, a similar approach is being adopted to control their abuse, and new solvents are being developed which it is hoped lack 'sniffing' appeal.

An interesting example of preventing drug abuse by tackling the drug itself comes from the USA, where there was a serious outbreak of pentazocine (Fortral, Talwin) abuse. Talwin tablets intended for oral use were crushed and injected together with tablets of the antihistamine tripelennamine, resulting in a 'high' said to be similar to that caused by heroin. The pharmacological response was to add naloxone, an opiate antagonist, to the preparation of pentazocine; if the drug was taken orally, as intended, its analgesic effect was unimpaired because naloxone is inactive by the oral route. If the drug were injected, however, the naloxone antagonized the effect of pentazocine and the drug abuser did not experience any 'high'.[23] A similar approach has been proposed for the reduction of buprenorphine abuse, with buprenorphine being mixed with naloxone.

Finally the use of the opiate antagonist naltrexone to prevent relapse in carefully selected patients (see Chapter 7) is another example of prevention utilizing pharmacological techniques.[24]

Clearly, measures such as these are peripheral to the main issues of prevention and can only be employed in occasional, circumscribed areas of the totality of drug abuse. Nevertheless, they may sometimes be of value.

Harm reduction

Harm reduction, which is discussed in more detail in Chapter 7 is a somewhat different approach to prevention which distinguishes between measures aimed at reducing the risk of engagement in substance abuse, and measures aimed at reducing the harm associated with drug abuse. In the present climate of anxiety about the wider risks of HIV and AIDS, more emphasis is now being placed on harm reduction.[25] This approach acknowledges that, as total eradication of drug abuse is impossible, every effort should be made to minimize its harmful consequences, both for the individual concerned and for society as a whole. A potential disadvantage of such measures is that they may give an impression of ambivalence in attitude towards substance abuse.

Conclusion

The prevention of drug abuse and drug dependence, like the treatment and the conditions themselves, is a chronic process. Once again, we see that there are no quick and easy solutions but a number of measures, none effective alone, but each making some contribution to the totality of a comprehensive programme. The preventive measures that seem likely to be most effective include reducing the availability of drugs by effective law enforcement, including the application of penalties severe enough to deter those who make huge profits by dealing in illicit drugs. Reduction of the availability of prescription drugs, however, relies less on law enforcement and much more on the education of doctors in rational prescribing. This is closely related to the problem of changing public attitudes towards medicine in general and psychoactive drugs in particular. Educating the public to reduce the demand for psychoactive drugs is a very long-term project. It probably offers the best hope for the prevention of drug abuse in years to come, but it will undoubtedly take a long time to reverse the trends of recent decades.[17]

In addition, this approach emphasizes the fact that effective prevention will never be brought about, or imposed on the community, by the actions of professionals and experts alone. On the contrary, it is absolutely essential that the whole community has a strong commitment to prevention. Unfortunately, it seems that the problem has to be severe before this kind of response is initiated, but it is reassuring that when a community is genuinely under threat it can and often does respond energetically.

Parallels can be drawn with what has happened and what is happening with cigarette smoking: community attitudes and responses to smoking now permit far more coercive and draconian measures to be taken than could have been contemplated 20 years ago, and the prevalence of cigarette smoking in the UK has declined steadily. In China, too, after liberation, fervent support on the part of the community enabled the total eradication of problems related to the use of opium. Continuing commitment to prevention has resulted in China remaining comparatively free of drug-related problems.[4]

It is to be hoped that the long-term, educational approaches outlined in this chapter will bear fruit in years to come and that pharmacological solutions to personal problems will cease to be the norm. In the meantime, the importance of indirect factors, such as improved housing, education, leisure opportunities and employment, that can all influence drug-taking significantly, should not be ignored.

Most of these preventive measures are neither dramatic nor newsworthy and it is difficult to evaluate their effectiveness. It is understandable that when governments are faced with an upsurge of drug abuse of one type or another, they require a more obvious response than a dogged perseverance with long-term programmes, however sound in principle they may be. In this situation, where they need to be seen to be responding to a crisis with some urgency, changes in the law or a strident advertising programme are often thought to be appropriate.

However, the effectiveness of these responses and of the other approaches outlined here must not be taken for granted. They should be carefully evaluated by means of ongoing epidemiological programmes, that can detect changes in drug abuse and monitor the effects of preventive approaches.[26]

12

The law and drug control policies

History of international drug control

The need for international measures to control drug abuse and dependence has long been recognized and the first conference was held in Shanghai, China, in 1909. There were delegates from 13 countries and, although they had no authority to introduce international legislation, they agreed on nine resolutions, some which were specifically addressed to those Governments that had concessions (i.e. territory) in China, following the Opium Wars. These resolutions requested governments to regulate the trade, distribution and consumption of opium in accordance with Chinese national legislation. In the other resolutions, which emphasized the need to suppress gradually opium smoking and to regulate the use of morphine to medical purposes, can be seen the germ of current international control measures (Table 12.1).

Perhaps the most important consequence of the Shanghai Conference was the organization at The Hague of another conference which led to the adoption of the first International Opium Convention in 1912 (The Hague Convention).[1] The main features of The Hague Convention were the gradual suppression of opium smoking, and limiting the use of morphine, other opiates and cocaine to medical and legitimate purposes, with their manufacture, trade and use made subject to an international system of permits and recording. There was a remarkable unanimity of international response to this convention, with 41 of the 46 nominally sovereign states that existed at that time signing the Convention and it was therefore agreed, on 25 June 1914, that the Convention would come into force by the end of that year. This was prevented by the outbreak of the First World War, but universal ratification of The Hague Convention took place immediately afterwards because all of the subsequent peace treaties required the parties to ratify and apply the 1912 Convention.

League of Nations

The momentum of The Hague Convention continued in the new League of Nations; the Advisory Committee on the Traffic in Opium and Other Dangerous

Table 12.1. Chronology of the development of the international drug control system

	Year	
I Control of plants		
Opium poppy	1953	
Coca bush	1953	
Cannabis plant	1961	
II Control of drugs		
A Plant materials		
Prepared opium	1925	(some measures in 1912)
Medicinal opium	1931	(some measures in 1925)
Raw opium	1931	(some measures in 1925)
Coca leaf	1953	(some measures in 1925)
Cannabis	1961	(some measures in 1925)
Cannabis resin	1961	(some measures in 1925)
Poppy straw		Some measures in 1961
B Natural (and semisynthetic compounds)		
Morphine and other opiates	1912	
Cocaine	1912	
Analogues of narcotic drugs	1931	
C Synthetic compounds		
Synthetic opioids	1948	
Some synthetic stimulants	1971	
Some synthetic sedatives	1971	
Some hallucinogens	1971	
III Control of substances used in the manufacture of drugs		
A Precursor compounds		
Cocaine precursors (ecgonine and its derivatives)	1925	
Precursors of other narcotic drugs (e.g. opiates)	1931	(some measures in 1925)
Some precursors of psychotropic substances	1988	
B Chemicals and solvents		
Some chemicals and solvents	1988	

Source: Bayer I & Ghodse H.[2]

Drugs (the predecessor of the Commission on Narcotic Drugs) was established and held its first meeting in 1921. At that time, opium smoking and cocaine abuse were the major drug problems, with unlimited production of opium in Asia and unlimited manufacture of opiates and cocaine in Europe.[2] The Conventions of 1925, 1931 and 1936 were all concerned with trying to address these issues.[3–5] However, it soon became apparent that little could be achieved without international monitoring and the League of Nations, through the International Opium Convention of 1925, established the Permanent Central Opium Board, which was the predecessor of the International Narcotics Control Board. This put an end to the wide-scale diversion of manufactured narcotic drugs from legal trade into the illicit market.

The 1925 Convention was important in other ways, too. It contained provisions for the control of coca leaf exports but also, significantly, the first provisions related to cannabis, prohibiting the export of cannabis resin to countries that prohibited its use and preventing illicit trade in Indian hemp. However, there was no attempt to control the traditional use of cannabis, coca chewing or opium eating and, with no limitations on the supply of raw materials for the manufacture of opiates and cocaine or the supply of manufactured drugs to consumer countries, it was impossible to reduce their use to that required for medical purposes.

The 1931 Convention responded to this by developing a system of 'estimates', requiring governments to identify their need for these drugs for medical and scientific purposes, permitting an annual statement of world requirements. Compliance with estimates was under the control of the Permanent Central Board, which could intervene if the agreed limits were not respected.

These drug control efforts were hampered, however, by a lack of cooperation between national authorities and by differences in their criminal justice systems, and a new Convention was agreed in 1936, initiated by the International Criminal Police Organization (Interpol), and containing provisions for the prosecution and extradition of traffickers and for direct police cooperation.

The United Nations

The transfer of functions from the League of Nations to the United Nations in relation to narcotic drugs was achieved by the 1946 Protocol which summarized the existing international treaties.[6] Subsequently, in 1948, there was another Protocol which brought synthetic narcotic drugs under the same sort of international control that already existed for those derived from natural raw materials. In addition, it extended controls to all drugs liable to the same kind of abuse and leading to the same harmful effects as those already specified in the Conventions. In other words, the 1948 Protocol articulated the principle of similarity, making it possible to bring under control not only new synthetic drugs but also any addiction-forming drug (whether already discovered or to be discovered in future).[7]

Although the manufacture and use of natural and semisynthetic opium alkaloids and synthetic narcotic drugs, had been controlled under earlier international legislation, prior to 1953, there were no such agreements limiting the production and nonmedical use of opium (except for the prohibition of opium smoking). This was addressed by the 1953 Protocol which specifically prohibited the nonmedical use of opium and required each producing country to establish a monopoly to control the cultivation of the opium poppy. The Protocol identified seven countries that were authorized to produce opium for export (Bulgaria, Greece, India, Iran, Turkey, USSR and Yugoslavia).[8]

Current international controls

It can be understood from the brief history above that the international system of control became very complicated and cumbersome. It was revised and modernized by the Single Convention on Narcotic Drugs, which was adopted in 1961 and was subsequently widened and strengthened by the 1972 Protocol.[9,10] Additional problems arose due to the introduction of new, synthetic psychoactive drugs which were widely used for the effective treatment of mental illness but which were often accompanied by the development of dependence and abuse. The Convention on Psychotropic Substances in 1971[11] extended the international drug control system to cover some of these new drugs, while the 1988 Convention against Illicit Traffic in Narcotic Drugs and Psychotropic Substances was introduced to hamper the activities of drug traffickers by depriving them of their ill-gotten gains and freedom of movement.[12]

These three conventions are designed to ensure the safe use of potentially dangerous psychoactive substances. They recognize that these substances often have legitimate scientific and medicinal uses that must be protected but that their abuse gives rise to public health, social and economic problems. Vigorous measures, involving close international cooperation, are required to restrict their use to legitimate purposes.

The Conventions list the controlled substances in different schedules with different levels of control, depending on the balance between therapeutic usefulness and the risk of abuse. Countries that ratify the Conventions are obliged to adopt appropriate legislation, introduce necessary administrative and enforcement measures and cooperate with international drug control agencies and with other parties to the Conventions. Internationally devised measures are thus translated into national controls by individual states within their own legal systems.

The Single Convention

The Single Convention puts strict controls on the cultivation of the opium poppy, coca bush and cannabis plant and their products, which for the purpose of the convention are described as 'narcotics' (although cocaine is a stimulant drug rather than one which induces sleep).[9] The Convention was amended by a further Protocol in 1972 which called for increased efforts to prevent illicit production of, traffic in, and use of narcotics. It also emphasized the need to provide treatment and rehabilitation services to drug abusers and to encourage their social reintegration.[10]

The substances covered by the Single Convention are classified in four schedules and a considerable number of opiate-like, dependence-producing drugs that are synthesized by scientific methods and manufactured industrially thereby come under varying degrees of control, according to their potential harmfulness and therapeutic usefulness.

Schedule I is the major schedule, roughly corresponding (except for heroin and cannabis) to Class A drugs of the UK Misuse of Drugs Act 1971. It includes the raw plant materials, such as opium, coca leaf and cannabis and many of their derivatives. These drugs are subject to all of the controls specified by the Convention.

Schedule II includes the drugs more commonly used for medical purposes that require less strict trade and distribution controls because there is a smaller risk of their abuse.

Schedule III drugs are the same as those in Schedule II but in lower concentrations and controlled proportions so that they are not liable to abuse.

Schedule IV includes a very few drugs which are subjected to extra controls because they have particularly dangerous properties and/or are of limited therapeutic use. Cannabis and heroin are both included in Schedule IV of the Single Convention.

Parties to the Single Convention undertake to limit the production, manufacture, export, import, distribution, stocks of, trade in, and use and possession of the controlled drugs so that they are used exclusively for medical and scientific purposes. The production and distribution of the drugs is licensed and supervised so that annual estimates and statistical returns can be made to the International Narcotics Control Board (INCB) of the quantities of drugs required, manufactured and utilized, and the quantities seized by police and customs officials. The accumulation of returns from many countries provides global information about the movement – licit and illicit – of these drugs.

As at 1 November, 2001, 176 states were party to the Single Convention on Narcotic Drugs or to the Convention as amended by the 1972 Protocol (162 were party to its amended form).[13]

The Psychotropic Convention

The Psychotropic Convention extends the same principles of control as those of the Single Convention to cover drugs such as central nervous system stimulants, sedative hypnotics and hallucinogens.[11] The drugs are listed in four schedules with different degrees of control:

Schedule I includes hallucinogens such as LSD which are dangerous drugs, causing serious risks to public health and with little, if any therapeutic use. They are therefore controlled very strictly to limit their use chiefly to research.

Schedule II contains the stimulant sympathomimetic drugs (e.g. amphetamine) which are of very limited therapeutic value. They are highly addictive drugs and are strictly controlled although the special provisions of Schedule I, limiting use to authorized individuals only, are omitted.

Schedule III covers fast- and medium-acting barbiturates that have been widely abused, but which are therapeutically useful.

Schedule IV includes a variety of hypnotics, tranquillizers and analgesic drugs that are widely used therapeutically (in some countries), but which have a marked dependence-producing liability.

All of these drugs are available only on medical prescription and parties to the Convention undertake to ensure that prescriptions are issued in accordance with sound medical practice and that labelling, packaging and advertising conform to certain rules.

As at 1 November 2001, 169 States were party to the Convention on Psychotropic Substances.[13]

1988 United Nations Convention against Illicit Traffic in Narcotic Drugs and Psychotropic Substances

This Convention defines drug trafficking activities, which now include money laundering, and illicit activities related to precursors, in a comprehensive and innovative manner.[12] States are required to establish these activities as criminal offences and provide for penalties adequate to their serious nature. To facilitate the tracing, freezing and confiscation of proceeds and property derived from drug trafficking, courts are empowered to make available or to seize bank, financial or commercial records, and bank secrecy cannot be invoked in such cases. Furthermore, the Convention bars all havens to drug traffickers, particularly through its provisions for: extradition of major drug traffickers; mutual legal assistance between States on drug-related investigations; and the transfer of proceedings for criminal prosecution. Another significant landmark is the commitment of parties to eliminate or reduce illicit demand for narcotic drugs and psychotropic substances.

As at 1 November 2001, 162 States and the European Community were party to the 1988 Convention, which came into force in 1990.[13]

Declaration on the Guiding Principles of Drug Demand Reductions

It can be seen from this brief history that, during most of the twentieth century, the traditional approach to drug misuse problems emphasized the suppression of supply and trafficking. It gradually became apparent, however, that such efforts, in isolation, will always be inadequate and it is now appreciated that demand fuels supply and that effective marketing can boost demand. The logical consequence is that, if the size of the total drug market is to be reduced, both supply and demand must be tackled vigorously and simultaneously.[14]

A major step forward in demand reduction was achieved in 1998 when the General Assembly of the United Nations adopted the Declaration on the Guiding Principles of Demand Reduction, which articulated the principle of a balanced approach between demand reduction and supply reduction in an integrated approach to solving the drug problem. With this Declaration, governments committed themselves to reducing demand for all substances of abuse and agreed a multistranded approach. This landmark Declaration offers a holistic approach to this complex problem, which will be interpreted and implemented differently in different countries so that culturally sensitive responses are developed.[15,16]

United Nations drug abuse control organs

The United Nations General Assembly is ultimately responsible for the control and supervision of international efforts to restrict the use of drugs to their proper medical purposes. It operates in this field through the Secretary General and the Economic and Social Council which is assisted and advised by the Commission on Narcotic Drugs (Fig. 12.1).

Recognizing the central role that must be played by the United Nations in fostering concerted international activity in this field, a special session of the General Assembly was convened in 1990, to consider, as a matter of urgency, the question of international cooperation against illicit production, supply, demand, trafficking and distribution of narcotic drugs, with a view to expanding the scope and increasing the effectiveness of such cooperation.[17] The General Assembly adopted a Global Programme of Action to achieve the goal of an international society free of illicit drugs and drug abuse and created the United Nations International Drug Control Programme (UNDCP), which integrated the structures and functions of the former United Nations drug units (i.e. the Division of

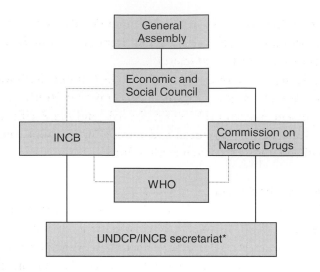

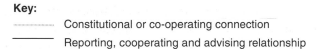

Key:

.... Constitutional or co-operating connection

———— Reporting, cooperating and advising relationship

* The INCB secretariat reports on substantive matters to INCB only.

Fig 12.1   United Nations system and drug control organs and their secretariat.

Narcotic Drugs (DND), the United Nations Fund for Drug Control (UNFDAC) as well as the secretariat of the International Narcotics Control Board (INCB)).

Commission on Narcotic Drugs (CND)

The Commission was established in 1946 and is the central policy-making body within the United Nations system for dealing with all questions related to the global effort of drug abuse control. It consists of representatives of 53 member states, elected by the Economic and Social Council and its annual meetings are also attended by observers from other governments, other United Nations organs and from agencies and organizations with an interest in drug control.

As well as planning and developing general strategies against drug abuse, a central function of the Commission is to advise on changes in the current system of international drug control, making proposals for new conventions and drug control instruments. More specifically, the Commission makes decisions on bringing new substances under the control of the Conventions and decides what level of control is required. To this end, it receives information and recommendations from the World Health Organization (WHO), which it may accept or reject (or sometimes amend) in the light of economic, social, legal and administrative factors that are considered relevant.

Subsidiary bodies of CND coordinate the Commission's work at regional level. There are regional groupings of the operational Heads of National Drug Law Enforcement Agencies (HONLEA) in Asia and the Pacific, as well as in Africa, Latin America, the Caribbean and Europe; interregional meetings of HONLEA strengthen international cooperation further.[18,19]

The International Narcotics Control Board (INCB)

The International Narcotics Control Board is an independent body created by the Single Convention. It reports to the Economic and Social Council through the Commission on Narcotic Drugs. There are 13 members of the Board who are proposed by the member states of the United Nations and elected by the Economic and Social Council but, once on the Board, they serve impartially in their personal capacities for periods of 5 years at a time. Three members, nominated by WHO, have medical, pharmacological or pharmaceutical experience.

The major responsibility of the INCB is to limit the cultivation, production, manufacture and utilization of the drugs that are controlled by the Conventions to the amounts that are necessary for medical and scientific purposes. Parties to the Conventions undertake to keep records of the flow and handling of the controlled substances so that they can provide the INCB with estimates of the total annual requirements of each controlled substance, and later with statistics about actual manufacture, international trade and consumption. The Board can then compare estimates with actual total use, to establish that the drugs available in each country for medical purposes are accounted for at the main stages of production, manufacture and trade. If there are discrepancies between consumption and statistically calculated available quantities, or between estimates and actual use, these can be investigated and the causes clarified. In this way the Board can assist governments to achieve the correct balance between supply and demand for controlled drugs. Under the 1988 Convention, traffic in precursor substances that are important for the illicit manufacture of narcotic drugs and psychotropic substances is also monitored and this, too, is the responsibility of INCB.

The INCB also receives information about illicit drug activity within national borders and uses this information, together with that about all aspects of the licit drug trade, to determine whether the aims of the conventions are being endangered by any country. If they are, it can make recommendations on remedial measures or, as a last resort, propose sanctions against defaulting countries. INCB maintains dialogues with Governments, both through regular consultations and by special missions, arranged in agreement with the Governments concerned. This type of 'quiet diplomacy' has brought about the strengthening of legislation in several countries which have acknowledged the need for coordination of national drug control efforts.

INCB's other activities include training programmes for drug control administrators and it also produces an annual report of the global situation on the working of the conventions and on illicit production and traffic of drugs. This report, which is submitted to the Economic and Social Council (ECOSOC) through the Commission on Narcotic Drugs, contains recommendations to Governments and is supplemented by technical reports on the licit movement of narcotic drugs and psychotropic substances.[18,19]

United Nations International Drug Control Programme (UNDCP)

Created in 1990, UNDCP has continued with the work of the Division of Narcotic Drugs and of the United Nations Fund for Drug Abuse Control, performing a variety of functions, deriving from the international drug control treaties and specific mandates of the General Assembly, ECOSOC and CND. It is therefore responsible for coordinating UN drug control activities, for promoting the implementation of the international conventions and for providing effective leadership in international drug control. In particular, it carries out the Secretary General's functions under the international conventions, assisting the Commission on Narcotic Drugs and the International Narcotics Control Board in implementing their treaty-based functions and promoting new instruments as necessary.[18,19]

UNDCP plays a very important role in providing technical assistance, through expertise and training, to help Governments set up adequate drug control structures and to define comprehensive national plans. These may encompass a wide range of activities such as integrated rural development and crop substitution, enforcement of drug-related laws, prevention, treatment and rehabilitation of drug addicts, as well as legislative and institutional reforms so that Governments are better able to fight drug abuse. New areas of concern for UNDCP include the damaging environmental effects of illicit cultivation and processing of drugs and the fight against 'money laundering'. Its 16 national and subregional field offices assist governments in the development of initiatives to enhance the concept of joint operations between different countries. The UNDCP had a budget of about US$70 million in the year 2000 but its important work is dependent on voluntary contributions to the Programme by donor countries.[20]

World Health Organization (WHO)

Because drug abuse constitutes a serious health hazard of steadily growing proportions in many countries, the World Health Organization, which is the competent international health authority, is closely involved on many fronts in the fight

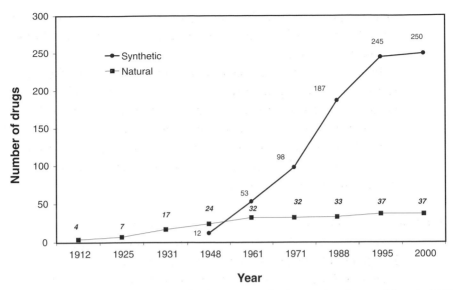

Fig. 12.2   Increase in the number of drugs and substances under international control (1912–2000). (Source: Bayer & Ghodse.[2])

against it. Within the field of control, for example, WHO is involved and concerned with regulations about the prescription of controlled drugs and their advertising. In addition, it has developed reporting programmes to monitor the adverse side effects of psychoactive drugs in relation to their risk of abuse and dependence potential, and programmes to establish the epidemiology of drug dependence.

The Conventions assign specific responsibilities to WHO in respect of changes in the control of substances and of placing them in appropriate schedules. WHO studies the medical and scientific characteristics of drugs in order to assess their therapeutic usefulness and dependence liability, and then evaluates the public health and social problems related to their abuse. To make these assessments, WHO relies on collaboration with member states. The fundamental research, whether biological, medical or epidemiological, is carried out in national universities and industrial laboratories which provide a steady flow of information to WHO, which in turn provides resources for research. Once the assessment is completed (by a group of experts), WHO communicates its findings to the Commission on Narcotic Drugs together with recommendations on control measures. The final decision about control is taken by the Commission, which also takes into account economic, social, legal and administrative factors which have been communicated to it from the United Nations International Drug Control Programme and the International Narcotics Control Board (Fig. 12.2). Research of this kind is always important, but its value is magnified many times over if several countries adopt standardized methodology. International comparisons then become possible and a truly global picture of patterns of drug abuse and dependence emerges, which permits appropriate international responses to be made.

Other WHO activities related to drug control include the promotion of the rational use of psychoactive substances, not just through regulations but through education. To this end, guidelines for rational use are being compiled together with a list of essential drugs for basic health needs, which serves as a guide for countries in identifying their own needs and priorities concerning drug availability. WHO is also involved in interregional training courses for health care professionals on prevention and on the treatment of drug dependence.[21]

Other United Nations organizations

Although drug abuse control is not their main function, a number of other United Nations organizations are actively involved in this area. They include:

- *United Nations Educational, Scientific and Cultural Organization (UNESCO)* which focuses on the prevention of drug abuse through public education and awareness and works to integrate preventive education concerning drug use into school curricula and out-of-school activities.
- *United Nations Children's Fund (UNICEF)* which is involved particularly in relation to the estimated 100 million 'street children' who are often drug abusers and drug sellers.
- The *International Maritime Organization*, the *International Civil Aviation Organization* and the *International Postal Union* which have all introduced measures aimed at combating the illicit transport of drugs while the *Food and Agriculture Organization* is involved in raising the income level of farmers so that the incentive to cultivate prohibited crops is reduced.
- Although it is not an agency of the United Nations, the *International Criminal Police Organization (ICPO/Interpol)*, which is composed of national law enforcement agencies, works with the United Nations to improve information about the flow of illicit drugs and illegally acquired assets across international borders.

Analysis of evolution of the international drug control policy clearly demonstrates the need for international collaboration in combating drug abuse and trafficking. The Conventions provide a mechanism for this and can act as a minimum common denominator; their universal ratification and implementation will prevent any serious loopholes in the system and offer the best chance of success. However, even 40 years after the Single Convention, complete success cannot be claimed.[22]

Control in the UK

Misuse of Drugs Act 1971

The Misuse of Drugs Act 1971, which came fully into operation in 1973, replaced earlier laws and is the principal legislation in the UK for controlling drug use and preventing misuse. It deals with nearly all drugs with abuse and/or dependence liability, laying down specific requirements for their prescription, safe custody and record-keeping and defining the offences related to their production, cultivation, supply and possession.[18]

The Act lists the drugs that are subject to control and classifies them in three categories according to their relative harmfulness when misused:

Class A includes alfentanil, carfentanil, cocaine, dextromoramide, dipipanone, heroin, lofentanil, LSD, methadone, morphine, opium, pethidine, phencyclidine (and injectable forms of Class B drugs).

Class B includes oral preparations of amphetamines, barbiturates, cannabis, cannabis resin, codeine, glutethimide, pentazocine, phenmetrazine and pholcodine.

Class C includes certain appetite suppressants such as phentermine, diethylpropion and mazindol, and sedatives such as meprobamate, methyprylone and most benzodiazepines.

The penalties for offences involving controlled drugs depend on the classification of the drug: penalties for misuse of Class A drugs are more severe than for Class B drugs which in turn are more severe than for Class C drugs. The Act also distinguishes, in terms of the penalties that may be imposed, between the crimes of possession and drug trafficking, with the latter receiving much more severe punishment.

An important part of the Misuse of Drugs Act is that the Home Secretary is empowered to make regulations to supplement the control of drugs. Many of these regulations have a direct effect on doctors and their work, although their clinical freedom to prescribe whatever drugs they consider necessary is largely unimpeded.

At the end of 2001, the Home Affairs Select Committee examined issues relating to drug control in the UK and the government indicated that, in accordance with its statutory duty, it would seek the advice of the Advisory Council on Misuse of Drugs (p. 399) about the reclassification of cannabis as a class C drug. The government made it quite clear that if reclassification of cannabis occurs, this would not amount to either legalization or decriminalization. Both possession and supply would remain criminal offences with a maximum penalty of 2 years imprisonment for possession and 5 years for supply. Although there is a power of arrest for supply and trafficking class C drugs, there is no power of arrest for possession. This change would therefore represent a relaxation of national drug control legislation and has led to increased debate on the advantages and disadvantages of the liberalization of drug legislation.

Misuse of Drugs Regulations 1985

These regulations define the classes of people (e.g. midwife, doctor, public laboratory analyst) who are authorized to possess or supply controlled drugs and the situation in which they are permitted to do so.[18]

As far as doctors are concerned the regulations provide a more practical classification of controlled drugs than that described earlier which was primarily for crimino-legal purposes. The regulations divide the drugs into five schedules with different requirements and rules governing prescribing, safe custody and record keeping for each schedule:

Schedule 1 includes drugs such as LSD, cannabis, raw opium and coca leaf for which there are no therapeutic indications. Special authorization is required from the Home Office for their possession and supply (which is usually for the purpose of research).

Schedule 2 includes drugs some of which are used in clinical medicine, but which have a high dependence liability, e.g. diamorphine (heroin), morphine, pethidine, dextromoramide, dipipanone, methadone, fentanyl, cocaine, amphetamine, secobarbital and glutethimide.

The regulations give specific instructions for the safe custody of these drugs which are usually kept in locked safes, cabinets or rooms which have to comply with precise specifications. Doctors (and others) should note that it is not considered safe to leave Schedule 2 drugs in a locked car (e.g. when visiting a patient). A register must be kept to record the use of these drugs.

Prescriptions for Schedule 2 drugs must conform to precise legal requirements. They must be hand-written in ink by the prescriber who must sign and date them and whose address must be stated (i.e. they cannot be produced by a printer from a computer or be typed). The prescription must state:

(a) The name and address of the patient;
(b) The drug and the form in which it is to be dispensed (e.g. tablets, mixture) and, if appropriate, the strength of the preparation (e.g. methadone mixture, x mg/ml);
(c) The dose;
(d) The total quantity or the number of dose units to be dispensed. This must be written in both words and figures.

All of this information is required by law. It is an offence for a doctor to issue an incomplete prescription for a drug controlled under Schedule 2, and it is an offence for a pharmacist to dispense the prescription if it is incomplete. 'Repeat' prescriptions for these drugs are not permitted, nor can they be issued as an 'emergency supply' by a pharmacist at the patient's request. Special arrangements exist when these drugs are prescribed to addicts in the course of treating their dependence.

Schedule 3 includes barbiturates (except secobarbital, which is in Schedule 2), buprenorphine, diethylpropion, flunitrazepam, mazindol, meprobamate, pentazocine phentermine and temazepam. These are all drugs that are known to cause dependence and that have been extensively abused. Prescriptions for Schedule 3 drugs (except for phenobarbitone and temazepam) must conform to the same legal requirements as those outlined above for Schedule 2 drugs, but there are no requirements for safe custody (except for buprenorphine, diethylpropion, flunitrazepam and temazepam), and there is no need to keep a register.

The term 'controlled drugs' is widely, although imprecisely, used as a collective description of the drugs in Schedules 2 and 3 of the Misuse of Drugs Regulations 1985, and has come to mean those drugs that are subject to the prescription requirements of the regulations. Strictly speaking, all drugs listed in the Act (or regulations) are 'controlled' drugs.

If phenobarbitone is the only drug from Schedule 2 or 3 on the prescription form, the requirement for a handwritten prescription does not apply. This exemption is a recognition of the role of phenobarbitone in the treatment of epilepsy when there is little risk of the development of drug abuse.

Schedule 4 includes 33 benzodiazepine drugs and pemoline in part II. They are, however, subject to only minimal control, and although they are 'prescription-only medicine', their prescriptions do not have to fulfil the requirements applicable to Schedule 2 and 3 drugs, nor are there any safe custody requirements. Part I of the schedule includes a number of androgenic and anabolic steroids as well as polypeptide hormones such as somatotropin (growth hormone).

Schedule 5 drugs are preparations which contain drugs listed in Schedules 2 or 3, but in such small quantities that they are harmless, or compounded in such a way that recovery of the drug in quantities that might be harmful is impossible or unlikely. For example, diphenoxylate is a Schedule 2 drug, but as Lomotil (2.5 mg diphenoxylate with atropine sulphate 25 µg), it is a schedule 5 drug and exempt from all controlled drug requirements except that of retaining invoices for a 2-year period.

Prescribing controlled drugs to addicts

If a decision is made to prescribe opiates or other drugs regularly to someone who is dependent upon them – either in the short term for detoxification, or in the long term for maintenance treatment – it is essential for the prescriptions to be dispensed on a daily basis. This is because it would be very unwise to give several days' supply of drugs to an addict all at once. As the prescription forms FP10 and FP10 HP are valid for supply on one occasion only, it follows that if these forms are used, six prescriptions must be written each week, with 2 days' prescription being dispensed on Sunday.

To facilitate prescribing for addicts, a new prescription form, FP10MDA1000, has been introduced to enable GPs to write a prescription for several days, treatment to be dispensed in instalments. Not more than 14 days' supply should be ordered on one form and the number of instalments to be dispensed and the interval between each instalment should be specified. Form FP10MDA1000 may only be used to prescribe Schedule 2 drugs to addicts and all other prescription-writing requirements for these drugs must be complied with. Since 1 April 2001, buprenorphine (which is a Schedule 3 drug) can also be prescribed in instalments, using these forms. It is the only Schedule 3 drug that can be prescribed in this way.

Whenever possible, the patient should be introduced to the particular pharmacist who has agreed to dispense the prescription, so that there is no confusion about the identity of the patient. It should be made clear to the patient that the prescription will not be dispensed in advance and cannot be collected 'in arrears'. The pharmacist should be encouraged to report back to the prescribing doctor if drugs are not collected, and always to check if the patient requests any alteration in the dispensing arrangements. Prescriptions are often posted directly to the pharmacist.

Special arrangements have also been made for doctors working in specialist DDTUs when they prescribe controlled drugs to addicts to save them from having to write six prescriptions per week for each patient on maintenance or detoxification treatment. They are provided with a different prescription form (FP10HP(AD)1000) which can only be used for prescribing cocaine, dextromoramide, diamorphine, dipipanone, methadone, morphine or pethidine and which permits these drugs to be dispensed in instalments so that only one prescription is needed each week. The quantity to be dispensed on each occasion and the interval between instalments must be stated. These doctors may also obtain exemption from the handwriting requirement for Schedule 2 and 3 drugs, so that prescriptions can be typed ready for them to sign. This exemption applies only to the named institutions in which they work.

Since 1 April 2001, buprenorphine (which is a Schedule 3 drug) can also be prescribed in instalments, using these forms. It is the only Schedule 3 drug that can be prescribed in this way.

Prescribing heroin, cocaine and dipipanone to addicts

Under the Misuse of Drugs (Notification of and Supply to Addicts) Regulations 1973 and 1997, only doctors who hold a special licence, issued by the Home Secretary, are permitted to prescribe heroin, dipipanone or cocaine for addicts for the purpose of treating their addiction. In practice, most doctors holding this licence work in the specialist clinics for treating drug dependence, where the prescription of these highly addictive (and therefore highly sought after) drugs is under scrutiny and discussion by members of a multidisciplinary team. It is hoped in this way to control and to restrict the prescription of these drugs to those cases for whom it is justified and necessary, and to prevent the re-emergence of a 1960s-type situation when some doctors prescribed unnecessarily large doses that contributed to the black market in drugs.

However, any doctor may prescribe heroin, dipipanone or cocaine to any patient (including addicts) if the drug is required for the treatment of organic disease. Thus an addict who needs heroin or morphine, for example, to provide analgesia after an abdominal operation, may be prescribed the necessary dose by the responsible doctor without recourse to a DDTU.

As at 1 May 2001, changes in the licensing provisions are being considered. Specifically, a number of additions to the current list of drugs subject to a licence requirement have been suggested. The changes proposed are:
- A licence requirement for prescribing any controlled drug in Schedules 2 or 3, with the exception of methadone liquid or mixture on a NHS prescription.
- A licence requirement for prescribing any controlled drug in Schedules 2 to 4 in injectable form.

The effect would be to place a licensing requirement on both NHS and private prescribing for any injectable controlled drugs and on private prescribing for all Schedule 2 and 3 controlled drugs in whatever form, but to leave the NHS prescribing of methadone liquid or mixture unaffected.

Obligation to notify

For many years in the UK, doctors were required to notify the Chief Medical Officer at the Home Office, in writing, of the personal particulars of any patient whom he or she considered (or had reasonable grounds to suspect) as addicted to certain controlled drugs. According to these regulations, a person was regarded as being addicted 'if, and only if, he has as a result of repeated administration become so dependent on the drug that he has an over-powering desire for the administration of it to be continued'.[18]

In May 1997, however, the Misuse of Drugs (Supply to Addicts) Regulations 1997 revoked this requirement and doctors and other professionals are now expected (but not legally required) to report cases of drug misuse to their local Drug Misuse Database, using a standard form (see Chapter 2). However, because the data are anonymized, it is not possible to use the Drug Misuse Databases in the way that the old Home Office Index could be used, to check whether a particular individual is already in receipt of a prescription.

Medicines Act 1968

It has been noted previously that some drugs with a potential for misuse are available without a prescription 'over the counter'. Under the Medicines Act there are two classes of such drugs:

Pharmacy Only medicines which can only be sold in a registered pharmacy; and

General Sales List medicines (GSL) which can also, under certain conditions, be sold in other shops – usually only in strictly limited quantities.

Medications with a potential for misuse (codeine, antihistamines, stimulant-like drugs) come within the former group.

Intoxicating Substances Supply Act 1985

Solvents, which are commercially available substances with a variety of uses, are not covered by the Misuse of Drugs Act, and the Intoxicating Substances Supply Act was therefore introduced in an attempt to deal with solvent sniffing. This act makes it an offence for a person to supply or offer to supply to someone under the age of 18 years, substances that the supplier knows, or has reason to believe, will be used 'to achieve intoxication'. The law is directed primarily at irresponsible shopkeepers, to deter them from selling solvents or volatile substances to youngsters who are going to sniff them. However, it is difficult to prove that a shopkeeper knows what the substance will be used for and there have been few prosecutions under this act. Nevertheless, the threat of legal action probably acts as a deterrent.

Health and Safety at Work Act 1974

Under this act, employers are required to ensure, as far as reasonably practicable, the health, safety and welfare of all their employees, and employees are required to take reasonable care of the health and safety of themselves and others who may be affected by their acts or omissions at work. This clearly has implications for substance abusers but, in addition, an employer, who knowingly allows a drug abuser to continue working without doing anything either to help the abuser or protect other employees, may also be liable to charges.

Drug Trafficking Act 1994

This legislation updated and consolidated the provisions of the earlier Drug Trafficking Offences Act 1986 which dealt with the tracing, freezing and confiscation of the proceeds of drug trafficking and the criminalization of drugs money laundering. The objectives of the legislation are to:

• Make it as difficult as possible for criminals to launder their proceeds through the UK banking and financial systems by a system of reporting suspicious transactions;

- Obtain useful intelligence on major criminals;
- Ensure that legislation has a maximum deterrent effect through prosecutions and by using confiscation orders to deprive offenders of the benefit of crimes.

It is anticipated that legislation will be further strengthened by a 'Proceeds of Crime Bill' which will enhance existing anti-money laundering measures by extending 'civil forfeiture' powers and strengthening confiscation laws so that it is harder for criminals to hang on to assets gained by illicit drug-related activities. A National Confiscation Agency is planned, to drive this approach forward.[23]

UK Anti-Drugs Coordinator

Several different Government departments are involved in dealing with drug-related issues and coordination between them is of paramount importance. The post of UK Anti-Drugs Coordinator was created in 1998, to provide leadership for the 10-year strategy 'Tackling Drugs to Build a Better Britain'. The Anti-Drug Coordinator, together with officials from the Anti-Drugs Coordination Unit (UKADCU), are responsible for monitoring the Strategy. They also advise the Ministerial Subcommittee on Drug Misuse, which is chaired by the Minister for the Cabinet Office, and which has overall responsibility for the Government's drugs strategy.[23]

National Treatment Agency

A new National Treatment Agency has been established (2001) to be responsible for drug treatment provision and for ensuring the delivery of high-quality services.

Advisory Council on Misuse of Drugs

The Advisory Council on Misuse of Drugs (ACMD) was set up under the Misuse of Drugs Act 1971. It is made up of at least 20 members who are appointed by the Home Secretary and who include representatives of the medical, veterinary, dental and pharmacy professions and of the pharmaceutical industry. Individuals with wide and recent experience of the social problems connected with drug misuse are also included.

The ACMD is responsible for advising the government about appropriate measures to educate the public about the dangers of drug misuse, about the best ways of treating drug misusers and helping their rehabilitation and about promoting research into drug misuse.

A particular and very important function of the ACMD is to review drugs which are being misused or which appear likely to be misused and to advise the government on measures to prevent this. Often this involves a drug being brought under control of the Misuse of Drugs Act, or of being put under stricter control because there is evidence that its misuse is increasing. Thus new controls can be initiated in response to changes in the drug scene without the need for a new Act of Parliament if a different drug becomes problematical. The potential for a (comparatively) swift response to changing trends of drug abuse is essential if new and perhaps dangerous patterns of drug abuse are to be dealt with effectively before the problem gets out of control.

In practice, of course, even swift responses depend on the gathering of relevant information and are slow in comparison with the rapid changes of the drug scene, so that 'solutions' are always late. Nevertheless, the ACMD reduces the duration of potentially damaging delays.

Appendix 1. Illicit manufacture of controlled substances

(a) Illicit manufacture of cocaine and heroin

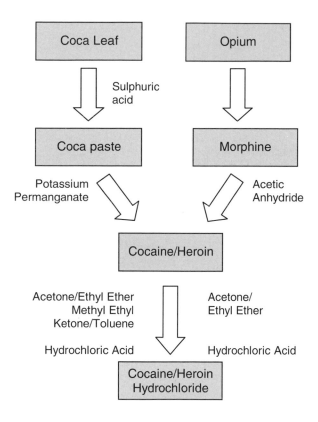

Adapted from INCB (UN) *Precursors Report 2001.*

(b) Illicit manufacture of amphetamine and methamphetamine

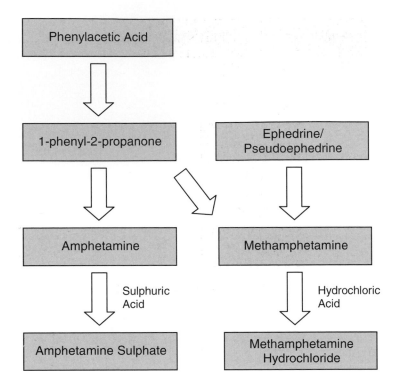

Adapted from INCB (UN) *Precursors Report 2001.*

(c) Illicit manufacture of LSD

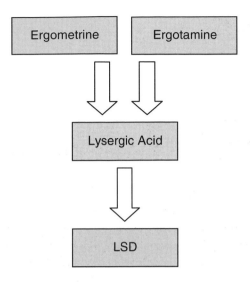

Adapted from INCB (UN) *Precursors Report 2001.*

(d) Illicit manufacture of MDMA and related drugs

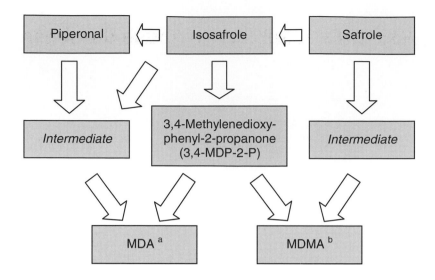

[a] MDA=3,4-methylenedioxyamphetamine.
[b] MDMA=3,4-methylenedioxymethamphetamine.

Adapted from INCB (UN) *Precursors Report 2001.*

Appendix 2. Substance Abuse Database

SUBSTANCE ABUSE MONITORING
COLLABORATIVE PROJECT

Interviewer's Name ....
Job Title ....
Agency Name ....

BASIC CLIENT DATA

Is this a new client to your agency? Y / N   (please circle)

	Female		Date of contact			Type of contact:	Face-to-face	
	Male						Telephone	
							Letter	
							Indirect	

Client's Initials [ ] [ ] OR code [ ]
Date of birth [ ] / [ ] OR age [ ]
Postcode [ ]

Client's Borough or Town [ ]

SUBSTANCE PROFILE:
substances used over last 12 months

STATE SUBSTANCE NAME BELOW
Put main substance first (including alcohol)
If alcohol is used, complete section below
as well

	Frequency of use over last 30 days							Most usual route over last 30 days							Source over last 30 days							Duration of this Episode of use	Age of first use
	No use	Less than once per week	Once per week or more	Once daily	2/3 times daily	4 or more times daily	Not known	Oral	Smoked	Injected	Sniffed / Snorted	Other routes	Not known	Illicit	Private Dr.	GP	Other Dr.	Other	Not known		
1.																					
2.																					
3.																					
4.																					

ALCOHOL: Type
(Beer, Wine, Spirits etc.)

Units consumed per week [ ]   Alcohol-free days per month [ ]

INJECTING DETAILS: (please circle)
Have you ever shared?   Y / N
Shared equipment in last 4 weeks?   Y / N
Have you ever injected?   Y / N

Has any HIV test ever been offered to you?   Y / N
Have you ever completed a Hep B vaccination course?   Y / N

REFERRAL DETAILS (tick any that apply)

Time between referral & assessment [ ] weeks

REFERRED BY:
Self
Family / friend
GP
Hospital
Probation
NHS Drug / Alcohol Team
Other, specify:

REASON FOR ATTENDANCE:
Financial
Legal
Job
Family / Relationships
Medical e.g. detoxification
Psychological
Other, specify:

SUBSTANCE-RELATED CONTACTS: (in last 6 months)
None
Non-statutory agency
GP / Practice nurse
NHS Drug / Alcohol Team
Probation Service
Social Services
Other, specify:

CLIENT DETAILS (tick only one in each section)

ETHNIC GROUP:

- British
- Irish
- Any other White background
- White and Black Caribbean
- White and Black African
- White and Asian
- Any other mixed background
- Indian
- Pakistani
- Bangladeshi
- Any other Asian background
- Caribbean
- African
- Any other Black background
- Chinese
- Any other*

*Specify

☐☐☐☐☐☐☐   ☐☐☐☐☐☐☐☐

Client lives with someone with substance use problem (please circle)   Y / N

There is a family history of substance use   Y / N

DEPENDANT CHILDREN:
How many?   ☐
Age of youngest   ☐

CURRENT / USUAL JOB:

EDUCATIONAL ATTAINMENT
- None
- GCSE
- A Level
- Diploma / Degree

☐☐☐☐

LIVING WITH:

- Alone
- Self & Children
- Partner/Spouse
- Partner/Spouse & Children
- Parents
- Friends
- Other, specify

☐☐☐☐☐☐☐

ACCOMMODATION:

- Parental home
- Owner occupied
- Private rented
- Council rented
- Housing Association
- Rehab/hostel
- No fixed abode
- Other, specify:

☐☐☐☐☐☐☐☐

OCCUPATIONAL STATUS:

- Unemployed
- Employed
- Self-employed
- Childcare / housewife
- Student
- Retired
- Invalidity / sickness
- Other, specify:

☐☐☐☐☐☐☐☐

TREATMENT & OUTCOMES

QUALITY OF LIFE MEASURE:

In the last month has the client:

Any legal problems   Y / N
Any work (inc. voluntary or education) Y / N

How is the client's

Sleep   poor ☐   good ☐
Appetite   poor ☐   good ☐

PROPOSED ACTION: (tick all that apply)
Referred to other agency, specify:

- Assessment
- Detoxification
- Long term prescribing (enter details below)
- Prescribing contract (enter details below)
- Counselling
- Family support
- Rehabilitation
- Other intervention, specify

☐☐☐☐☐☐☐☐☐☐

PRESCRIBING INTENTIONS: (if known)
Specify all drugs you plan to prescribe:

Probable duration of prescribing (weeks) ☐

Will this be a reducing dose?   Y / N
(please circle)   not
    known

Guidelines on completion of the form

The S.A.M. Collaborative Project

The aim of the project is to give service providers who participate, good quality information on the utilization of services by clients, paying particular attention to the effectiveness of treatment interventions, by measuring outcomes in terms of the clients' quality of life. Resulting data will also be of great benefit to purchasers and commissioners of substance misuse services.

As well as providing quality data at a local level, the data can be forwarded and included in the Department of Health regional and national statistics.

The project is supervised by the Addiction Resource Agency for commissioners at the Centre for Addiction Studies, St George's Hospital Medical School.

WHO the form is about

Any client with whom you have contact who has a recent substance problem of any kind. A broad view of substance use is adopted, including all psychoactive drugs with the exclusion only of tobacco. Prescribed drugs (such as benzodiazepines) should be included as well as over-the-counter preparations (such as codeine linctus). Alcohol use should also be recorded in the appropriate slot provided in the Substance Profile table.

WHEN to complete the form

Please complete a form when the client first presents to your agency, and whenever a new episode of substance use starts. A new episode starts when a person with substance-related problems *either* goes to a particular agency for the first time, *or* returns to a particular agency after an interval of 6 months or more.

WHO completes the form

This form is intended for completion by a staff member who has interviewed a client. It is *not* intended as a self-completion form for drug users. Please ensure that you complete the initial section which asks for basic information about you (the interviewer) and the agency for which you work.

WHERE does it go

Please send all completed forms to the S.A.M. Project at the end of each month.

Confidentiality and anonymity

All data entered onto the Database is password protected. The password is known only to the Project Manager and the data-entry clerk. Summarized information only is contained in reports to third parties and this *never* contains client information (such as initials, date of birth or *full* postcode).

Different levels of personal identification may be chosen according to client/agency preferences. A code (allocated by your agency) may be submitted in place of initials and an age in place of date of birth.

This means that it is not possible to check for double-counting at agency level. It is therefore *essential* that each new episode is only reported once by your agency to the Database.

Data Protection Act

The database is registered with the Data Protection Registrar. It is considered good practice to inform clients about the purposes of the database, that it is confidential and that their rights are protected under the Data Protection Act.

Forms (top copy) should be returned to:

Appendix 3. The European Substance Use Database

The European Substance Use Database (EuroSUD) is a brief initial assessment instrument collecting basic demographic data about drug users who present to services, as well as information about their current drug using behaviour and the types of treatment intervention offered to them. The information contained on the EuroSUD may be used for either clinical or research purposes. The Database itself is a valuable epidemiological tool at local, national and international levels. EuroSUD computer programs, written in shareware software, enable data entry and report generation at local level at minimal cost. The EuroSUD is currently in use in treatment centres in 10 European countries.

Interviewer's name ....

Job title ....

Agency name ....

European Substance Use Database

BASIC CLIENT DATA

1 CLIENT DATA

Client's Initials [ ] [ ]   OR code [ ] [ ] [ ] [ ]   OR age [ ] [ ] [ ]

Date of birth / /

Postcode OR postal district

Female [ ]
Male [ ]

2 CONTACT DATA

Date of contact / /

Type of contact: Face-to-face [ ]
Telephone [ ]
Letter [ ]
Indirect [ ]

3 SUBSTANCE PROFILE:
substances used over last 12 months

STATE SUBSTANCE NAME BELOW
Put main substance first. If alcohol is
used at all, fill in final slot on table.

	Frequency of use over last 30 days							Most usual route over last 30 days						Source over last 30 days						Duration of this Episode of use	Age of first use
	No use	Less than once per week	Once per week or more	Once daily	2 / 3 times daily	4 or more times daily	Not known	Oral	Smoked	Injected	Sniffed / Snorted	Other routes	Not known	Illicit	Private Dr.	Own Doctor	Other Dr.	Other	Not known		
1.																					
2.																					
3.																					
4.																					

ALCOHOL:		Units consumed per week	

4 INJECTING DETAILS:

Have you ever injected? Y / N
Have you ever shared? Y / N

Has a HIV test ever been offered to you? Y / N
Have you ever completed a Hep B vaccination course? Y / N

How long ago was most recent sharing .... years ...... months .... days

5 REFERRED BY:
(tick one only)

Self [ ]
Dr [ ]
Hospital [ ]
Social Services [ ]
Voluntary agency [ ]
Legal services [ ]
Police [ ]
Other, specify: [ ]

6 REASON FOR ATTENDANCE:
(tick up to 4)

Financial [ ]
Job [ ]
Family / Relationships [ ]
Medical [ ]
Psychological [ ]
Housing [ ]
Pregnancy [ ]
Casualty [ ]
Needle exchange [ ]
Others, specify

7 DRUG-RELATED CONTACTS:
(in last 6 months)
(tick up to 3)

Non-statutory agency [ ]
Doctor [ ]
NHS Drug Team [ ]
Legal Services [ ]
Social Services [ ]
Accident & Emergency [ ]
Other, specify: [ ]

8 ETHNIC GROUP:
(tick one only)

British [ ]
Irish [ ]
Any other White background [ ]
White and Black Caribbean [ ]
White and Black African [ ]
White and Asian [ ]
Any other mixed background [ ]
Indian [ ]

Pakistani [ ]
Bangladeshi [ ]
Any other Asian background [ ]
Caribbean [ ]
African [ ]
Any other Black background [ ]
Chinese [ ]
Any other* [ ]

*Specify

9 EDUCATIONAL ATTAINMENT
(tick one only)

No qualifications [ ]
High school quals [ ]
Professional quals [ ]
Degree / Diploma [ ]

10 LIVING WITH:
(tick one only)

Alone [ ]
Self & children [ ]
Partner / spouse [ ]
Partner / spouse & children [ ]
Parents [ ]
Friends [ ]
Other, specify: [ ]

Client lives with someone with substance use problem (please circle)   Y / N

There is a family history of substance use   Y / N

11 DEPENDENT CHILDREN:

How many? [ ]
Age of youngest [ ]

12 TYPE OF ACCOMMODATION:
(tick one only)

Parental home [ ]
Owner occupied [ ]
Private rented [ ]
Council rented [ ]
Housing Association [ ]
Squat [ ]
Rehab / hostel [ ]
Hospital [ ]
Prison [ ]
No fixed abode [ ]
Other, specify: [ ]

13 OCCUPATIONAL STATUS:
(tick one only)

Unemployed [ ]
Employed [ ]
Self-employed [ ]
Childcare / housewife [ ]
Student [ ]
Armed forces [ ]
National service [ ]
Retired [ ]
Voluntary work [ ]
Other, specify: [ ]

14 CURRENT / USUAL JOB:
(BLOCK LETTERS please)

15 PROPOSED ACTION:
(tick up to 3)

Referred to other agency: [ ]
Assessment [ ]
Detoxification [ ]
Long-term prescribing [ ]
Prescribing contract [ ]
Counselling [ ]
Family support [ ]
Rehabilitation [ ]
No action [ ]
Other intervention specify: [ ]

16 REFERRED TO:
(tick up to 3)

Outpatient drug facility [ ]
Inpatient drug facility [ ]
NHS Doctor [ ]
Private Doctor [ ]
Non-statutory agency [ ]
Accident & Emergency [ ]
Psychiatric services [ ]
Social Services [ ]
Other, specify: [ ]

Appendix 4. Substance Abuse Assessment Questionnaire

Part I   Preliminary Assessment

Name of interviewer: ....

INDEX NO.	[ ] [ ] [ ] [ ] [ ] [ ]	1–5
STUDY NO.	[ ] [ ]	6–7
CARD NO.	[0] [1]	8–9

Section I (a)   INITIAL INFORMATION (General assessment)

1.   Date of interview: [ ] [ ] [ ] [ ] [ ] [ ]   10–15

2.   Place of interview: [ ]   –16
            1   Treatment centre
            2   Hospital
            3   Home
            4   Other (specify): ....

3.   Date of referral: [ ][ ][ ][ ][ ][ ]   17–22

4.   Client's name: ....[ ][ ]   23–24

5.   Client's address: ....

                                       [ ][ ][ ][ ][ ][ ]   25–30
      Tel No: ....
      Post Code: ....

6.   Client's sex   [ ]   –31
            1   Male   2   Female

7.   Client's date of birth: [ ][ ][ ][ ][ ][ ]   32–37

For example, 1 September, 1963=[0][1] [0][9] [6][3]

99 99 99 = Not known

8.   Client's age: [ ][ ]   38–39

9.   Ethnic group: [ ][ ]   40–41

    01   British   09   Pakistani

    02   Irish   10   Bangladeshi

    03   Any other White background   11   Any other Asian background

    04   White and Black Caribbean   12   Caribbean

    05   White and Black African   13   African

    06   White and Asian   14   Any other Black background

    07   Any other mixed background   15   Chinese

    08   Indian   16   Any other*

                                     99   Not known

    *Specify...

10.   Marital status: [ ]   –42

    1   Single

    2   Married/Cohabiting

    3   Separated

    4   Divorced

    5   Widowed

    9   Not known

11.   Number of children: [ ][ ]   43–44

12.   Ages of children to nearest whole year: [ ][ ]   45–46

                                                                     [ ][ ]   47–48

                                                                     [ ][ ]   49–50

                                                                     [ ][ ]   51–52

                                                                     [ ][ ]   53–54

> Should the client have more than 5 children please place the youngest child's age in the first two boxes and the eldest child's age in the last two boxes.

13.   Does client have a . . .

    1   Yes   2   No   8   Not applicable   9   Not known

    Family Doctor   [ ]   –55

    Social Worker   [ ]   –56

    Probation Officer   [ ]   –57

    Other Professional Care Worker,   [ ]   –58

    Please Specify ....

    Name and address of key person:

    ....

    ....

    Tel: ....

14.   Source of Referral: [ ][ ]   59–60

    01   Self

    02   Family/Friend/Cohabitee

    03   Family Doctor/Community Health Centre

    04   Accident & Emergency/Hospital

05   Other Drug Clinic
06   Psychiatric Service
07   Police
08   Probation/Courts/Lawyer
09   Social Services
10   Voluntary Agency/Hostel
11   Other (Specify) ....
99   Not known

15.   Current Living Arrangements: [ ][ ]   −61
01   Alone
02   With Spouse or partner
03   With Spouse/Partner and children
04   Self and children
05   Friends/Hostel
06   Parents
07   Other (Specify) ....
99   Not known

16.   Type of accommodation at address: [ ][ ]   62–63
01   Parental home
02   Owned by Client and/or his/her spouse/partner
03   Rented house/flat
04   Squat
05   Hospital
06   Therapeutic Community
07   Probation Hostel
08   Prison
09   No fixed abode
10   Other (Specify) ....
99   Not known

17.   Education – Number of years of schooling completed   [ ][ ]   64–65
88   Still attending
99   Not known

18.   Schooling: [ ]   −66
1   No formal education
2   Special Educational Needs
3   No Qualifications
4   High School Qualifications
5   Professional Qualifications
6   Degree/Diploma

19.   Occupational Status: [ ][ ]   67–68
01   Unemployed
02   Employed
03   Self-employed
04   Child care/Housewife
05   Student
06   Armed Forces

    07   National Service

    08   Retired

    09   Voluntary Work

    10   Other (Specify) ....

    99   Not known

20.   Current/usual job .... *[ ][ ]   69–70

    Local Coding System to be used

21.   Longest period of unemployment:

	years	months	
	[ ][ ]	[ ][ ]	71–74

    88   Not applicable (still at school/college)

    99   Not known

22.   Longest period in same job:

	years	months	
	[ ][ ]	[ ][ ]	75–78

    88   Not applicable (still at school/never employed)

    99   Not known

INDEX NO.	[ ][ ][ ][ ][ ]	1–5
STUDY NO.	[ ][ ]	6–7
CARD NO.	[0][2]	8–9

23.   How many jobs has Client had since leaving school?

    number   [ ][ ]   10–11

    88   Not applicable (still at school/college)

    99   Not known

    00   Never employed

24.   Reason for attendance

    1   Yes   2   No   8   Not applicable   9   Not known

Financial	[ ]	–12
Job	[ ]	–13
Family/Relationships	[ ]	–14
Medical	[ ]	–15
Psychological	[ ]	–16
Housing	[ ]	–17
Pregnancy	[ ]	–18
Accident and Emergency	[ ]	–19
Needle Exchange	[ ]	–20
Other (Specify)	[ ]	–21

25.   Are there any other Agencies involved with the Client?

                                                     [ ]   –22

    1   Yes   2   No   8   Not applicable   9   Not known

    If Yes, specify ....

              ....

              ....

26.   Has Client received treatment for their drug use before?   [ ]   –23

    1   Yes   2   No   8   Not applicable   9   Not known

Section I (b) DRUG USE ASSESSMENT

1. Substance Profile:

Substance Profile	Ever used	Age at first use	Duration of use	Frequency of use over last 30 days	Most usual route over last 30 days	Source over last 30 days	Box Code
	1 Yes	88 Never used	1. Once or twice	1. No use	1. Oral	1. Illicit	
	2 No	90 Has used, but age unknown	2 <6 mths	2 Less than once per week	2 Smoked	2 Private doctor	
	3 Not known	99 Not known	3 7 mths–1 yr	3 Once per week or more	3 Injected	3 Family doctor	
			4 2–5 yrs	4 2/3 times daily	4 Sniffed/Snorted	4 Hospital doctor	
			5 6–10 yrs	5 Once daily	5 Other routes	5 Other doctor	
			6 >10 yrs	4 2/3 times daily	8 N/A	6 OTC/Legal purchase*	
			8 N/A	5 4 or more times daily	9 Not known	8 N/A	
			9 Not known	8 N/A		9 Not known	
				9 Not known			
01 Heroin	[ ]	[ ][ ]	[ ]	[ ]	[ ]	[ ]	10–16
02 Methadone	[ ]	[ ][ ]	[ ]	[ ]	[ ]	[ ]	17–23
03 Other Opiates Specify:	[ ]	[ ][ ]	[ ]	[ ]	[ ]	[ ]	24–30
04 Barbiturates	[ ]	[ ][ ]	[ ]	[ ]	[ ]	[ ]	31–37
05 Benzodiazepines	[ ]	[ ][ ]	[ ]	[ ]	[ ]	[ ]	38–44

						Col.
06	Other Sedatives Specify:	[ ]	[ ]	[ ]	[ ][ ]	[ ]	45–51
07	Antidepressants major tranquillizers Specify:	[ ]	[ ]	[ ]	[ ][ ]	[ ]	52–58
08	Cocaine	[ ]	[ ]	[ ]	[ ][ ]	[ ]	59–65
09	Amphetamines	[ ]	[ ]	[ ]	[ ][ ]	[ ]	66–72
10	Other Stimulants Specify:	[ ]	[ ]	[ ]	[ ][ ]	[ ]	72–78

INDEX NO. [ ][ ][ ][ ][ ][ ]   1–5
STUDY NO. [ ][ ]   6–7
CARD NO. [0][4]   8–9

						Col.
11	Cannabis	[ ]	[ ]	[ ]	[ ][ ]	[ ]	10–16
12	Hallucinogens	[ ]	[ ]	[ ]	[ ][ ]	[ ]	17–23
13	Solvent/Inhalants	[ ]	[ ]	[ ]	[ ][ ]	[ ]	24–30
14	Alcohol	[ ]	[ ]	[ ]	[ ][ ]	[ ]	31–37
15	Tobacco	[ ]	[ ]	[ ]	[ ][ ]	[ ]	38–44
16	Other, specify:	[ ]	[ ]	[ ]	[ ][ ]	[ ]	45–51

* OTC = *Over the Counter Medications*

2.   How were you introduced to drug taking?   [ ]   −52
          1   Partner
          2   Sibling
          3   Friend or acquaintance
          4   Parent or relative
          5   Drug dealer
          6   Doctor (include therapeutic addicts)
          7   Other (please specify) ....
          9   Not known

3.   How long do you consider that you have had a 'drug problem'?
                        years   months   53–56
                        [ ][ ]   [ ][ ]
          99   Not known

          For example, four and a half years = [0][4]   [0][6]

---

4.   Have you experienced any of the following symptoms over the last six months?
          1   Yes   2   No   9   Not known

Opiate Withdrawals	[ ]	−57
Sedative Withdrawals	[ ]	−58
Convulsions	[ ]	−59
Hallucinations	[ ]	−60
Paranoid State	[ ]	−61
Depersonalization	[ ]	−62
Derealization	[ ]	−63
Flashbacks	[ ]	−64

5.   How soon after you wake up in the morning do you use drugs?   [ ]   −65
          1   Immediately
          2   After breakfast/a few hours
          3   After several hours
          4   Not known

6.   How much money do you estimate you spend in an average week on drugs?
          Please state currency: ....
                                                          [ ][ ][ ][ ][ ][ ][ ]   66–73

7.   Have you been absent from work for more than 2 days in last month because
          of drug use?   [ ]   −74
          1   Yes   2   No   8   Not applicable   9   Not known

8.   In last 12 months how many weeks have you been totally drug free?

　　　　Insert number of weeks　　　　　　　　　　　　　　　　[ ][ ]　　75–76

　　　　99　Not known

For example, Seven weeks = [0][7], No weeks = [0][0]

INDEX NO.	[ ][ ][ ][ ][ ]	1–5
STUDY NO.	[ ][ ]	6–7
CARD NO.	[0][5]	8–9

9.   Have you ever received any of the following treatments for your drug use?

　　　　1　Yes　　2　No　　9　Not known

Through voluntary/self-help group	[ ]	–10
Through your Family Doctor	[ ]	–11
Private Practice	[ ]	–12
Substance Misuse Team (outpatient/community)	[ ]	–13
As inpatient	[ ]	–14
As resident in rehabilitation	[ ]	–15
Other (please specify):	[ ]	–16

Please state when and where treatment took place, if known:

Date	Place		
[ ][ ]/[ ][ ]/[ ][ ]		[ ]	17–22
[ ][ ]/[ ][ ]/[ ][ ]		[ ]	23–28
[ ][ ]/[ ][ ]/[ ][ ]		[ ]	29–34
[ ][ ]/[ ][ ]/[ ][ ]		[ ]	35–40

10.   How many cigarettes (tobacco) do you smoke in a day?

　　　　　　　　　　　　　　　　　　　　　　　　　　　　　　　　[ ][ ]　　41–42

　　　　98　Occasional smoker

　　　　88　Does not smoke

　　　　99　Not known

11.   How soon after you wake up in the morning do you smoke?

　　　　　　　　　　　　　　　　　　　　　　　　　　　　　　　　[ ]　　–43

1	Immediately	5	Within six hours
2	Within the first hour	8	Not applicable
3	Within three hours	9	Not known
4	Evening only (i.e. 6 p.m. onwards)		

12.   ASSESSMENT RATING (Drug Use)

(1) Do you see your present 'drug use' as: [ ]   −44
    0 No problem   1 Limited problem   2 Moderate problem
    3 Serious problem

(2) Do you think you need help because of your drug use   [ ]   −45
    0 No need   1 Limited need   2 Moderate need   3 Serious need

(3) Does interviewer think Client's drug use is: [ ]   −46
    0 No problem   1 Limited problem   2 Moderate problem
    3 Serious problem

(4) Does interviewer assess Client's need for help with drug problem as: [ ]   −47
    0 No need   1 Limited need   2 Moderate need   3 Serious need

NOTES:

Section I (c) **ALCOHOL USE**		
	INDEX NO. [ ][ ][ ][ ][ ]	1–5
	STUDY NO. [ ][ ]	6–7
	CARD NO. [0][6]	8–9

1.   Do you consider you have ever had problems with alcohol?
    1   Yes   2   No   9   Not known   [ ]   −10

2.   Do you consider you have current problems with alcohol (within the last 12 months)?
    1   Yes   2   No   9   Not known   [ ]   −11

3.   Have you ever been convicted of alcohol related offences?
    1   Yes   2   No   9   Not known   [ ]   −12

For example, drink/driving, drunk and disorderly, breach of the peace

4.   Are you suffering financial hardship due to the amount you spend on alcohol?
    1   Yes   2   No   9   Not known   [ ]   −13

5.   Do you think your relationships are suffering due to the amount of alcohol you drink?
    1   Yes   2   No   9   Not known   [ ]   −14

6.   Have you been absent from work for more than two days in the last month because of drink?
    1   Yes   2   No   8   Not applicable   9   Not known   [ ]   −15

7.   Number of standard drinks consumed in an average week:
    grams   [ ][ ][ ]   16–18
    or units   [ ][ ][ ]   19–21

Calculation Formula: 1 Unit of alcohol = 8 g of absolute alcohol No. of alcohol units = % Alcohol By Volume (ABV) × amount of beverage (in ml)

8.   Have you experienced any of the following symptoms over the last six months related to alcohol consumption?
    1   Yes   2   No   9   Not known

Morning drinking	[ ]	−22
Morning nausea/vomiting	[ ]	−23
Shakes	[ ]	−24
Sweating	[ ]	−25
Anxiety/panic attacks	[ ]	−26
Depression	[ ]	−27
Loss of memory	[ ]	−28
Blackouts	[ ]	−29
Delirium Tremens	[ ]	−30
Convulsions	[ ]	−31
Hallucinations	[ ]	−32

9. On average how many days in a week do you consume alcohol? [ ] −33
    9   Not known

10. What is your usual style of drinking? [ ] −34
    1   Weekend/other short episodes
    2   Bouts of more than two days
    3   Steady, daily
    4   Other, specify ....
    8   Not applicable
    9   Not known

11. If you drink in bouts what is their average duration?
    days   weeks   months
    [ ][ ]   [ ][ ]   [ ][ ]   35–40

12. What is the average length of time between bouts?
    days   weeks   months
    [ ][ ]   [ ][ ]   [ ][ ]   41–46

13. In the last year how many weeks have you been alcohol free?

                                                                  [ ][ ] 47–48
    88 Not applicable
    99 Not known

14. How long do you think you have had a problem with alcohol?
    years   months
    [ ][ ]   [ ][ ]   49–52
    88 Not applicable
    99 Not known

15. Have you ever had treatment for your problem with alcohol? [ ] −53
    1   Yes
    2   No
    8   Not applicable (i.e. no alcohol problem)

9   Not known

If the answer to question 15 is no treatment leave all boxes blank and go to next question.

---

16.   Treatment received:
           1   Yes   2   No   9   Not known
           Family Doctor treatment   [ ]   –54
           As hospital out-patient   [ ]   –55
           As hospital in-patient   [ ]   –56
           Community Alcohol Team   [ ]   –57
           Non-statutory/Voluntary agency   [ ]   –58
           Other (specify):   [ ]   –59

Please state when and where treatment took place, if known:

Date	Place	
[ ][ ]/[ ][ ]/[ ][ ]		[ ]60–65
[ ][ ]/[ ][ ]/[ ][ ]		[ ]66–71

17.   ASSESSMENT RATING (Alcohol)

(1) How do you rate your alcohol use?   [ ]   –72
     0 No problem   1 Limited problem   2 Moderate problem
     3 Serious problem
(2) Do you think you need help with an alcohol problem?   [ ]   –73
     0 No need   1 Limited need   2 Moderate need   3 Serious need
(3) How does interviewer rate Client's alcohol problem?   [ ]   –74
     0 No problem   1 Limited problem   2 Moderate problem
     3 Serious problem
(4) Does interviewer think Client needs help with alcohol problem?   [ ]   –75
     0 No need   1 Limited need   2 Moderate need   3 Serious need

NOTES:

Section I (d)   SUMMARY OF REQUESTS AND REQUIREMENTS

INDEX NO.   [ ][ ][ ][ ][ ]   1–5
STUDY NO.   [ ][ ]   6–7
CARD NO.   [0][7]   8–9

1.   What treatment is Client asking for?

   1   Yes   2   No   9   Not known

Out-patient Programmes		
Programme	Client requests	Interviewer's initial recommendation
Out-patient Detox Programme		
• Opiate	[ ]	[ ] 10–11
• Sedative	[ ]	[ ] 12–13
• Stimulants	[ ]	[ ] 14–15
• Alcohol	[ ]	[ ] 16–17
Out-patient Maintenance Programme		
• Opiate	[ ]	[ ] 18–19
• Sedative	[ ]	[ ] 20–21
• Stimulants	[ ]	[ ] 22–23
In-patient Assessment Prior to any of the above		[ ] –24

In-patient Programmes

Programme	Client requests	Interviewer's initial recommendation
In-patient Detox Programmes		
• Opiate	[ ]	[ ] 25–26
• Sedative	[ ]	[ ] 27–28
• Stimulant	[ ]	[ ] 29–30
• Alcohol	[ ]	[ ] 31–32
In-patient treatment other (specify)	[ ]	[ ] 33–34
Residential Recovery/Rehab	[ ]	[ ] 35–36

Day Care		
Programme	Client requests	Interviewer's initial recommendation
Day Care	[ ]	[ ] 37–38
Other Options		
Treatment for physical health (specify)	[ ]	[ ] 39–40
Treatment for psychiatric health problem (specify)	[ ]	[ ] 41–42
Naltrexone	[ ]	[ ] 43–44
Disulfiram	[ ]	[ ] 45–46
NET	[ ]	[ ] 47–48
Acupuncture	[ ]	[ ] 49–50
Needle Exchange	[ ]	[ ] 51–52
HIV Counselling/Testing	[ ]	[ ] 53–54
Psychological Interventions	[ ]	[ ] 55–56
Other, please specify:	[ ]	[ ] 57–58
....	[ ]	[ ] 59–60
Social Work assistance	[ ]	[ ] 61–62
Court report	[ ]	[ ] 63–64

2.   At the time of this interview was the client: [ ]   –65

   1   Sober   2   Intoxicated   3   Withdrawing   9   Not known

3.   SUMMARY RATING (General Preliminary Assessment: Sections 1a, 1b, 1c and 1d)

(1) Does Client perceive their present situation as: [ ]   –66
     0 No problem   1 Limited problem   2 Moderate problem
     3 Serious problem
(2) Does Client perceive their present need for help as: [ ]   –67
     0 No need   1 Limited need   2 Moderate need   3 Serious need
(3) Does interviewer perceive Client's present situation as: [ ]   –68
     0 No problem   1 Limited problem   2 Moderate problem
     3 Serious problem
(4) Does interviewer perceive Client's need for help as: [ ]   –69
     0 No need   1 Limited need   2 Moderate need   3 Serious need

NOTES:

Part II   Comprehensive Assessment

> **Section II   MEDICAL AND MENTAL HEALTH ASSESSMENT**
>
> INDEX NO.   [ ][ ][ ][ ][ ]   1–5
> STUDY NO.   [ ][ ]   6–7
> CARD NO.   [0][8]   8–9

> **Section II (a)   PHYSICAL HEALTH**

1.   Have you any complaints about your present state of physical health and/or do you suffer any disability?

    1   Yes   2   No   9   Not known   [ ]   –10

    If Yes, specify: ....

    ....

2.   What is your appetite like?

    1   Good   2   Poor   9   Not known   [ ]   –11

3.   How do you sleep?

    1   Well   2   Poorly   9   Not known   [ ]   –12

4.   Are you presently receiving any treatment for a physical illness and/or disability?

    1   Yes   2   No   9   Not known

    From Family Doctor: [ ]   –13

    From Hospital, Out-patient: [ ]   –14

    From Hospital, In-patient: [ ]   –15

    Other (specify) ....   [ ]   –16

    What is the illness/disability?   *[ ][ ][ ][ ][ ]   17–21

    Local Coding System to be used

    ....

    What is the treatment?   *[ ][ ]   22–23

    Local Coding System to be used

    ....

    If receiving prescribed drugs (apart from methadone) please give names:

    Local Coding System to be used

    ....*[ ][ ][ ]   24–26

    ....

5.   Have you ever been hospitalized in the last two years for a physical illness?

    1   Yes   2   No   8   Not applicable   9   Not known   [ ]   –27

> If Yes, specify:

Nature of illness	Age at which it occurred	Length of admission (months)

6.   Have you ever injected?   [ ]   −28
       1   Yes   2   No   9   Not known

If No, go to question 11

7.   Which method(s) of injecting do you use?
       1   Yes   2   No   9   Not known
       Intravenous (I.V.)   [ ]   −29
       Intramuscular (I.M.)   [ ]   −30
       Subcutaneous (Skin-popping)   [ ]   −31

8.   Which sites do you use?
       1   Yes   2   No   9   Not known
       Arm   [ ]   −32
       Groin   [ ]   −33
       Feet   [ ]   −34
       Neck   [ ]   −35
       Other (specify): ....   [ ]   −36

9.   Have you ever shared?   [ ]   −37
       1   Yes   2   No   9   Not known

10.   How long ago was most recent sharing?

                                              years   months   days
                                             [ ][ ]   [ ][ ]   [ ][ ]   38–43

11.   Has an HIV test ever been offered to you?   [ ]   −44
       1   Yes   2   No   9   Not known

12.   Did you take up the offer of testing?   [ ]   −45
       1   Yes   2   No   9   Not known

13.   Have you ever completed a Hep B vaccination course?   [ ]   −46
       1   Yes   2   No   9   Not known

14.   Have you ever had any of the following?
       1   Yes   2   No   9   Not known
       HIV   [ ]   −47
       Hepatitis B   [ ]   −48

Hepatitis C	[ ]	–49
Septicaemia	[ ]	–50
Abscesses	[ ]	–51
Endocarditis	[ ]	–52
Over-dose (deliberate)	[ ]	–53
Over-dose (accidental)	[ ]	–54
Other (specify):	[ ]	–55

Female Clients Only

Amenorrheoa	[ ]	–56
Miscarriage/spontaneous abortion	[ ]	–57
Termination of pregnancy	[ ]	–58

15. PHYSICAL EXAMINATION

(a) General Physical Examination

1   Yes   2   No   9   Not known

Poor dental care	[ ]	–59
Injection marks on skin	[ ]	–60
Tattoos	[ ]	–61
Abscesses	[ ]	–62
Anaemia	[ ]	–63
Malnutrition	[ ]	–64
Lymphadenopathy	[ ]	–65
Jaundice	[ ]	–66

(b) Systems Examination

1   Normal   2   Abnormal (specify)   9   Not known

	Specify	Code	
Cardiovascular System		[ ]	–67
Respiratory		[ ]	–68
Alimentary		[ ]	–69
Urogenital		[ ]	–70
Endocrine		[ ]	–71
Nervous System		[ ]	–72
Locomotor		[ ]	–73

INDEX NO.	[ ][ ][ ][ ][ ]	1–5
STUDY NO.	[ ][ ]	6–7
CARD NO.	[0][9]	8–9

16. Blood Pressure:

Systolic	[ ][ ][ ]	10–12
Diastolic	[ ][ ][ ]	13–15
Pulse	[ ][ ][ ]	16–18

17.   LABORATORY INVESTIGATIONS:

(a) Hepatitis Screen	1 Positive 2 Negative 8 Not done 9 Not known	
Type	Date of result	Code
B antibody B antigen C antibody C antigen	[ ][ ]/[ ][ ]/[ ][ ] [ ][ ]/[ ][ ]/[ ][ ] [ ][ ]/[ ][ ]/[ ][ ] [ ][ ]/[ ][ ]/[ ][ ]	[ ] 19–25 [ ] 26–32 [ ] 33–39 [ ] 40–46

(b) HIV Screen	1 Positive 2 Negative 8 Not done 9 Not known	
	Date of result	Code
	[ ][ ]/[ ][ ]/[ ][ ]	[ ] 47–53

(c) Electrolytes and Urea	1 Normal 2 Abnormal 8 Not done 9 Not known	
Date of result	If abnormal, specify:	Code
[ ][ ]/[ ][ ]/[ ][ ]		[ ] 54–60

(d) Liver Function Test	1 Normal 2 Abnormal 8 Not done 9 Not known	
Date of result	If abnormal, specify:	Code
[ ][ ]/[ ][ ]/[ ][ ]		[ ] 61–67

(e) Full Blood Count	1 Normal 2 Abnormal 8 Not done 9 Not known	
Date of result	If abnormal, specify:	Code
[ ][ ]/[ ][ ]/[ ][ ]		[ ] 68–74

INDEX NO.   [ ][ ][ ][ ][ ]   1–5
STUDY NO.   [ ][ ]   6–7
CARD NO.   [1][0]   8–9

(f) X-rays	1 Normal 2 Abnormal 8 Not done 9 Not known	
Date of result	If abnormal, specify:	Code
[ ][ ]/[ ][ ]/[ ][ ]		[ ] 10–16

18.   URINE RESULTS

1   Positive   2   Negative   8   Not done   9   Not known

	Date: //	Date: //	Date: //	Date: // 17–40

Drug	result	result	result	result
Morphine	[ ]	[ ]	[ ]	[ ] 41–44
Methadone	[ ]	[ ]	[ ]	[ ] 45–49
Other Opiates	[ ]	[ ]	[ ]	[ ] 50–54
Amphetamines	[ ]	[ ]	[ ]	[ ] 55–59
Cocaine	[ ]	[ ]	[ ]	[ ] 60–64
Barbiturates	[ ]	[ ]	[ ]	[ ] 65–69
Benzodiazepines	[ ]	[ ]	[ ]	[ ] 70–74
Cannabis	[ ]	[ ]	[ ]	[ ] 75–79

INDEX NO.   [ ][ ][ ][ ][ ]   1–5
STUDY NO.   [ ][ ]   6–7
CARD NO.   [1][1]   8–9

Alcohol Other (specify)	[ ] [ ]	[ ] [ ]	[ ] [ ]	[ ] 10–14 [ ] 15–19

19.   ASSESSMENT RATING (Physical Health)

(1) How would you rate your physical health at present?   [ ]   –20
    0   No problem   1 Limited problem   2 Moderate problem
    3 Serious problem

(2) Do you think you need help with physical health
    problems?   [ ]   –21
    0   No need   1 Limited need   2 Moderate need   3 Serious need

(3) How does interviewer rate Client's physical health?   [ ]   –22
    0   No problem   1 Limited problem   2 Moderate problem
    3 Serious problem

(4) Does interviewer think Client needs help with physical health problems?[ ]   –23
    0   No need   1 Limited need   2 Moderate need   3 Serious need

NOTES:

INDEX NO. [ ][ ][ ][ ][ ]   1–5
STUDY NO. [ ][ ]   6–7
CARD NO.   [1][2]   8–9

Section II (b)   MENTAL HEALTH

18.   Are you presently receiving treatment for a mental health problem? (Except drug/alcohol use):

1   Yes   2   No   9   Not known

From Family Doctor	[ ]	–10
Hospital (Out-patient/Day patient)	[ ]	–11
Hospital (In-patient)	[ ]	–12
Community Mental Health Team	[ ]	–13
Other (specify): .... [ ]		–14

What is the illness/problem?   *[ ][ ][ ][ ][ ]   15–19
*Local Coding System to be used

....
....

What is the treatment?   *[ ][ ]   20–21
*Local Coding System to be used

....
....

If receiving prescribed drugs please give names:
*Local Coding System to be used

                                                *[ ][ ][ ]   22–24

....
....

19.   Have you ever been a hospital in-patient because of mental illness?   [ ]   –25

1   Yes   2   No   9   Not known

If Yes, please specify

Nature of illness	Age	Date	
	[ ][ ]	[ ][ ]/[ ][ ]/[ ][ ] ...	26–33
	[ ][ ]	[ ][ ]/[ ][ ]/[ ][ ] ...	34–41
	[ ][ ]	[ ][ ]/[ ][ ]/[ ][ ] ...	42–50

20.   What is your sexual orientation?   [ ]   –51

1   Exclusively heterosexual
2   Mainly heterosexual

3 Mainly homosexual

4 Bisexual

5 Exclusively homosexual

9 Not known

21. Do you consider you have any problem with your sexual functioning?   [ ]   −50

1 Yes (secondary to drug/alcohol use)

2 Yes (other reason)

3 No

9 Not known

If Yes, please specify

....

22. Mental State

1 Normal   2 Abnormal (specify)   9 Not known

	Specify abnormality	Code
Appearance		[ ] −51
Behaviour		[ ] −52
Mood		[ ] −53
Talk		[ ] −54
Thought		[ ] −55
Perception		[ ] −56
Insight		[ ] −57
Cognitive function		[ ] −58
Orientation		[ ] −59
Concentration		[ ] −60
Memory		[ ] −61
Intelligence		[ ] −62
Other		[ ] −63

23. At the time of the mental state being carried out, was client   [ ]   −64

1 Sober   2 Intoxicated   3 Withdrawing   9 Not known

24.   ASSESSMENT RATING (Mental Health)

(1) How would you rate your mental health at present?   [ ]   –65
      0   No problem   1 Limited problem   2 Moderate problem
      3 Serious problem

(2) Do you think you need help with mental health problems?   [ ]   –66
      0   No need   1 Limited need   2 Moderate need   3 Serious need

(3) How does interviewer rate Client's mental health?   [ ]   –67
      0   No problem   1 Limited problem   2 Moderate problem
      3 Serious problem

(4) Does interviewer think Client needs help with mental health?   [ ]   –68
      0   No need   1 Limited need   2 Moderate need   3 Serious need

NOTES:

Section III FORENSIC ASSESSMENT		
	INDEX NO. [ ][ ][ ][ ][ ]	1–5
	STUDY NO. [ ][ ]	6–7
	CARD NO. [1][3]	8–9

1. Have you ever been involved in any criminal activity?   [ ]   –10
    1   Yes   2   No   9   Not known

> If answer to this question is No: STOP HERE, leave all intervening boxes blank, and go to question 11.

2. At what age did you first become involved in criminal activity?   [ ][ ]   –11
    99   Not known

3. Do you at present have any court cases pending?   [ ][ ]   –12
    1   Yes   2   No   9   Not known

> If answer is Yes, please specify for what offence(s):
> *Local Coding System to be used.

    ....
    .... *[ ][ ]   13–14

4. Are you at present on: . . .
    1   Yes   2   No   9   Not known
    Condition of treatment   [ ]   –15
    Probation   [ ]   –16
    Suspended sentence   [ ]   –17
    Deferred sentence   [ ]   –18
    Parole   [ ]   –19
    Other (specify) .... [ ]   –20

5.

> If answer is yes, please specify for what offence(s)
> *Local Coding System to be used

    ....
    .... *[ ][ ]   21–22

6. Which of the following types of offences have you ever
    committed, and number of convictions?
    1   Yes   2   No   9   Not known

Offences	Committed before drug use began	Committed after drug use began	Number of convictions	
Drug related	[ ]	[ ]	[ ] [ ]	23–26
Driving	[ ]	[ ]	[ ] [ ]	27–30
Public disorder	[ ]	[ ]	[ ] [ ]	31–34
Violence against property	[ ]	[ ]	[ ] [ ]	35–38
Crimes of acquisition	[ ]	[ ]	[ ] [ ]	39–42
Sex offences	[ ]	[ ]	[ ] [ ]	43–46
Violence against the person	[ ]	[ ]	[ ] [ ]	47–50

7.   Have you had any periods of imprisonment?   [ ][ ]   51–52

> If yes, code number of times, i.e. three times = [0][3]
>
> 99 = Not known
>
> 88 = Never been in prison

8.   If you have been in prison, what was the longest sentence served?

days   months   years

[ ][ ]   [ ][ ]   [ ][ ]   53–58

99   Not known

9.   Whilst in prison did you continue to use drugs?

1   Yes, frequently   3   Yes, occasionally

2   No   9   Not known   [ ]   –59

10.   Of the crimes committed since the onset of drug use, what percentage do you estimate were committed whilst intoxicated?

                percentage %

                [ ][ ]   60–61

99   Not known

11.   ASSESSMENT RATING (Forensic/Legal)

> (1) How severe would you rate your legal problems as being at the moment?   [ ]   –62
>   0 No problems   1 Limited problems   2 Moderate problems
>   3 Serious problems
> (2) Do you think you need help with your legal problems at present?   [ ]   –63
>   0 No need   1 Limited need   2 Moderate need   3 Serious need [ ]
> (3) Does the interviewer think the Client's present legal problems are: [ ]   –64
>   0 No problems   1 Limited problems   2 Moderate problems
>   3 Serious problems
> (4) How much help does the interviewer think the Client needs with legal problems?   –65
>   0 No need   1 Limited need   2 Moderate need   3 Serious need [ ]

NOTES:

Section IV	PSYCHOSOCIAL AND FAMILY ASSESSMENT	
	INDEX NO. [ ][ ][ ][ ][ ]	1–5
	STUDY NO. [ ][ ]	6–7
	CARD NO. [1][4]	8–9

1. Do you have a Social Worker already involved with yourself or your family   [ ]   –10
    1   Yes   2   No   9   Not known
    Name and address ....
    ....
    Tel: ....

2. Number of siblings
        Male   [ ][ ]   11–12
        Female   [ ][ ]   13–14
    88   None
    99   Not known

3. What position are you in birth order?   [ ][ ]   15–16
    01   First
    02   Second (etc.)
    99   Not applicable (only child)

4. Are you a twin?   [ ]   –17
    1   Yes, identical twin
    2   Yes, non-identical twin
    3   No
    9   Not known

5. Father's occupation/last job   [ ]   18–19
    Please specify
    Local Coding System to be used

    ....

6. Father's age   [ ][ ]   20–21
    or age at death?   [ ][ ]   21–22
    10   Not applicable (i.e. father unknown)
    99   Not known

7. Mother's occupation/last job: [ ][ ]*   23–24
    Please specify
    Local Coding System to be used

    ....

8. Mother's age   [ ][ ]   25–26
    or age at death?   [ ][ ]   27–28
    10   Not applicable(i.e. mother unknown)
    99   Not known

9.   Are members of the immediate family aware of drug use?

       1 Yes   2 No   8 Not applicable   9 Not known

       Parents   [ ]   −29

       Partner   [ ]   −30

       Children   [ ]   −31

10.   Are members of the immediate family aware of alcohol problem?

       1 Yes   2 No   8 Not applicable   9 Not known

       Parents   [ ]   −32

       Partner   [ ]   −33

       Children   [ ]   −34

11.   If you are married or have a regular partner, what is partner's occupation?   [ ][ ]   35–36

       Please specify

       Local Coding System to be used

       ....

12.   Are you worried about your children in any of the following areas?

       1 Yes   2 No   8 No children   9 Not known

	Code
Problems at home	[ ] −37
Problems at school	[ ] −38
Problems with police	[ ] −39
Using drugs/alcohol	[ ] −40
Physical health/handicap	[ ] −41
Mental health/handicap	[ ] −42

13.   Are any of your children, under the age of 16 years, living away from you at present?

       1 Yes   2 No   8 No children   9 Not known

       With other parent/family member   [ ]   −43

       Under the care of Statutory Supervision   [ ]   −44

       Other reasons (please specify):

       .... [ ]   −45

Include here, e.g. attending special school, children have left home, children in hostel, etc.

14.   Are any of your children on a Statutory Protection Register (i.e. At Risk Register)

       1 Yes   2 No   8 No children   9 Not known

       If Yes, please specify *Local Coding System to be used*

       .... [ ][ ]*   46–47

15.   Have any of your children been on a Statutory Protection Register (i.e. At Risk Register) in the past?

1   Yes   2   No   8   No Children   9   Not known

If Yes, please specify* *Local Coding System to be used*

....   [ ][ ]*   48–49

16.   Do you usually use drugs: [ ]   −50

     1   Alone

     2   With others

     8   Not applicable (never uses drugs)

     9   Not known

17.   What proportion of friends/associates take drugs?

                   percentage %   [ ][ ]   51–52

     88   Not applicable (never uses drugs)

     99   Not known

18.   What percentage of your time is spent in drug seeking/drug using?

                   percentage %   [ ][ ]   53–54

     88   Not applicable (never uses drugs)

     99   Not known

19.   Over the last 12 months have any of the following caused you particular concern?

     1   Yes, serious concern   2   Yes, moderate concern

     3   Yes, slight concern   4   No concern

     9   Not known

Event	Code	
Problems at work	[ ]	−55
Financial hardship	[ ]	−56
Housing difficulties	[ ]	−57
Partner's drug/alcohol abuse	[ ]	−58
Ill health in the family	[ ]	−59
Relationship/marital discord	[ ]	−60
Violence in the family	[ ]	−61
Separation from children	[ ]	−62
Separation from partner/spouse	[ ]	−63
Bereavement	[ ]	−64
Other, specify	[ ]	−65

INDEX NO.   [ ][ ][ ][ ][ ]   1–5

STUDY NO.   [ ][ ]   6–7

CARD NO.   [1][5]   8–9

20.   Have any members of your family suffered from a psychiatric illness/dependency on drugs and/or alcohol?

   1   Yes   2   No   8   Not applicable   9   Not known

Member of family	Psychiatric illness	Dependency on drugs	Dependency on alcohol	
Father	[ ]	[ ]	[ ]	10–12
Mother	[ ]	[ ]	[ ]	13–15
Sibling(s)	[ ]	[ ]	[ ]	16–18
Children	[ ]	[ ]	[ ]	19–21
Partner	[ ]	[ ]	[ ]	22–24
Other, specify				
....	[ ]	[ ]	[ ]	25–27
If yes, please give details	....	....	....	

21.   Do any members of your family have a criminal record?

   1   Yes   2   No   8   Not applicable   9   Not known

		Criminal details	
Father	[ ]		−28
Mother	[ ]		−29
Sibling(s)	[ ]		−30
Partner	[ ]		−31
Children	[ ]		−32
Other (specify)			
....	[ ]		−33
....	[ ]		−34

22.   During childhood or adolescence, was your family life disrupted by any of the following events?

1   Yes   2   No   3   Not known

Event	Childhood (0–12 years)	Adolescence (13–20 years)	
Client went into care/fostered/adopted	[ ]	[ ]	35–36
Frequent relocation	[ ]	[ ]	37–38
Financial hardship	[ ]	[ ]	39–40
Violence against Client	[ ]	[ ]	41–42
Sexual assault	[ ]	[ ]	43–44
Incest	[ ]	[ ]	45–46
Marital discord between parents	[ ]	[ ]	47–48
Violence between parents	[ ]	[ ]	49–50
Separation/Divorce of parents	[ ]	[ ]	51–52
Imprisonment of parent	[ ]	[ ]	53–54
Hospitalization of parent for over 3/12	[ ]	[ ]	55–56
Death of sibling	[ ]	[ ]	57–58
Death of father	[ ]	[ ]	59–60
Death of mother	[ ]	[ ]	61–62
Family joined by step-parent/step-siblings	[ ]	[ ]	63–64

23.   ASSESSMENT RATING (Psychosocial/Family)

(1) How concerned are you about social/family problems?   [ ]   –65

   0   No concern   1 Limited concern   2 Moderate concern

   3   Serious concern

(2) Do you think you need help with social/family problems?   [ ]   –66

   0   No need   1 Limited need   2 Moderate need

   3   Serious need

(3) How concerned is interviewer about Client's social/family problems?   [ ]   –67

   0   No concern   1 Limited concern   2 Moderate concern

   3   Serious concern

(4) Does interviewer think Client needs help with social/family problems?   [ ]   –68

   0   No need   1 Limited need   2 Moderate need   3 Serious need

NOTES:

Section V   ASSESSMENT PROFILE

INDEX NO.	[ ][ ][ ][ ][ ]	1–5
STUDY NO.	[ ][ ]	6–7
CARD NO.	[1][6]	8–9

1.   Did the Client complete assessment?

    1   Yes   2   No   9   Not known   [ ]   –10

    If Client failed to complete assessment, please state reason for dropping out

    *Local Coding System to be used

    .... [ ][ ][ ][ ]   11–14

    ....

    ....

    ....

3.   Principal Substance of Misuse

> Please list in rank order, for example;
> 1= primary substance
> 8= not a problem now, or never used
> 9= not known

Opiates   [ ]   –15

Barbiturates   [ ]   –16

Benzodiazepines   [ ]   –17

Amphetamine   [ ]   –18

Cocaine   [ ]   –19

Other stimulants   [ ]   –20

Psychotropics (including LSD & Cannabis)   [ ]   –21

Alcohol   [ ]   –22

Solvents/Inhalants   [ ]   –23

4.   Overall Assessment Rating Scores

Insert corresponding scores from assessment ratings for each section

	Client's Perception		Care Worker's Perception		
	Problem	Need	Problem	Need	Box codes
Drug	[ ]	[ ]	[ ]	[ ]	24–27
Alcohol	[ ]	[ ]	[ ]	[ ]	40–43
General/Preliminary	[ ]	[ ]	[ ]	[ ]	28–31
Physical	[ ]	[ ]	[ ]	[ ]	32–35
Mental	[ ]	[ ]	[ ]	[ ]	36–39
Legal/Forensic	[ ]	[ ]	[ ]	[ ]	44–47
Psychosocial/Family	[ ]	[ ]	[ ]	[ ]	48–51

The maximum problem/need score in each of the dimensions is 12.
Overall scoring is not deemed appropriate.

5. Diagnosis
    Record as many coexisting mental disorders, general medical conditions and other factors that are relevant to the care and treatment of the individual. The primary diagnosis should be listed first. Please specify the classification system used (DSM III-R/DSM-IV/ICD-9/ICD-10)

ICD.../DSM...Name	ICD.../DSM...CODE	Box Code
	[ ] [ ] [ ] [ ] . [ ] [ ]	49–53
	[ ] [ ] [ ] [ ] . [ ] [ ]	54–58
	[ ] [ ] [ ] [ ] . [ ] [ ]	59–63
	[ ] [ ] [ ] [ ] . [ ] [ ]	64–68

FOR EXAMPLE ICD.../DSM...Name	ICD.../DSM...CODE	Box Code
Alcohol Abuse (DSM-IV)	[3] [0] [5] . [0] [0]	
Dependent personality Disorder (DSM-III-R)	[3] [0] [1] . [6] [0]	
Hypothyroidism (ICD-9-CM)	[2] [4] [4] . [9] [ ]	

6.   Client's requirements (as perceived by Centre)

(a) Drug Problem	Code	
1 Requires in-patient treatment	[ ]	−69
2 Requires out-patient treatment	[ ]	−70
3 Requires in-patient treatment in DDU	[ ]	−71
4 Other (please specify):		
	[ ]	−72
8 Not applicable	[ ]	−73
9 Not known	[ ]	−74

INDEX NO.   [ ][ ][ ][ ][ ]   1–5
STUDY NO.   [ ][ ]   6–7
CARD NO.   [1][7]   8–9

(b) Physical Health Problem	Code	
1 Requires in-patient treatment in another hospital department	[ ]	−10
2 Requires in-patient treatment in drug treatment centre	[ ]	−11
3 Requires out-patient treatment in another hospital department	[ ]	−12
4 Requires out-patient treatment in drug treatment centre	[ ]	−13
5 Other (please specify)	[ ]	−14
8 Not applicable	[ ]	−15
9 Not known	[ ]	−16

(c) Mental health problem	Code	
1 Requires formal in-patient psychiatric treatment	[ ]	−54
2 Requires formal out-patient psychiatric treatment in another hospital department	[ ]	−55
3 Requires out-patient treatment in this Centre	[ ]	−56
4 Other (please specify)	[ ]	−57
8 Not applicable	[ ]	−58
9 Not known	[ ]	−59

Social problems	Code	
1 Requires referral to other agency	[ ]	−60
2 Requires help from this Centre	[ ]	−61
3 Other (please specify)	[ ]	−62
8 Not applicable	[ ]	−63
9 Not known	[ ]	−64

Section VI   TREATMENT PROFILE

INDEX NO.	[ ][ ][ ][ ][ ]	1–5
STUDY NO.	[ ][ ]	6–7
CARD NO.	[1][8]	8–9

1. What type of treatment was offered to the Client?   [ ]   −10
    1   Out-patient
    2   Community Intervention
    3   In-patient
    4   Day Care
    5   Residential Rehabilitation

2. Place of treatment   [ ][ ]   11–12
    1   Specialized Out-Patient Drug Treatment Centre
    2   General Out-Patient clinic
    3   Client's home
    4   Community Health Centre/Family Doctor's surgery
    5   Specialized In-Patient Drug Treatment Unit
    6   General In-Patient Psychiatric Unit
    7   General Medical/Surgical In-Patient Unit
    8   Specialized Drug Day Programme
    9   General Day Care Programme
    10 Other (specify)

    ....

3. Was medication prescribed?
   1. Yes 2. No

*If yes, please give details: *Local Coding System to be used*

Dependency	Drug Prescribed	Dose in mg over a 24 hr period	Length of proposed detox*/ maintenance*. Please indicate days*/weeks*/months* by deletion	Starting Date	Box Codes
Opiate/Opioid	Specify: .... [ ][ ][ ][ ][ ]	[ ][ ][ ]	[ ][ ]	[ ][1/][1/][1/][ ][ ]	11–26
Benzodiazepines/ sedative	Specify: .... [ ][ ][ ][ ][ ]	[ ][ ][ ]	[ ][ ]	[ ][1/][1/][1/][ ][ ]	27–42
Alcohol	Specify: .... [ ][ ][ ][ ][ ]	[ ][ ][ ]	[ ][ ]	[ ][1/][1/][1/][ ][ ]	43–58
Stimulant	Specify: .... [ ][ ][ ][ ][ ]	[ ][ ][ ]	[ ][ ]	[ ][1/][1/][1/][ ][ ]	59–74

Other, specify	Specify: .... [ ][ ][ ][ ][ ]	[ ][ ][ ]	[ ][ ]	[ ][1/][1/][1/][ ][ ]	10–25

4.   Were any of the following General Treatment Measures offered?
      1 Yes   2 No   9 Not known

	Code	
Counselling	[ ]	–26
Individual psychotherapy	[ ]	–27
Behaviour therapy	[ ]	–28
Relaxation therapy	[ ]	–29
Family therapy	[ ]	–30
Joint marital therapy	[ ]	–31
Group therapy	[ ]	–32
Alcohol Support Group	[ ]	–33
Drug Use Support Group	[ ]	–34
Other, please state:	[ ]	–35
....		

Treatment Plan

A précis of the treatment plan agreed by the client and keyworker should be documented. It should include:

a) The nature of treatment
b) The order of interventions and their proposed duration
c) The ways in which treatment will be implemented

....
....
....
....
....
....
....
....
....
....
....
....
....
....
....
....

Section VII **SUMMARY OF ASSESSMENT AND TREATMENT**

This summary should provide an adequate basis for letters to family doctors, formal reports and referrals and should include:

1. Reason and source of referral.
2. Date of assessment and discipline(s)of professionals involved.
3. Major substance(s) of use including the duration and pattern of use.
4. Previous treatment history and agencies involved.
5. Major problem areas and need for intervention.
6. Patient's personality, motivation and other psychological factors.
7. Treatment goals (short-, medium- and long-term) and plan of action.
8. Formulation of the case.

....
....
....
....
....
....
....
....
....
....
....
....
....
....
....
....
....
....
....
....
....
....
....
....
....
....
....
....
....
....
....

Section VIII	GUIDELINES ON SCORING THE SAAQ RATING SCALE

1. Problems Rating Score

Domain		Score Category
1.1 Drug use	0	Abstinence or near abstinences from prescribed and illicit drugs
	1	Prescribed drugs or only occasional illicit drug use
	2	Illicit drug use – no injecting or only occasional injecting
	3	Chaotic or regular injecting or sharing injecting equipment
1.2 Alcohol use	0	Abstinent or moderate alcohol use (M<=21 F<=14 u/week)
	1	Heavy drinking (M 22–50 u/week; F14–35 u/week)
	2	Excessive drinking (M>50; F>35 u/week) and moderate alcohol dependence
	3	Severe alcohol dependence (e.g. severe withdrawal or morning relief drinking) or regular/prolonged binges
1.3 General/Preliminary	0	Abstinence or near abstinence from all substances – no need for significant intervention
	1	Moderate problems with substance misuse which has been acknowledged by the client and/or noted by others – need for brief intervention
	2	Significant substance misuse problems – need for specialist intervention
	3	Serious substance misuse problems with significant risk of harm to the client and/or others – need for intensive interventions
1.4 Physical health	0	No physical health problems
	1	Limited problems (e.g. weight loss, poor physical care, poor diet)
	2	Moderate problems (disabilities related to use, no acute illness, abscesses, ODs (non-DSH), asymptomatic HIV, hepatitis)
	3	Serious problems (serious physical illness e.g. symptomatic HIV, hepatitis, endocarditis, septicaemia, DVT)
1.5 Mental Health	0	No mental health problems
	1	Limited problems (e.g. mild depression/anxiety)
	2	Moderate problems (e.g. moderate depression/anxiety, suicidal ideation, impulsive DSH attempt)
	3	Serious problems (e.g. psychoses, severe depression, serious DSH attempt)

1.6 Forensic/legal	0	No forensic or legal problems
	1	Limited (e.g. shoplifting, occasional petty crime, no serious offences, possession)
	2	Moderate (e.g. nonviolent crime, probation, fines, drunk driving, or pending, possession with intent to supply)
	3	Serious (e.g. violent offences, sexual assault, rape, possible imprisonment, trafficking)
1.7 Social/Family	0	No problems (no threat e.g. stable relationships, accommodation, job)
	1	Limited problems(threat e.g. threats to job, relationship, housing)
	2	Moderate problems (serious threat e.g. unstable relationships, housing, work)
	3	Serious problems (breakdown e.g. relationship breakdown, violence, loss of job, eviction, homelessness, or threat of)

At intake score refers to the 6 month period before assessment
At reassessment refers to the previous 3 month period

2. Treatment need rating score

Scores on each domain are based upon the interviewer's and client's rating of treatment need. This refers to the patient's need for continued or additional treatment at the time of assessment. Refers to the need for treatment with a specialist drug agency or, in addition, a mental health team (in the case of mental health) or a medical service (in the case of physical health).

0	No treatment need:	No further treatment required.
1	Limited need:	Further treatment desirable but not essential.
2	Moderate need:	Needs further ongoing intensive treatment, in-patient admission or residential rehabilitation.
3	Serious need:	Needs ongoing intensive treatment, in-patient admission or residential rehabilitation.

Appendix 5. Np-SAD

Reporting Form

NOTIFICATION OF DRUG RELATED DEATH

Section 1. Demographic Information

Deceased Forename(s) _____ Gender: Male   Female

Family Name _____

Known Aliases: _____

Date of Birth _____/_____/_____   Place of Birth _____

Usual Address _____

Postcode

Ethnicity (tick one):

British	Pakistani
Irish	Bangladeshi
Any other White background	Any other Asian background
White and Black Caribbean	Caribbean
White and Black African	African
White and Asian	Any other Black background
Any other mixed background	Chinese
Indian	Any other*

*Specify _____

Occupational Status (tick one):

Employed (manual)	Unemployed	Retired	Student
Employed (non-manual)	Childcare/Houseperson	Not known	Self-employed
Invalidity/sick	Other, specify _____		

Living Arrangements (tick one):

Alone	Self & children	No fixed abode
With partner	With parent(s)	Not known
Partner & children	With friend(s)	Other, specify _____

Section II. Circumstances of Death

Date of death _____/_____/_____   Place of death: _____

Was the deceased on prescribed medication?   Yes   No/Not known
If yes, please list drugs: 1. _____ 2. _____ 3. _____
4. _____ 5. _____

Was the deceased a drug addict or known drug abuser?
Yes   No   Not known
Please list drugs present at post mortem (including alcohol) which were implicated in the death:
1. _____ 2. _____ 3. _____
4. _____ 5. _____

Section III. Causes of Death

_____
1(a) _____
1(b) _____
2. _____
Coroner's Verdict (if verdict is accident or misadventure, please <u>also</u> complete
Section IV) _____

Section IV. Accidental Deaths and Misadventure

Place where accident occurred (tick one only):
☐ Home   ☐ Mine or quarry   ☐ Residential institution
☐ Farm   ☐ Street or highway   ☐ Place of recreation/sport
☐ Industrial place   ☐ Educational institution   ☐ Other specified place
Details of accident:

_____
_____
_____

Section V. Any other relevant information

Section VI. Coroner's Details

Coroner's Name: _____ Date of Inquest: _____/_____/_____
Jurisdiction: _____ Office: _____
Signature: _____ Date: _____/_____/_____

Appendix 6. Narcotics Anonymous

The Twelve Steps

1. We admitted that we were powerless over our addiction, that our lives had become unmanageable.
2. We came to believe that a Power greater than ourselves could restore us to sanity.
3. We made a decision to turn our will and our lives over to the care of God *as we understood God*.
4. We made a searching and fearless moral inventory of ourselves.
5. We admitted to God, to ourselves, and to another human being the exact nature or our wrongs.
6. We were entirely ready to have God remove all these defects of character.
7. We humbly asked God to remove our shortcomings.
8. We made a list of all persons we had harmed, and became willing to make amends to them all.
9. We made direct amends to such people wherever possible, except when to do so would injure them or others.
10. We continued to take personal inventory and when we were wrong promptly admitted it.
11. We sought through prayer and meditation to improve our conscious contact with God *as we understood God*, praying only for knowledge of God's will for us and the power to carry that out.
12. Having had a spiritual awakening as a result of these steps, we tried to carry this message to addicts, and to practice these principles in all our affairs.

The Twelve Traditions

We keep what we have only with vigilance, and just as freedom for the individual comes from the Twelve Steps, so freedom for the group springs from our Traditions. As long as the ties that bind us together are stronger than those that would tear us apart, all will be well.

1. Our common welfare should come first: personal recovery depends on NA unity.
2. For our group purposes there is but one ultimate authority – a loving God as He may

457

express Himself in our group conscience. Our leaders are but trusted servants, they do not govern.

3. The only requirement for membership is a desire to stop using.

4. Each group should be autonomous except in matters affecting other groups or NA as a whole.

5. Each group has but one primary purpose – to carry the message to the addict who still suffers.

6. An NA group ought never to endorse, finance, or lend the NA name to any related facility or outside enterprise, lest problems of money, property or prestige divert us from our primary purpose.

7. Every NA group ought to be fully self-supporting, declining outside contributions.

8. Narcotics Anonymous should remain forever non-professional, but our service centres may employ special workers.

9. NA, as such, ought never be organized, but we may create service boards or committees directly responsible to those they serve.

10. Narcotics Anonymous has no opinion on outside issues; hence the NA name ought never be drawn into public controversy.

11. Our public relations policy is based on attraction rather than promotion: we need always maintain personal anonymity at the level of press, radio and films.

12. Anonymity is the spiritual foundation of all our Traditions, ever reminding us to place principles before personalities.

The Twelve Steps of Alcoholics Anonymous

1. We admitted we were powerless over alcohol – that our lives had become unmanageable.

2. Came to believe that a Power greater than ourselves could restore us to sanity.

3. Made a decision to turn our will and our lives over to the care of God *as we understood Him.*

4. Made a searching and fearless moral inventory of ourselves.

5. Admitted to God, to ourselves, and to another human being the exact nature of our wrongs.

6. Were entirely ready to have God remove all the defects of character.

7. Humbly asked Him to remove our shortcomings.

8. Made a list of all persons we had harmed, and became willing to make amends to them all.

9. Made direct amends to such people wherever possible, except when to do so would injure them or others.

10. Continued to take personal inventory and when we were wrong promptly admitted it.

11. Sought through prayer and meditation to improve our conscious contact with God *as we understood Him,* praying only for knowledge of His will for us and the power to carry that out.

12. Having had a spiritual awakening as the result of these steps, we tried to carry this message to alcoholics, and to practice these principles in all our affairs.

Reprinted and adapted with permission of AA World Services, Inc.

Appendix 7. Opiate withdrawal

Opiate Withdrawal Symptom Questionnaire

Patient's name: _____ Patient study no. [   ]

Please rate the absence or presence of the following symptoms over the past 24 hours using the following scale at approximately the same time each day.

Scale   0= none/not at all   1= slightly/little/occasionally
            2= moderately   3= very much/a great deal/continuously

Over the last 24 hours to   Enter date [   ]
what extent have you: Enter time [am/pm   ]

1	Been yawning		10	Felt sick	
2	Had muscle cramp		11	Had stomach cramps	
3	Had pounding heart		12	Had difficulty sleeping	
4	Had a runny nose		13	Felt aches in bones or muscles	
5	Been sneezing		14	Felt twitching and shaking	
6	Experienced pins and needles		15	Felt irritable/bad tempered	
7	Had hot/cold flushes		16	Been sweating	
8	Had diarrhoea		17	Had runny eyes	
9	Had gooseflesh		18	Felt craving *Total score* (leave blank)	

Appendix 8. Opiate Withdrawal Scoring Sheet

Patient's name: _____ Patient study no. |_____|

Before each dose of opiate please complete a set of observations, filling in the results below. At the same time give patient a symptom questionnaire to fill in.

Date and time of admission _____

	Date								
	Time (24 hour)								
*Signs**									
1	Yawning								
2	Lacrimation								
3	Rhinorrhoea								
4	Perspiration								
5	Tremor								
6	Piloerection								
7	Restlessness								
8	Pupil size (mm)								
9	Anorexia								
10	Vomiting								
11	Diarrhoea								
12	Insomnia								
13	Drug seeking								

continued overleaf

Date									
Time (24 hour)									
Observations†									
Temperature									
Respiration rate									
Pulse									
Blood pressure									
Weight									
Drugs									
Dose of opiates									
Other treatments									
Adverse effects									
Comments									
Other investigations									

* Signs 1–13 should be determined as either: present =2; not sure =1; or absent =0.

† Observations (+sign 8): record actual measurements.

Appendix 9. Attendance Record

Name: Key worker: Doctor:

Date							
Seen by							
Reason for attendance*							
Drug use in past 24 hours							
Clinical state:							
Intoxicated†	sedated						
	elated						
Sober							
Withdrawing†	opiate						
	sedative						
Urine result lab no.							
Amphetamine							
Barbiturate							
Benzodiazepine							
Cannabis							
Codeine							
Cocaine							
Methadone							
Morphine							
Other							

*e.g. follow-up (f/u): daily attendance (d/a); assessment, blood test; special visit.

†Score: +, ++, +++.

Note: This record is to be maintained at *every* attendance. To be completed by member of team who formally sees the patient: key worker, doctor, clinic nurse, social worker, etc.

References and further reading

Introduction: further reading

Advisory Committee on Drug Dependence (1968). *Cannabis. The Wootton Report.* London: HMSO.

Austin GA (1978). *Perspective on the History of Psychoactive Substance Use.* Rockville, MD: National Institute of Drug Abuse.

Bayer I & Ghodse AH (1999). Evolution of International drug control 1945–1995. *Bulletin on Narcotics,* **LI,** nos 1 and 2.

Berridge V & Edwards G (1987). *Opium and the People: Opiate Use in Nineteenth Century England.* New Haven, CT: Yale University Press.

Bucknell P & Ghodse AH (1996). *Misuse of Drugs,* 3rd edn. London: Sweet and Maxwell.

Department of Health (1999). *Drug Misuse and Dependence: Guidelines on Clinical Management.* London: The Stationery Office.

Edwards G & Busch C (eds) (1981). *Drug Problems in Britain: A Review of Ten Years.* London: Academic Press.

Edwards G, Marshall EJ & Cook CCH (1997) *The Treatment of Drinking Problems.* Cambridge: Cambridge University Press.

Ghodse AH & Maxwell D (eds.) (1990). *Substance Abuse and Dependence: An Introduction for the Caring Professions.* London: Macmillan Press.

Ghodse AH & Kreek M-J (eds.) (1998). Substance misuse. *Current Opinion in Psychiatry,* **11,** 245–93.

Ghodse AH (ed.) (1999). Substance misuse. *Current Opinion in Psychiatry,* **12,** 265–310.

Ghodse AH & Ricaurte GA (eds.) (2000). Substance misuse. *Current Opinion in Psychiatry,* **13,** 281–3.

Ghodse AH & Ricaurte GA (eds.) (2001). Substance misuse. *Current Opinion in Psychiatry,* **14,** 163–211.

Jaffe J, Petersen R & Hodgson R (1980). *Addiction Issues and Answers.* London: Harper & Row.

Murray R, Ghodse AH, Harris C, Williams D & Williams P (eds.) (1981). *The Misuse of Psychotropic Drugs.* London: Gaskell, Royal College of Psychiatrists.

Orford J (1985). *Excessive Appetites: A Psychological View of Addiction.* Chichester: Wiley.

Platt JJ (1986). *Heroin Addiction: Theory, Research and Treatment,* 2nd edn. Malabar: Robert E. Krieger.

Royal College of Psychiatrists (1987). *Drug Scenes.* London: Gaskell.

Royal College of Psychiatrists and Royal College of Physicians (2000). *Drugs Dilemmas and Choices.* London: Gaskell.

Royal College of Psychiatrists (2000). Joint Report of the Royal College of Psychiatrists, the Royal College of General Practitioners and Association of Police Surgeons. *Substance Misuse Detainees in Police Custody: Guidelines for Clinical Management.* London: Royal College of Psychiatrists.

World Health Organization (1993). *WHO Expert Committee on Drug Dependence. Twenty-Eighth Report.* (Technical report series 836.) Geneva: WHO.

World Health Organization (1998). *WHO Expert Committee on Drug Dependence. Thirtieth Report.* (Technical report series 873). Geneva: WHO.

Chapter 1

1. World Health Organization (1969). *WHO Expert Committee on Drug Dependence. Sixteenth Report.* (Technical report series 407.) Geneva: WHO.

2. World Health Organization (1994). *Lexicon of Alcohol and Drug Terms.* Geneva: WHO.

3. World Health Organization (1993). *WHO Expert Committee on Drug Dependence. Twenty-eighth Report.* (Technical report series 836). Geneva: WHO.

4. World Health Organization (1992). *The ICD-10 Classification of Mental and Behavioural Disorders. Clinical Descriptions and Diagnostic Guidelines.* Geneva: WHO.

5. Eddy NB, Halbach H, Isbell H & Seevers MH (1965). Drug dependence: its significance and characteristics. *Bulletin of the World Health Organization*, **32**, 723.

6. O'Brien CP (1996). Drug addiction and drug abuse. In *Goodman and Gilman's The Pharmacological Basis of Therapeutics*, 9th edn, ed. JG Hardman and LE Limbird. New York: McGraw-Hill.

7. Murray RM (1973). Dependence on analgesics in analgesic nephropathy. *British Journal of Addiction*, **68**, 265–72.

8. Marrow, LP, Overton PG, Brain PF & Clark D (1999). Encounters with aggressive con-specifics enhance the locomotor activating effect of cocaine in the rat. *Addiction Biology*, **4**, 437–41.

9. Miczek KA & Mutschler NH (1996). Activational effects of social stress on IV cocaine self-administration. *Psychopharmacology*, **128**, 256–64.

10. Koob GF (1992). Neural mechanisms of drug reinforcement. *Annals of the New York Academy of Science*, **654**, 171–91.

11. Nutt DJ (1993). Neurochemistry of drugs other than alcohol. *Current Opinion in Psychiatry*, **3**, 395–402.

12. Sudbury P & Ghodse AH (1991). Substance abuse and antisocial behaviour. *Current Opinion in Psychiatry*, **4**, 440–7.

13. Ghodse AH (1995). Substance misuse and personality disorders. *Current Opinion in Psychiatry*, **8**, 177–9.

14. Oyefeso A (1995). Psychological, social and behavioural correlates of substance use and misuse. *Current Opinion in Psychiatry*, **8**, 184–8.

15. Preble E & Casey JJ Jr (1969). Taking care of business: the heroin user's life on the street. *The International Journal of the Addictions*, **4**, 1–24.

16. Wieder H & Kaplan E (1969). Drug use in adolescents. In *The Psychoanalytic Study of the Child*, vol. 24, ed. A. Freud, et al., pp. 399–431. London: Hogarth Press.

17. Fischman VS (1968). Stimulant users in the Californian Rehabilitation Center. *International Journal of the Addictions*, **3**, 113–30.

18. Shedler J & Block J (1990). Adolescent drug use and psychological health: a longitudinal inquiry. *American Psychologist*, **45**, 612–30.

19. Boys A, Marsden J, Fountain J, Griffiths P, Stillwell G & Strang J (1999). What influences young people's use of drugs? A qualitative study of decision making. *Drugs: Education, Prevention and Policy*, **6**, 373–87.

20. Andrados J-LR (1995). The influence of family, school and peers on adolescent drug misuse. *The International Journal of the Addictions*, **30**, 1407–23.

21. Plant M & Plant M (1992). *Risk-Takers. Alcohol Drugs Sex and Youth*. London: Tavistock/Routledge.

22. Carvalho V, Pinsky I, De Souza e Silva R, et al. (1995). Drug and alcohol use and family characteristics: a study among Brazilian high school students. *Addiction*, **90**, 65–72.

23. Kandel D, Yamaguchi K & Chen K (1992). Stages of progression in drug involvement from adolescence to adulthood: further evidence for the gateway theory. *Journal of Studies on Alcohol*, **53**, 447–57.

24. Sloboda Z, Baker O, Mounteney J & Neaman R (eds) (1998). *State of the Art of Prevention Research in the United States. Evaluating Drug Dependence in the European Union*, pp. 31–44. Luxembourg: Office for Official Publications of the European Communities.

25. Brook JS, Balka EB & Whiteman M (1999). The risks for late adolescence of early adolescence marijuana use. *American Journal of Public Health*, **89**, 1549–54.

26. Schuckit MA (1992). Advances in understanding the vulnerability to alcoholism. In *Addictive States*, ed. CP O'Brien & J Jaffe. New York: Raven Press.

27. Heath AC, Whitfield PAF, Madden KK, et al. (2001). Towards a molecular epidemiology of alcohol dependence: analysing the interplay of genetic and environmental risk factors. *British Journal of Psychiatry*, **178** (Suppl. 40), S33–S40.

28. Nutt DJ (1993).Neurochemistry of drugs other than alcohol. *Current Opinion in Psychiatry*, **3**, 395–402.

29. Goldstein A. (1991). Heroin addiction: neurobiology, pharmacology and policy. *Journal of Psychoactive Drugs*, **23**, 123–33.

30. Merton RK (1957). *Social Theory and Social Structure*, rev.edn. New York: The Free Press of Glencoe.

31. Ghodse AH (1977). Casualty departments and the monitoring of drug dependence. *British Medical Journal*, **i**, 1381–2.

Chapter 2

1. Berridge V (1979). Morality and medical science: concepts of narcotic addiction in Britain, 1820–1926. *Annals of Science*, **36**, 67.

2. Anderson S & Berridge V (2000). Opium in twentieth-century Britain: pharmacists, regulation and people. *Addiction*, **95**, 23–36.

3. Spear HB (1969). The growth of heroin addiction in the United Kingdom. *British Journal of Addiction*, **64**, 245–56.

4. Departmental Committee (1926). *Report of the Departmental Committee on Drug Dependence.* (Rolleston Committee.) London: HMSO.

5. Ministry of Health and Department of Health for Scotland (1961). *Drug Addiction: Report of the Interdepartmental Committee.* London: HMSO.

6. Frankau IM & Stanwell PM (1961). The treatment of heroin addiction. *Lancet*, **i**, 1377–8.

7. Spear HB & Glatt MM (1971). The influence of Canadian addicts on heroin addiction in the United Kingdom. *British Journal of Addiction*, **66**, 141–9.

8. Zacune J (1971). A comparison of Canadian narcotic addicts in Great Britain and Canada. *Bulletin on Narcotics*, **23**, 41.

9. Ministry of Health and Department of Health for Scotland (1965). *Drug Addiction: The Second Report of the Interdepartmental Committee.* London: HMSO.

10. Home Office. *Statistics on the Misuse of Drugs in the United Kingdom.* London: Home Office (published annually).

11. Miller PM & Plant M (1996). Drinking smoking and illicit drug use among 15 and 16 year olds in the United Kingdom. *British Medical Journal*, **313**, 394–7.

12. Webb E, Ashton CH, Kelly PH, et al. (1996). Alcohol and drug use in UK university students. *Lancet*, **348**, 922–5.

13. Williams P (1981). Trends in the prescribing of psychotropic drugs. In *The Misuse of Psychotropic Drugs*, ed. R Murray, H Ghodse, C Harris, D Williams & P Williams. London: Gaskell, Royal College of Psychiatrists.

14. Das Gupta S (1990). Identifying the problem. In *Substance Abuse and Dependence*, ed. Ghodse AH & Maxwell D, pp. 53–79. London: Macmillan Press.

15. Connell PH (1958). *Amphetamine Psychosis.* (Maudsley monograph 5.) London: Oxford University Press.

16. Hawks D, Mitcheson M, Ogborne A & Edwards G (1969). Abuse of methylamphetamine. *British Medical Journal*, **ii**, 715–21.

17. Ghodse AH, Sheehan M, Taylor C & Edwards G (1985). Death of drug addicts in the United Kingdom 1967–1981. *British Medical Journal*, **290**, 425–8.

18. Lewis R, Hartnoll R, Bryer S, Daviaud E & Mitcheson M (1985). Scoring smack: the illicit heroin market in London 1980–1983. *British Journal of Addiction*, **80**, 281–90.

19. Power R (1994). Drug trends since 1968. In *Heroin Addiction and Drug Policy*, ed. J Strang & M Gossop; pp. 29–39. Oxford: Oxford University Press.

20. Advisory Council on the Misuse of Drugs (1982). *Treatment and Rehabilitation.* London: HMSO.

21. Department of Health, The Scottish Office Department of Health, Welsh Office, Department of Health and Social Services, Northern Ireland (1991). *Drug Misuse and Dependence: Guidelines on Clinical Management.* London: HMSO.

22. Department of Health, The Scottish Office Department of Health, Welsh Office, Department of Health and Social Services, Northern Ireland (1999). *Drug Misuse and Dependence: Guidelines on Clinical Management.* London: HMSO.

23. *Tackling Drugs Together: A Strategy for England 1995–98* (1995). London: HMSO.

24. Cabinet Office (1998). *Tackling Drugs to Build a Better Britain: The Government's 10-Year Strategy for Tackling Drug Misuse.* London: The Stationery Office.

25. Department of Health, The Scottish Office Home and Health Department and Welsh Office (1994). *Substance Misuse Detainees in Police Custody. Guidelines for Clinical Management. Report of a Medical Working Group.* London: HMSO.

26. Royal College of Psychiatrists and Association of Police Surgeons (2000). *Substance Misuse Detainees in Police Custody: Guidelines for Clinical Management,* 2nd ed. *Report of a Medical Working Group.* (Council report CR81). London: Royal College of Psychiatrists.

27. Center on Addiction and Substance Abuse at Columbia University (CASA) (1995). Legalisation: Panacea or Pandora's Box. (White paper 1.) New York: CASA.

28. Abou-Saleh MT & Miller J (1999). The management of drug misuse in primary care. *Primary Care Psychiatry,* **5**(2), 49–56.

29. Glanz A & Taylor C (1986). Findings of a national survey of the role of general practitioners in the treatment of opiate misuse: extent of contact. *British Medical Journal,* **293**, 427–30.

30. Glanz A (1994). The fall and rise of the general practitioner. In *Heroin Addiction and Drug Policy,* ed. J Strang & M Gossop, pp. 151–66. Oxford: Oxford University Press.

31. Edmunds M, May T, Hearnden I, et al. (1998). *Arrest Referral: Emerging Lessons from Research.* London: The Stationery Office.

32. Cabinet Office (2000). *The United Kingdom Anti-Drug Co-ordinator's Annual Report 1999/ 2000.* London: Cabinet Office.

33. Singleton N, Meltzer H, Gatward R, Coid J & Deasy D (1998). *Psychiatric Morbidity Among Prisoners in England and Wales.* London: Office for National Statistics.

34. Thomson LDG (2000). Substance abuse and criminality. *Current Opinion in Psychiatry,* **12**, 653–7.

35. HM Prison Service (1998). *Tackling Drugs in Prison: The Prison Service Drug Strategy.* London: HM Prison Service.

36. Home Office (2000). *Statistical Bulletin: Drug Seizure and Offender Statistics. United Kingdom, 1998.* London: Home Office Research and Statistics Directorate.

37. Parker H & Bottomley T (1996). *Crack-Cocaine and Drugs-Crime Careers.* London: Home Office Publications Unit.

38. Bennett T (1998). *Drugs and Crime: The Results of Research on Drug Testing and Interviewing Arrestees.* (Home Office research study 183). London: Home Office Research and Statistics Directorate.

39. Bennett T (2000). *Drugs and Crime: The Results of the Second Developmental Stage of the NEW-ADAM Programme* (Home Office research study 205). London: Home Office Research and Statistics Directorate.

40. Department of Health Statistical Division 1E, Prescription Cost Analysis System.

41. Corkery JM (1997). *Statistics of Drug Addicts Notified to the Home Office, United Kingdom 1996.* (Home Office statistical bulletin 22/1997.) London: Governmental Statistical Service.

42. Department of Health Statistical Bulletin (2000/30). *Statistics from the Regional Drug Misuse Databases for Six Months ending March 2000.* London: Department of Health.

43. Ghodse H, Oyefeso A & Kilpatrick B (1998). Mortality of drug addicts in the United Kingdom 1967–1993. *International Journal of Epidemiology,* **27**, 473–8.

44. Advisory Council on the Misuse of Drugs (2000). *Reducing Drug-Related Deaths.* London: Advisory Council on the Misuse of Drugs.

45. Ghodse AH, Sheehan M, Stevens, Taylor C & Edwards G (1978). Mortality among addicts in Greater London. *British Medical Journal*, **ii**, 1742–4.

46. Oyefeso A, Ghodse H, Clancy C & Corkery JM (1999). Suicide among drug addicts in the UK. *British Journal of Psychiatry*, **175**, 277–82.

47. ONS (2000). Drug-related deaths database: first results for England and Wales 1993–97. *Health Statistics Quarterly*, **5**, 57–60.

48. Taylor JC. Field Smith ME, Norman CL, et al. (2000). *Trends in Deaths Associated with Abuse of Volatile Solvents 1971–1998*. London: Department of Public Health Sciences and the Toxicology Unit Department of Cardiological Sciences, St George's Hospital Medical School.

49. Ghodse H, Oyefeso A, Hunt M, et al. (2001). *Drug-related Deaths as reported by Coroners in England and Wales*. (Annual review 2000 and np-SAD surveillance report 7.) London: Centre for Addiction Studies, St George's Hospital Medical School.

50. Ramsay M & Partridge S (1999). *Drug Misuse Declared in 1998: Results from the British Crime Survey*. (Home Office research study 197.) London: Research Development and Statistics Directorate.

51. Health Education Authority (1996). *Drug Realities: National Drugs Campaign Survey: Summary of Key Findings*. London: Health Education Authority.

52. McKeganey N & Norrie J (1999). Pre-teen drug misuse in Scotland. *Addiction Research*, **7**, 371–5.

53. Aldridge J, Parker H & Measham F (1999). *Drug Trying and Drug Use Across Adolescence: A Longitudinal Study of Young People's Drug Taking in Two Regions of Northern England*. (DPAS paper 1.) London: Home Office Drugs Prevention Advisory Service.

54. Flood-Page C, Campbell S, Harrington V & Miller J (2000). *Youth Crime Findings from the 1998/99 Youth Lifestyles Survey*. (Home Office research study 209.) London: Home Office Research Development and Statistics Directorate.

55. Office of Applied Studies (2000). *Drug Abuse Warning Network: Annual Medical Examiner Data, 1998*. Washington, DC: Department of Health and Human Services.

56. Ghodse AH, Stapleton J, Edwards G, Bewley T & A-Samarrai M (1986). A comparison of drug-related problems in London accident and emergency departments, 1975–1982. *British Journal of Psychiatry*, **148**, 658–62.

57. Cabinet Office (2000). *The United Kingdom Anti-Drug Co-ordinator's Second National Plan*. London: Cabinet Office.

58. Idanpaan-Heikkila J, Ghodse AH & Khan I (eds.) (1987). *Psychoactive Drugs and Health Problems*. Helsinki: National Board of Health.

59. PHLS and SCIEH (2000). *AIDS/HIV Quarterly Surveillance Tables: UK Data to end June 2000*. (No. 47;00/2.) London: Public Health Laboratory Service AIDS Centre and the Scottish Centre for Infection and Environmental Health.

60. European Monitoring Centre for Drugs and Drug Addiction (1999). *Annual Report on the State of the Drugs Problem in the European Union*. Luxembourg: Office for the Official Publications of the European Communities.

61. Kaplan CD (1992). What works in drug abuse epidemiology in Europe. *Journal of Addictive Disease*, **11**, 47–59.

62. International Narcotics Control Board (INCB) (2001). *Narcotic Drugs: Estimated World Requirements for 2001; Statistics for 1999.* New York: United Nations Publications. (Sales no. E/F/S.01.XI.2.)

63. INCB (2000). *Report of the INCB for 1999.* New York: United Nations Publications.

64. INCB (2001). *Report of the INCB for 2000.* New York: United Nations Publications.

65. INCB (2001). *Psychotropic Substances Statistics for 1999. Assessment of Medical and Scientific Requirements for Substances in Schedule, II, III & IV.* New York: United Nations Publications.

66. INCB (2002). *A Report of INCB for 2001.* New York: United Nations Publications.

67. United Nations (2000). *World Drug Report 2000.* New York: Oxford University Press.

68. United Nations (2000). *Global Illicit Drug Trends 2000.* ODCCP Studies on Drugs and Crime Statistics. New York: United Nations Publications.

69. United Nations (2001). *Global Illicit Drug Trends 2001.* ODCCP Studies on Drugs and Crime Statistics. New York: United Nations Publications.

Chapter 3

1. Reisine T & Pasternak G (1996). Opioid analgesics and antagonists. In *Goodman and Gilman's The Pharmacological Basis of Therapeutics*, 9th edn, ed. JG Hardman & LE Limbird, pp. 521–55. New York: McGraw-Hill.

2. Tucker C (1990). Acute pain and substance abuse in surgical patients. *Journal of Neuroscience Nursing*, **22**, 339–50.

3. Gold MS & Johnson CR (1998). Psychological and psychiatric consequences of opiates. In *Handbook of Substance Abuse. Neurobehavioural Pharmacology*, ed. RE Tarter, RT Ammerman & PJ Ott, pp. 363–77. New York: Plenum.

4. Pert CB & Snyder SH (1973). Opiates receptor: demonstration in nervous tissue. *Science*, **179**, 1011–14.

5. Pasternak GW (1993). Pharmacological mechanisms of opioid analgesics. *Clinical Neuropharmacology*, **16**, 1–18.

6. Jaffe JH & Martin WR (1991). Opioid analgesics and antagonists. In *Goodman and Gilman's The Pharmacological Basis of Therapeutics*, 8th edn, ed. AG Gilman, et al. New York: Pergamon.

7. Goldstein A (1983). Some thoughts about endogenous opioids and addiction. *Drug and Alcohol Dependence*, **11**, 11–14.

8. Childers SR (1991). Minireview: opioid receptor-coupled second messenger systems. *Life Science*, **48**, 1991–2003.

9. Randall T (1993). Morphine receptor cloned: improved analgesics, addiction therapy expected. *JAMA*, **270**, 1165–6.

10. Glanz M, Klawansky S, McAullife W & Chalmers T (1997). Methadone vs L-alpha-acetylmethadol (LAAM) in the treatment of opiate addiction. A meta-analysis of the randomized controlled trials. *American Journal of Addiction*, **6**, 339–49.

11. Madden S (1990). Effects of drugs of dependence. In *Substance Abuse and Dependence*, ed. AH Ghodse & D Maxwell, pp. 30–52. London: Macmillan Press.

12. Jasinski D, Fudala PJ & Johnson RE (1989). Sublingual versus subcutaneous buprenorphine in opiate abusers. *Clinical Pharmacology and Therapeutics*, **45**, 513–19.

13. Walsh SL, Preston KL, Stitzer ML, Cone EJ & Bigelow GE (1994). Clinical pharmacology of buprenorphine: ceiling effect of high doses. *Clinical Pharmacology and Therapeutics*, **55**, 569–80.

14. Johnson RE, Jaffe JH, Fudala PJ (1992). A controlled trial of buprenorphine treatment for opioid dependence. *JAMA*, **267**, 2750–5.

15. King MB, Gabe J, Williams P & Rodrigo EK (1990). Long term use of benzodiazepines: the views of patients. *British Journal of General Practice*, **40**, 194–6.

16. Lader M (1983). Dependence on benzodiazepines. *Journal of Clinical Psychiatry*, **44**, 121–7.

17. Pétursson H & Lader M (1984). *Dependence on Tranquillizers*. New York: Oxford University Press.

18. Pétursson H (1994). The benzodiazepine withdrawal syndrome. *Addiction*, **89**, 1455–9.

19. Woods JH, Katz JL & Winger G (1992). Benzodiazepines: use, abuse, and consequences. *Pharmacological Reviews*, **44**, 151–347.

20. Juergens SM (1993). Benzodiazepines and addiction. *Psychiatric Clinics of North America*, **16**, 75–86.

21. Rush CR, Hayes CA & Higgins ST (1998). Behavioral pharmacology of sedatives, hypnotics, and anxiolytics. In *Handbook of Substance Abuse. Neurobehavioural Pharmacology*, ed. RE Tarter, RT Ammerman & PJ Ott, pp. 435–70. New York: Plenum.

22. Dåderman AM & Lidberg L (1999). Flunitrazepam (Rohypnol) abuse in combination with alcohol causes premeditated grievous violence in male juvenile offenders. *Journal of American Academy of Psychiatry and Law*, **27**, 83–9.

23. Saum CA & Inciardi JA (1997). Rohypnol misuse in United States. *Substance Use and Misuse*, **32**, 723–31.

24. Anglin D, Spears KL & Hutson HR (1997). Flunitrazepam and its involvement in date or acquaintance rape. *Academy of Emergency Medicine*, **4**, 323–6.

25. Gallager DW & Primus RJ (1993). Benzodiazepine tolerance and dependence: $GABA_A$ receptor complex locus of change. In *Neurochemistry of Drug Dependence*, ed. S Wonnacott & G Glunt, pp. 135–51. London: Portland.

26. Hobbs WR, Rall, TW & Verdoorn TA (1996). Hypnotics and sedatives: ethanol. In *Goodman and Gilman's The Pharmacological Basis of Therapeutics*, 9th edn, ed. JG Hardman & LE Limbird. New York: McGraw-Hill.

27. Wilens TE & Biederman J (1992). The stimulants. *Psychiatric Clinics of North America*, **15**, 191–222.

28. King GR & Ellingwood EH (1992). Amphetamines and other stimulants. In *Substance Abuse: A Comprehensive Textbook*, 2nd edn, ed. JH Lowinson, P Ruiz, RD Millman & JG Langrod, pp. 247–70. Baltimore, MD: Williams & Wilkins.

29. Jaffe JH (1991). Drug addiction and drug abuse. In *Goodman and Gilman's The Pharmacological Basis of Therapeutics*, 8th edn, ed. AG Gilman et al. New York: Pergamon.

30. Gawin FH, Khalsa ME & Ellingwood E (1994). Stimulants. In *Textbook of Substance Abuse Treatment*, ed. M Galanter & HD Kleber, pp. 111–39. Washington, DC: American Psychiatric Press.

31. Ghodse AH (1999). Dramatic increase in methylphenidate consumption. *Current Opinion in Psychiatry*, **12**, 265–8.

32. Ghodse AN & Kreek M-J (1998). Resurgence of abuse of amphetamine-type stimulants. *Current Opinion in Psychiatry*, **11**, 245–7.

33. National Institute for Clinical Excellence (NICE) (2000). *Guidance on the Use of Methylphenidate for ADHD in Childhood.* (Technology appraisal guidance 13.) London: NICE, www.nice.org.uk

34. Van Dyke C & Byck R (1983). Cocaine use in man. In *Advances in Substance Abuse*, vol 3, ed. NK Mello, pp. 1–24. Greenwich, CT: JAI Press.

35. Grinspoon L & Bakalar JB (1981). Coca and cocaine as medicines: a historical review. *Journal of Ethnopharmacology*, **3**, 149–59.

36. Middleton RM & Kirkpatrick MB (1993). Clinical use of cocaine: a review of the risks and benefits. *Drug Safety*, **9**, 212–17.

37. McEvoy AW, Kitchen ND & Thomas DGT (2000). Intracerebral haemorrhage in young adults: the emerging importance of drug misuse. *British Medical Journal*, **320**, 1322–4.

38. Schifano F (1996). Cocaine misuse and dependence. *Current Opinion in Psychiatry*, **9**, 225–30.

39. Gawin FH & Ellingwood EH (1990). Consequences and correlates of cocaine abuse: clinical phenomenology. In *Cocaine and the Brain*, ed. ND Volkow & AC Swan, pp. 155–78. New Brunswick, NJ: Rutgers University Press.

40. Margolin A, Avants SK & Kosten TR (1996). Abstinence symptomatology associated with cessation of chronic cocaine abuse among methadone-maintained patients. *American Journal of Drug and Alcohol Abuse*, **22**, 377–88.

41. Grabowski J (ed.) (1984). *Cocaine: Pharmacology, Effects and Treatment Abuse.* (NIDA research monograph.) Rockville, MD: Department of Health & Human Services.

42. Johanson C-E, Balster RL & Bonese K (1976). Self-administration of psychomotor stimulant drugs: the effects of unlimited access. *Pharmacology, Biochemistry & Behaviour*, **4**, 45–51.

43. Mitchell J & Vierkant AD (1991). Delusions and hallucinations of cocaine abusers and paranoid schizophrenics: a comparative study. *Journal of Psychology*, **125**, 301–10.

44. Satel SL, Southwick SM & Gawin FH (1991). Clinical features of cocaine-induced paranoia. *American Journal of Psychiatry*, **148**, 495–8.

45. Serper MR, Chou JC, Allen MH, Czobor P & Cancro R (1999). Symptomatic overlap of cocaine intoxication and acute schizophrenia at emergency presentation. *Schizophrenic Bulletin*, **25**, 387–94.

46. Kennedy J, Teague J, Rrokaw W & Cooney E (1983). A medical evaluation of the use of qat in North Yemen. *Social Science and Medicine*, **17**, 783–93.

47. Alem A, Kebede D & Kullgren G (1999). The prevalence and socio-demographic correlates of khat chewing in Butajira, Ethiopia. *Acta Psychiatrica Scandinavica (Suppl)*, **100**, 84–91.

48. Alem A & Shibbe T (1997). Khat induced psychosis and its medico-legal implication: a case report. *Ethiopian Medical Journal*, **35**, 137–41.

49. Getahun A & Krikorian AD (1983). The economic and social importance of khat and

suggested research and services. In *Proceedings of the International Conference on Khat*, January 17–21, Antannarivo, Madagascar.

50. Kalix P (1987). Khat: scientific knowledge and policy issues. *British Journal of Addiction*, **82**, 47–53.

51. Kalix P (1990). Pharmacological properties of the stimulant khat. *Pharmacology & Therapeutics*, **48**, 397–416.

52. Griffiths P, Gossop M, Wickenden S, Dunworth J, Harris K & Lloyd C (1997). A transcultural pattern of drug use: qat (khat) in the UK. *British Journal of Psychiatry*, **170**, 282–4.

53. Strassman RJ (1984). Adverse reactions to psychedelic drugs: a review of the literature. *Journal of Nervous and Mental Disease*, **171**, 577–95.

54. Glennon RA (1994). Classical hallucinogens: an introductory overview. In *Hallucinogens: An Update*. (NIDA monograph series 146.) ed. GC Lin & RA Glennon, pp. 4–32. Washington, DC: US Department of Health and Human Services.

55. Seymour RB & Smith DE (1998). Psychological and psychiatric consequences of hallucinogens. In *Handbook of Substance Abuse. Neurobehavioural Pharmacology*, ed. RE Tarter, RT Ammerman & PJ Ott. pp. 241–51. New York: Plenum.

56. McKim WA (1997). *Drugs and Behavior: An Introduction to Behavioral Pharmacology*, 3rd edn. Upper Saddle River, NJ: Prentice-Hall.

57. Brecher M, Wang B-W, Wong H & Morgan JP (1988). Phencyclidine and violence: Clinical and legal isssues. *Journal of Clinical Psychopharmacology*, **8**, 397–401.

58. Ghodse AH (1986). Cannabis psychosis. *British Journal of Addiction*, **81**, 473–8.

59. Hawks RL (1982). The constituents of cannabis and the disposition and metabolism of cannabinoids. In *The Analysis of Cannabinoids in Biological Fluids*, ed. RL Hawks, pp. 125–37. (NIDA research monograph 42.) Rockville, MD: US Department of Health and Human Services.

60. Compton DR, Harris LS, Lichtman AH & Martin BR (1996). Marihuana. In *Pharmacological Aspects of Drug Dependence: Toward an Integrated Neurobehavioral Approach*, ed. CR Schuster & MJ Kuhar, pp. 83–158. Berlin: Springer-Verlag.

61. Hall W, Solowij N & Lemon J (1994). *The Health and Psychological Consequences of Cannabis Use*. (National drug strategy monograph series 25.) Canberra: Australian Government Publishing Service.

62. Shiloh R, Nutt D & Weizman A (1999). *Atlas of Psychiatric Pharmacotherapy*. London: Martin Dunitz.

63. Goldberg S, Munzar P & Tanda G (2000). *Nature Neuroscience*, **3**, 1073–4.

64. Chopra G & Smith J (1974). Psychotic reactions following cannabis use in East Indians. *Archives of General Psychiatry*, **30**, 24–7.

65. Johnson BA (1990). Psychopharmacological effects of cannabis. *British Journal of Hospital Medicine*, **43**, 114–22.

66. Chaudry HR, Moss HB, Bashir A & Suliman T (1991). Cannabis psychosis following bhang ingestion. *British Journal of Addiction*, **86**, 1075–81.

67. Linszen, DH, Dingemans PM & Lenior ME (1994). Cannabis abuse and the course of recent-onset schizophrenic disorders. *Archives of General Psychiatry*, **51**, 273–9.

68. Mathers DC, Ghodse AH, Cann AW & Scott SA (1991). Cannabis use in a large sample of acute psychiatric admissions. *British Journal of Addiction*, **86**, 779–84.

69. Mathers DC & Ghodse AH (1992). Cannabis and psychotic illness. *British Journal of Psychiatry*, **161**, 648–53.

70. Sudbury PR & Ghodse AH.(1990). Solvent misuse. *Current Opinion in Psychiatry*, **3**, 388–92.

71. Ramsey J, Taylor J, Anderson R, & Flanagan RJ (1995). Volatile substance abuse in the United Kingdom. In *Epidemiology of Inhalant Abuse: An International Perspective* (NIDA research monograph 148), ed. N Kozel, Z Sloboda & M De La Rosa, pp. 205–49. Rockville, MD: NIDA.

72. Rosenberg NL & Sharp CW (1992). Solvent toxicity: A neurological focus. In *Inhalant Abuse: A volatile research agenda* (NIDA research monograph 129), ed. CW Sharp, F Beauvas & R Spence, pp. 117–71. Rockville, MD: NIDA.

73. Siegel E & Wasson S (1990). Sudden death caused by inhalation of butane and propane. *New England Journal of Medicine*, **323**, 1638.

74. Evans EB (1998). Pharmacology of inhalants. In *Handbook of Substance Abuse. Neurobehavioral Pharmacology*, ed. RE Tarter, RT Ammerman & PJ Ott, pp. 255–62, New York: Plenum.

75. Ricaurte GA, McCann UD, Szabo Z & Scheffel U (2000). Toxicodynamics and long-term toxicity of the recreational drug, 3.4-methylenedioxymethamphetamine (MDMA, 'Ecstasy'). *Toxicology Letters*, **112–13**, 143–6.

76. Ghodse AH & Kreek M-J (1997). A rave of ecstasy. *Current Opinion in Psychiatry*, **10**, 191–3.

77. Solowij N (1993). Ecstasy C3, 4-methylenedioxymethamphetamine. *Current Opinion in Psychiatry*, **6**, 411–15.

78. Rochester JA & Kirchner JT (1999). Ecstasy (3,4-methylenedioxymethamphetamine): history, neurochemistry, and toxicology. *Journal of American Board of Family Practice*, **12**, 137–42.

79. United Nations International Drug Control Program (1996). *Amphetamine-Type Stimulants: A Global Review*. Vienna: UNDCP.

80. Bahrke MS, Yesalis CE & Brower KJ (1998). Anabolic-androgenic steroid abuse and performance-enhancing drugs among adolescents. *Child & Adolescent Psychiatric Clinics of North America*, **7**, 821–38.

81. Haupt HA & Rovere GD (1984). Anabolic steroids: a review of the literature. *American Journal of Sports Medicine*, **12**, 469–84.

82. Middleman AB & Du Rant RH (1996). Anabolic steroid use and associated health risk behaviours. *Sports Medicine*, **21**, 251–5.

83. Whelton A (1995). Renal effects of over-the-counter analgesics. *Journal of Clinical Pharmacology*, **35**, 454–63.

84. Ghodse AH (1994). Combined use of drugs and alcohol. *Current Opinion in Psychiatry*, **7**, 249–51.

85. Cami J, Bigelow GE, Griffiths RR & Drummond DC (eds.) (1991). Clinical testing of drug abuse liability. (Special issue.) *British Journal of Addiction*, **86**, 1525–652.

Chapter 4

1. Royal Colleges of Physicians, Psychiatrists and General Practitioners (1995). *Alcohol and the Heart in Perspective. Sensible Limits Reaffirmed. Report of a Joint Working Group.* London: Royal Colleges.

2. Department of Health (1995). *Sensible Drinking. The Report of an Inter-Departmental Working Group.* London: Department of Health.

3. Edwards G & Gross MM (1976). Alcohol dependence: provisional description of a clinical syndrome. *British Medical Journal*, i, 1058–61.

4. Drummond DC (2000). UK Government announces first major relaxation in the alcohol licensing laws for nearly a century. *Addiction*, **95**, 997–8.

5. Harkin AM, Anderson P & Goos C. (1997). Smoking, drinking and drug taking in the European Region. Alcohol, drugs and tobacco programme. Copenhagen: WHO Regional Office for Europe.

6. Harkin AM, Anderson P & Lehto J. (1995). Alcohol in Europe: a health perspective. Copenhagen: WHO Regional Office for Europe.

7. Office of National Statistics (1998). *Living in Britain: Results from the 1996 General Household Survey.* London: The Stationery Office.

8. Goddard E (1997). Young teenagers and alcohol in 1996, vol. 1, England. London: Office for National Statistics.

9. Mayfield D, McLeod G & Hall P (1974). The CAGE questionnaire: validation of a new alcoholism screening instrument. *American Journal of Psychiatry*, **131**, 1121–3.

10. Selzer ML (1971). The Michigan alcoholism screening test: the quest for a new diagnostic instrument. *American Journal of Psychiatry*, **127**, 1653–8.

11. Saunders JP, Aasland OG, Amundsen A, et al. (1993). Alcohol consumption and related problems among primary health care patients: WHO collaborative project on early detection of persons with harmful alcohol consumption. Geneva: WHO.

12. Drummond C & Ghodse H (1999). Use of investigations in the diagnosis and management of alcohol use disorders. *Advances in Psychiatric Treatment*, **5**, 366–75.

13. Anderson P (1995). Alcohol and the risk of physical harm. In *Alcohol and Public Policy: Evidence and Issues*, ed. HD Holder & G Edwards. Oxford: Oxford University Press.

14. Jacobson JL & Jacobson SW (1994). Prenatal alcohol exposure and neurobehavioural development: where is the threshold? *Alcohol and Health Research World*, **18**, 30–6.

15. Jones KL & Smith DW (1973). Recognition of the fetal alcohol syndrome in early infancy. *Lancet*, ii, 999–1001.

16. Chick JD (1999). Management of alcohol dependence. *Proceedings of the Royal College of Physicians of Edinburgh*, **29**, 43–50.

17. Drummond DC (1997). Alcohol interventions: do the best things come in small packages? *Addiction*, **92**, 375–9.

18. Nuffield Institute for Health, Centre for Health Economics, Royal College of Physicians (1993). Brief interventions and alcohol use. *Effective Health Care*, **1**, 1–14.

19. Bien TH, Miller WR & Tonigan JS (1993). Brief interventions for alcohol problems: a review. *Addiction*, **88**, 315–36.

20. Edwards G, Marshall EJ & Cook CCH (1997). Working towards normal drinking.

In *The Treatment of Drinking Problems*, 3rd edn. Cambridge: Cambridge University Press.

21. Garbutt JC, West SL, Carey TS, Lohr KN & Crews FT (1999). Pharmacological treatment of alcohol dependence. A review of the evidence. *JAMA*, **281**, 1318–25.

22. Whitworth A, Fischer F, Lesch OM, et al. (1996). Acamprosate versus placebo in the long term treatment of patients with alcohol dependence. *Lancet*, **347**, 1438–42.

23. Chick J, Anton R, Checinski K, et al. (2001). A multicentre, randomised, double-blind, placebo-controlled trial of naltrexone in the treatment of alcohol dependence. *Alcohol and Alcoholism*, **35**, 593–7.

24. Moncrieff J & Drummond DC (1997). New drug treatments for alcohol problems: a critical appraisal. *Addiction*, **92**, 939–47.

25. Drummond DC (2000). Treatment services for alcohol use disorders. In *New Oxford Textbook of Psychiatry*, ed. M Gelder et al. Oxford: Oxford University Press.

26. Godfrey C (1997). Nature and extent of the problem. In *Alcohol Dependence: A Clinical Problem*, ed. J Chick, C Godfrey, B Hore, J Marshall & T Peters. London: Mosby-Wolfe Medical Communications.

27. Denney R (1997). *None for the Road: Understanding Drink-Driving*. London: Shaw and Sons.

28. Alcohol Concern (1999). *Proposals for a National Alcohol Strategy for England*. London: Alcohol Concern.

29. Edwards G, Anderson P, Babor TF, et al. (1994). *Alcohol Policy and the Public Good*. Oxford: Oxford University Press.

30. Hansbro J, Bridgewood A, Morgan A & Hickman M (1996). *Health in England: What People Know, What People Think, What People Do*. London: HMSO.

31. Leon DA (2001). Alcohol: the changing face of a perennial problem. *International Journal of Epidemiology*, **30**, 653–4.

32. Marmot MG (2001). Reflections on alcohol and coronary heart disease. *International Journal of Epidemiology*, **30**, 729–34.

Chapter 5

1. Reisine T & Pasternak G (1996). Opioid analgesics and antagonists. In *Goodman and Gilman's The Pharmacological Basis of Therapeutics*, 9th edn, ed. JG Hardman and LE Limbird. New York: McGraw-Hill.

2. Ghodse AH, Bewley TH, Kearney MK & Smith SE (1986). Mydriatic response to topical naloxone in opiate abusers. *British Journal of Psychiatry*, **148**, 44–6.

3. Ghodse H, Taylor DR, Greaves JL, Britten AJ & Lynch D (1995). The opiate addiction test: a clinical evaluation of a quick test for physical dependence on opiate drugs. *British Journal of Clinical Pharmacology*, **39**, 257–9.

4. Ghodse AH, Greaves JL & Lynch D (1999). Evaluation of the opioid addiction test in an out-patient drug dependency unit. *British Journal of Psychiatry*, **175**, 158–62.

5. Wyatt SA & Ziedonis D (1998). Psychological and psychiatric consequences of amphetamines. In *Handbook of Substance Abuse. Neurobehavioural Pharmacology*, ed. RE Tarter, RT Ammerman & PJ Ott, pp. 529–44. New York: Plenum.

6. Churchill AC, Burgess P, Pead J & Gill T (1993). Measurement of the severity of amphetamine dependence. *Addiction*, **88**, 1335–40.

7. Ashton H (1991). Protracted withdrawal syndromes from benzodiazepines. *Journal of Substance Abuse Treatment*, **8**, 19–28.

8. Department of Health (2000). *Hepatitis C: Guidance for Those Working with Drug Users.* London: Department of Health. www.drugs.gov.uk

9. General Medical Council (1997). *Serious Communicable Diseases.* London: GMC Publications.

10. Sherman MF & Bigelow, GE (1992). Validity of patients' self-reported drug use as a function of treatment status. *Drug and Alcohol Dependence*, **30**, 1–11.

11. Kilpatrick B, Howlett M, Sedgwick P & Ghodse AH (2000). Drug use, self report and urinalysis. *Drug & Alcohol Dependence*, **58**, 111–16.

12. Magura S, Freeman RC, Siddiqi Q & Lipton DS (1992). The validity of hair analysis for detecting cocaine and heroin use among addicts. *International Journal of the Addictions*, **27**, 51–6.

13. Cook RF, Bernstein AD, Aarrington TL, Andrew CM & Marshall GA (1995). Methods of assessing drug use prevalence in the workplace: a comparison of self-report, urinalysis and hair analysis. *International Journal of the Addictions*, **30**, 403–26.

14. World Health Organization (1993). *Health Promotion in the Work Place: Alcohol and Drug Abuse.* (WHO expert committee. Technical report series 833.) Geneva: WHO.

15. World Health Organization (1992). *The ICD-10 Classification of Mental and Behavioural Disorders. Clinical Descriptions and Diagnostic Guidelines.* Geneva: WHO.

16. American Psychiatric Association (1987). *Diagnostic and Statistical Manual of Mental Disorders*, 3rd edn. (DSM-III-R). Washington, DC: APA.

17. American Psychiatric Association (1994). *Diagnostic and Statistical Manual of Mental Disorders*, 4th edn. (DSM-IV). Washington, DC: APA.

18. Peachey JE & Loh E (1994). Validity of alcohol and drug assessment. *Current Opinion in Psychiatry*, **7**, 252–8.

19. Bucknell P & Ghodse H (1996). *Misuse of Drugs*, 3rd edn. London: Sweet and Maxwell.

Chapter 6

1. Prochaska JO & DiClemente CC (1986). Toward a comprehensive model of change. In *Treating Addictive Behaviors: Process of Change*, ed. WR Miller & N Healther, pp. 3–27. New York: Plenum Press.

2. Gossop M & Strang J (1990). Psychological treatments. In: *Substance Abuse and Dependence*, ed. AH Ghodse & D Maxwell, pp. 131–48. London: Macmillan Press.

3. Woody GE, Luborsky L, McLellan AT, et al. (1983). Psychotherapy for opiate addicts: does it help? *Archives of General Psychiatry*, **40**, 639–45.

4. Getter H, Litt MD, Kadden RM and Cooney NL (1992). Measuring treatment process in coping skills and interactional group therapies for alcoholism. *International Journal of Group Psychotherapy*, **42**, 419–30.

5. Kaufman E & Kaufman P (eds.) (1979). *Family Therapy of Drug and Alcohol Abuse.* New York: Gardner Press.

6. Diamond GS & Liddie HA (1996). Resolving a therapeutic impasse between parents and adolescents in multidimensional family therapy. *Journal of Consulting and Clinical Psychology*, **64**, 481–8.

7. Liddle HA & Dakof GA (1995). Efficacy of family therapy for drug abuse: promising but not definitive. *Journal of Marital Family Therapy*, **21**, 511–43.

8. Farmer R & Ghodse AH (1993). Therapies for substance misuse. In *Recent Advances in Clinical Psychiatry*, ed. K. Granvill-Grossman. Edinburgh: Churchill Livingstone.

9. McLellan AT, Woody GE, Luborsky L & O'Brien CP (1988). Is the counselor an 'active ingredient' in substance abuse treatment? *Journal of Nervous and Mental Disease*, **176**, 423–30.

10. McLellan AT, Arndt I, Metzger DS, Woody GE & O'Brien CP (1993). The effects of psychosocial services in substance abuse treatment. *JAMA*, **269**, 1953–9.

11. Miller WR (1983). Motivational interviewing with problem drinkers. *Behavioural Psychotherapy*, **1**, 147–72.

12. Miller WR (1996). Motivational interviewing: research, practice and puzzles. *Addictive Behaviors*, **21**, 835–42.

13. Rotgers F (1996). Behavioral theory of substance abuse treatment: bringing science to bear on practice. In *Treating Substance Abusers: Theory and Technique*. ed. F Rotgers, D Keller & J Morgenstern, pp. 174–201. New York: Guilford Press.

14. Melamed BG & Siegell J (eds.) (1980). *Behavioural Medicine: Practical Applications in Health Care*. New York: Springer-Verlag.

15. Pinkerton SS, Hughes H & Wenrich WW (eds.) (1982). *Behavioural Medicine: Clinical Applications*. Chichester: Wiley.

16. Beck AT & Aaron T (1993). *Cognitive Therapy of Substance Abuse*. New York: Guilford Press.

17. Marlatt GA & George W (1984). Relapse prevention: introduction and overview of the model. *British Journal of Addiction*, **79**, 261–73.

18. Marlatt GA & Gordon JR (1985). *Relapse Prevention: Maintenance Strategies in the Treatment of Addictive Behaviours*. New York: Guilford Press.

19. Powell J, Bradley B & Gray J (1992). Classical conditioning and cognitive determinants of subjective craving for opiates: an investigation of their relative contributions. *British Journal of Addictions*, **87**, 1133–44.

20. Saxon AJ, Clasyn DA, Kivlahan DR & Roszell DK (1993). Outcome of contingency contracting for illicit drug use in a methadone maintenance program. *Drug and Alcohol Dependence*, **31**, 205–14.

21. Stitzer ML, Iguchi MY & Felch LJ (1992). Contingent take-home incentive: effects on drug use of methadone maintenance patients. *Journal of Consulting and Clinical Psychology*, **60**, 927–34.

22. Stitzer ML, Iguchi MY, Kidorf M & Bigelow GE (1993). Contingency management in methadone treatment: the case for positive incentives. In *Behavioral Treatments for Drug Abuse and Dependence* (NIDA research monograph series 137), ed. LS Onken, JD Blaine & JJ Boren, pp. 19–36. Rockville, MD: NIDA.

23. Silverman K, Higgins ST, Brooner RK, et al. (1996). Sustained cocaine abstinence in

methadone maintenance patients through voucher-based reinforcement therapy. *Archives of General Psychiatry*, **53**, 409–15.

24. Boudin HM, Valentine VE, Ruiz MR & Regan EJ (1980). Contingency contracting for drug addiction: an outcome evaluation. In *Evaluating Alcohol and Drug Abuse Treatment Effectiveness*, ed. L Sobell, MC Sobell & E Ward. New York: Pergamon.

25. Stitzer ML, Bigelow GE & McCaul ME (1985). Behaviour therapy in drug abuse treatment: review and evaluation. In *Progress in the Development of Cost-Effective Treatment for Drug Abusers* (NIDA research monograph series 58), ed. RS Asher. Rockville, MD: Department of Health & Human Services.

26. Callahan EJ, Price KA & Dahlkoetter J (1980). Behavioural treatment of drug abuse. In Daitzman R (ed.) *Clinical Behaviour Therapy and Behaviour Modification*, ed. R. Daitzman. New York: Garland Press.

27. Mattick RP & Heather N (1993). Developments in cognitive and behavioural approaches to substance misuse. *Current Opinion in Psychiatry*, **6**, 424–9.

28. Childress AR, Hole AV, Ehrman RN, Robbins SJ, McLellan AT & O'Brien CP (1993). Cure reactivity and cure reactivity interventions in drug dependence. In *Behavioral Treatments of Drug Abuse and Dependence* (NIDA research monograph series 137), ed. LS Onken, JD Blaine & JJ Boren. Rockville, MD: NIDA.

29. Platt JJ & Metzer D (1985). The role of employment in the rehabilitation of heroin addicts. In: *Progress in the Development of Cost-Effective Treatment of Drug Abusers*, ed. RS Ashery, pp. 111–21. (NIDA research monograph series 58.) Rockville, MD: Department of Health & Human Services.

30. De Leon G (1995). Therapeutic communities for addictions: a theoretical framework. *International Journal of the Addictions*, **30**, 1603–49.

31. De Leon G & Rosenthal MS (1979). Therapeutic communities. In *Handbook on Drug Abuse*. ed. RL Dupont, A Goldstein & J O'Donnell. Washington, DC: National Institute of Drug Abuse.

32. Wells (1990). Psychosocial Interventions. In *Substance Abuse and Dependence*, ed. AH Ghodse & D Maxwell, pp. 149–75. London: Macmillan Press.

33. National Institute on Drug Abuse (1999). *Drug Abuse Treatment Outcome Studies* (DATOS) www.datos.org/background.html

34. Landry M (1995). *Overview of Addiction Treatment Effectiveness*. Rockville, MD: SAMHSA, Office of Applied Studies, 116.

35. WHO Expert Committee on Drug Dependence (1988). *Thirtieth Report*. (Technical report series 873.) Geneva: WHO.

36. Kaplan SR & Razin AM (1978). The psychological substrate of self-help groups. *Journal of Operational Psychiatry*, **9**, 57.

37. Narcotics Anonymous (1987). *Narcotics Anonymous*, 4th edn. Van Nuys. California: World Service Office.

38. Emrick C (1989). Alcoholics Anonymous: membership characteristics and effectiveness as treatment. In *Recent Developments in Alcoholism: Treatment and Research*, ed. M Galanter, pp. 37–53. New York: Plenum.

39. Anderson DJ, McGovern JP and DuPont RL (1999). The origins of the Minnesota Model of addiction treatment: a first person account. *Journal of Addictive Diseases*, **18**, 107–14.

40. Cook CH (1988). The Minnesota model in the management of drug and alcohol dependency: miracle, method or myth? *British Journal of Addiction*, **83**, 625–34.

41. Winters KC, Stinchfield RD, Opland E, Weller C & Latimer WW (2000). The effectiveness of the Minnesota Model approach in the treatment of adolescent drug abusers. *Addiction*, **95**, 601–12.

42. Jameson A, Glanz A & Macgregor S (1984). *Dealing with Drug Misuse. Crisis Intervention in the City*. London: Tavistock.

43. Mott J (1981). Criminal involvement and penal response. In *Drug Problems in Britain: A Review of Ten Years*, ed. G Edwards & C Busch. London: Academic Press.

44. Cabinet Office (2000). *Tackling Drugs to Build a Better Britain. UK Anti-Drugs Co-ordinator's Second National Plan*. London: Cabinet Office.

45. Jaffe AJ, Rounsaville B, Chang G, et al. (1996). Naltrexone, relapse prevention and supportive therapy with alcoholics: an analysis of patient treatment matching. *Journal of Consulting and Clinical Psychology*, **64**, 1044–53.

Chapter 7

1. Department of Health, The Scottish Office Department of Health, Welsh Office & Department of Health and Social Services, Northern Ireland (1999). *Drug Misuse and Dependence: Guidelines on Clinical Management*. London: HMSO.

2. Kleber HD, Riordan CE, Rounsaville BJ, et al. (1985). Clonidine in outpatient detoxification from methadone maintenance. *Archives of General Psychiatry*, **42**, 391–4.

3. Ghodse H, Myles J & Smith SE (1994). Clonidine is not a useful adjunct to methadone gradual detoxification in opioid addiction. *British Journal of Psychiatry*, **165**, 370–4.

4. Carnwath T & Hardman J (1998). Randomised double-blind comparison of lofexidine and clonidine in the out-patient treatment of opiate withdrawal. *Drug and Alcohol Dependence*, **50**, 251–4.

5. Kahn A, Mumford JP, Rogers GA & Beckford H (1997). Double-blind study of lofexidine and clonidine in the detoxification of opiate addicts in hospital. *Drug and Alcohol Dependence*, **44**, 57–61.

6. Rosen MI, McMahon TJ, Hameedi FA, et al. (1996). Effect of clonidine pretreatment on naloxone-precipitated withdrawal. *Journal of Pharmacology & Experimental Therapeutics*, **276**, 1128–35.

7. Riordan CE & Kleber HD (1980). Rapid opiate detoxification with clonidine and naloxone. *Lancet*, **i**, 1079–80.

8. O'Connor PG & Kosten TR (1998). Rapid and ultra-rapid opioid detoxification techniques. *JAMA*, **279**, 229–34.

9. Strang J, Bearn J & Gossop M (1997). Opiate detoxification under anaesthesia: enthusiasm must be tempered with caution and scientific scrutiny. *British Medical Journal*, **315**, 1249–50.

10. Wen HI & Cheung SY (1973). Treatment of drug addiction by acupuncture and electrical stimulation. *Asian Journal of Medicine*, **9**, 138–41.

11. Moner SE (1996). Acupuncture and addiction treatment. *Journal of Addictive Behaviour*, **15**, 79–100.

12. Timofeev MF (1999). Effects of acupuncture and an agonist of opiate receptors on heroin dependent patients. *American Journal of Chinese Medicine*, **27**, 143–8.

13. Patterson MA (1975). *Addictions Can be Cured. The Treatment of Drug Addiction by Neuro-electric Stimulation*. Berkhamsted: Lion Publishing.

14. Dole VP & Nyswander MA (1965). Medical treatment for diacetylmorphine (heroin) addiction. *JAMA*, **193**, 645–56.

15. Ghodse AH, Creighton FJ & Bhatt AV (1990). Comparison of oral preparations of heroin and methadone to stabilise opiate misusers as inpatients. *British Medical Journal*, **300**, 719–20.

16. Morgan JR (1990). Treatment and management. In *Substance Abuse and Dependence*, ed. AH Ghodse & D Maxwell, pp. 98–130. London: Macmillan Press.

17. Arif A & Westermeyer J (eds.) (1990). *Methadone Maintenance in the Management of Opioid Dependence: an International Review*. New York: Praeger.

18. Ball JC & Ross A (1991). *The Effectiveness of Methadone Maintenance Treatment: Patients, Programmes, Services and Outcome*. New York: Springer-Verlag.

19. Newman RG (1979). Double-blind comparison of methadone and placebo maintenance treatments of narcotic addicts in Hong Kong. *Lancet*, **ii**, 485–8.

20. Zador D (2001). Injectable opiate maintenance in the UK: is it good clinical practice? *Addiction*, **96**, 547–53.

21. Jaffe JH (2001). Injectable opiate maintenance in the United Kingdom: a view from the United States. *Addiction*, **96**, 557–60.

22. Rawson RA, Hasson AL, Huber AM, et al. (1998). A 3-year progress report on the implementation of LAAM in the United States. *Addiction*, **93**, 533–40.

23. Walsh SL, Johnson RE, Cone EJ & Bigelow GE (1998). Intravenous and oral L-alpha acetylmethadol: pharmacodynamics and pharmacokinetics in humans. *Journal of Pharmacology and Experimental Therapeutics*, **285**, 71–82.

24. Glanz M, Klawansky S, McAuliffe W & Chalmers T (1997). Methadone vs L-alpha-acetylmethadol in the treatment of opioid addiction. *American Journal of Addiction*, **6**, 339–49.

25. Houtsmuller, EJ, Walsh SL, Schuh KJ et al. (1998). Dose-response analysis of opioid cross-tolerance and withdrawal suppression during LAAM maintenance. *Journal of Pharmacology and Experimental Therapeutics*, **285**, 387–96.

26. Ling W, Charuvastra C, Collins JF et al. (1998). Buprenorphine maintenance treatment of opiate dependence: a multicenter randomised clinical trial. *Addiction*, **93**, 475–86.

27. Fudala PJ, Yu E, Macfadden W et al. (1998). Effects of buprenorphine and naloxone in morphine stabilised opioid addicts. *Drug and Alcohol Dependence*, **50**, 1–8.

28. Sellers EM (1984). Diazepam tapering in detoxification for high dose benzodiazepine abuse. *Clinical Pharmacology and Therapeutics*, **36**, 410–16.

29. Sellers EM (1988). Alcohol, barbiturate and benzodiazepine withdrawal syndromes: clinical management. *Canadian Medical Association Journal*, **139**, 113–18.

30. Marks J (1988). Techniques of benzodiazepine withdrawal in clinical practice. A consensus workshop report. *Medical Toxicology*, **3**, 324–33.

31. Gawin FH (1988). Chronic neuropharmacology of cocaine: progress in pharmacotherapy. *Journal of Clinical Psychiatry* (Suppl), **49**, 11–16.

32. Leshner JL (1996). Molecular mechanisms of cocaine addiction. *New England Journal of Medicine*, **335**, 128–9.

33. O'Brien CP (1997). A range of research-based pharmacotherapies for addiction. *Science*, **278**, 66–70.

34. Cornish JW & O'Brien CP (1998). Developing medications to treat cocaine dependence: a new direction. *Current Opinion in Psychiatry*, **11**, 249–51.

35. Stimson GV (1995). AIDS and injecting drug use in the United Kingdom 1987–1993: the policy response and the prevention of the epidemic. *Social Science Medicine*, **5**, 699–716.

36. Klee H & Morris J (1995). The role of needle exchanges in modifying sharing behaviour: cross-study comparisons 1989–1993. *Addiction*, **90**, 1635–45.

37. Crawford V (1997). Injecting drug use. *Current Opinion in Psychiatry*, **10**, 215–19.

38. Ghodse AH, Tregenza G & Li M (1987). Effect of fear of AIDS on sharing of injection equipment among drug abusers. *British Medical Journal*, **ii**, 698–9.

Chapter 8

1. Maxwell D (1990). Clinical complications of substance abuse. In *Substance Abuse and Dependence*, ed. AH Ghodse & D Maxwell, pp. 176–203. London: Macmillan Press.

2. Frontera JA & Gradon JD (2000). Right-side endocarditis in injection drug users: review of proposed mechanisms of pathogenesis. *Clinical Infectious Diseases*, **30**, 374–9.

3. Libman H & Witzburg RA (1993). *HIV Infection: A Clinical Manual*, 2nd edn. Boston, MA: Little, Brown.

4. World Health Organization (1994). *Multi-City Study on Drug Injecting and HIV Infection*. Geneva: WHO.

5. Des Jarlais DC, Hagan H, Friedman SR, et al. (1995). Maintaining low seroprevalence in populations of injecting drug users. *JAMA*, **274**, 1226–31.

6. Department of Health (1999). Unlinked anonymous prevalence monitoring programme. Prevalence of HIV and hepatitis infections in the United Kingdom. London: Department of Health. www.doh.gov.uk/hivhepatitis99.htm

7. McCoy CB, Metsch LR, Inciardi JA, et al. (1996). Sex drugs and the spread of HIV/AIDS in Belle Glade, Florida. *Medical Anthropology Quarterly*, **10**, 83–93.

8. AIDS and HIV infection in the United Kingdom: monthly report (1999). *Communicable Disease Report*, **9**, 277–80.

9. Advisory Council on the Misuse of Drugs (1993). *AIDS and Drug Misuse Update*. London: HMSO.

10. General Medical Council (undated). *Serious Communicable Diseases*. London: General Medical Council. www.gmc-uk.org

11. HIV in pregnancy and early childhood (1999). *Drug and Therapeutics Bulletin*, **37** (9), 65–7.

12. Thomas HC (1996). Clinical features of viral hepatitis. In *Oxford Textbook of Medicine*, 3rd edn, ed. DJ Weatherall, JGG Ledingham & DA Warrell, pp. 2061–9. Oxford: Oxford University Press.

13. Stark K (1996). Frontloading: a risk factor for HIV and hepatitis C virus infection among drug users in Berlin. *AIDS*, **10**, 311–17.

14. Department of Health (2001). Hepatitis C: guidance for those working with drug users. London: Department of Health. www.doh.gov.uk

15. Ghodse H & Ricaurte GA (2000). Hepatitis C: bad news for substance misusers. *Current Opinion in Psychiatry*, **13**, 281–3.

16. European Association for the Study of the Liver, Consensus Panel (1999). EASL International Consensus Statement on hepatitis C. *Journal of Hepatology*, **30**, 956–61.

17. Best D, Noble A, Finch E et al. (1999). Accuracy of perceptions of hepatitis B and C status: cross sectional investigation of opiate addicts in treatment. *British Medical Journal*, **319**, 290–1.

18. Serfaty MA, Lawrie A, Smith B et al.(1997). Risk factors and medical follow-up of drug users tested for hepatitis C. Can the risk of transmission be reduced? *Drug and Alcohol Review*, **16**, 339–47.

19. Allwright S, Bradley F, Long J et al. (2000). Prevalence of antibodies to hepatitis B, hepatitis C and HIV and risk factors in Irish prisoners: results of a national cross-sectional survey. *British Medical Journal*, **321**, 78–82.

20. National Institute for Clinical Excellence (2000). *Guidance on the Use of Combination Therapy for Hepatitis C*. London: NICE. www.nice.org.uk

21. Mangtani P, Kovats S & Hall A (1995). Hepatitis B vaccination policy in drug treatment services. *British Medical Journal*, **311**, 1500.

22. Johns A (2001). Psychiatric effects of cannabis. *British Journal of Psychiatry*, **178**, 116–22.

23. Ghodse AH & Creighton FJ (1984). Opioid analgesics and narcotic antagonists. In *Meyler's Side Effects of Drugs*, 11th edn, ed. MNG Dukes, pp. 137–55. Amsterdam: Elsevier.

24. Hobbs WR, Rall, TW & Todd AV (1996). Hypnotics and sedatives: ethanol. In *Goodman and Gilman's The Pharmacological Basis of Therapeutics*, 9th edn, ed. JG Hardman & LE Limbird. New York: McGraw-Hill.

Chapter 9

1. Ghodse AH (1990). Problems of maternal substance abuse. In *Substance Abuse and Dependence*, ed. AH Ghodse & D Maxwell, pp. 16–231. London: Macmillan Press.

2. Riley D (1987). Management of the pregnant drug addict. *Bulletin of the Royal College of Psychiatrists*, **11**, 362–5.

3. Zuckerman B, Frank D & Brown E (1995). Overview of the effects of abuse and drugs on pregnancy and offspring. In *Medications Development for the Treatment of Pregnant Addicts and their Infants*, ed. CN Chiang & LP Finnegan, pp. 16–38 (NIDA research monograph 149). Rockville, MD: NIDA.

4. Zuckerman B & Brown E (1993). Maternal substance abuse and infant development. In *Handbook of Infant Mental Health*, ed. R Tsang, pp. 143–58. New York: Guilford Press.

5. Finnegan LP & Kaltenbach K (1992). Neonatal abstinence syndrome. In *Primary Pediatric Care*, 2nd edn, ed. RA Hoekelman & NM Nelson. St Louis: Mosby Year Book.

6. Ghodse AH, Reed JL & Mack JW (1977). The effect of maternal narcotic addiction on the newborn infant. *Psychological Medicine*, **7**, 667–75.

7. The European Collaborative Study (1999). Maternal viral load and vertical transmission of HIV-1: an important factor but not the only one. *AIDS*, **13**, 1377–85.

8. HIV in pregnancy and early childhood (1999). *Drug and Therapeutics Bulletin*, **37**(9), 65–7.

9. Department of Health (2001). *Hepatitis C: Guidance for Those Working with Drug Users.* London: Department of Health. www.drugs.gov.uk

10. Kaltenbach K & Finnegan L (1997). Children of maternal substance misusers. *Current Opinion in Psychiatry*, **10**, 220–4.

11. Brewster JM (1986). Prevalence of alcohol and other drug problems among physicians. *JAMA*, **255**, 1913–20.

12. Ghodse H (2000). Doctors and their health. Who heals the healers? In *Doctors and Their Health*, ed. H Ghodse, S Mann & P Johnson. Sutton, Surrey: Reed Healthcare.

13. General Medical Council (1995). *Good Medical Practice.* London: General Medical Council. www.gmc.uk.org

14. Johns A (2000). Sick doctors and the law. In *Doctors and their Health*, ed. H Ghodse, S Mann & P Johnson. Sutton, Surrey: Reed Healthcare.

15. Krausz M (1996). Old problems – new perspectives. *European Addiction Research*, **2**, 1–2.

16. Lehmann AF, Meyers CP & Corty E (1989). Classification of patients with psychiatric and substance abuse syndromes. *Hospital and Community Psychiatry*, **40**, 1019–25.

17. Kessler RI (1995). Epidemiology of psychiatric comorbidity. In *Textbook of Psychiatric Epidemiology*, ed. M Tsuang, M Tohen & GEP Zahner. New York: Wiley.

18. Kessler R, Crum RM, Warner LA, et al. (1997). Lifetime co-occurrence of DSM-iii-R psychiatric disorders in the United States. *Archives of General Psychiatry*, **54**, 313–21.

19. Glass IB & Jackson P (1988). Maudsley Hospital Survey: prevalence of alcohol problems and other psychiatric disorders in a hospital population. *British Journal of Addiction*, **83**, 1105–11.

20. Ross HE, Swinson, R, Larkin EJ & Doumani S (1994). Diagnosing comorbidity in substance abusers: computer assessment and clinical validation. *Journal of Nervous and Mental Disorders*, **182**, 556–63.

21. Anthenelli RM (1994). The initial evaluation of the dual diagnosis patient. *Psychiatric Annals*, **24**, 427–31.

22. Farrell M, Howes S, Bebbington P, et al. (2001). Nicotine, alcohol and drug dependence and psychiatric comorbidity. *British Journal of Psychiatry*, **179**, 432–7.

23. Degenhardt L, Hall, W & Lynskey M (2001). Alcohol, cannabis and tobacco use among Australians: a comparison of their associations with other drug use and use disorders, affective and anxiety disorders, and psychosis. *Addiction*, **96**, 1603–14.

24. Mueser KT, Drake RE & Wallach MA (1998). Dual diagnosis: a review of etiological theories. *Addictive Behaviour*, **23**, 7217–34.

25. Crawford V (1996). Comorbidity of substance misuse and psychiatric disorders. *Current Opinion in Psychiatry*, **9**, 231–4.

26. Williams H, Salter M & Ghodse AH (1996). Management of substance misusers on the general hospital ward. *British Journal of Clinical Practice*, **50**, 94–8.

27. Ghodse AH, Stapleton J, Edwards G & Edeh J (1987). Monitoring changing patterns of drug dependence in accident and emergency departments. *Drug and Alcohol Dependence*, **19**, 265–9.

28. Richmond RL & Anderson P (1994). Research in general practice for smokers and excessive drinkers in Australia and the UK. *Addiction,* **89**, 35–62.

29. Williams H & Ghodse AH (1996). The prevention of alcohol and drug misuse. In *The Prevention of Mental Illness in Primary Care.* ed. A Kendrick, A Tylie & P Freeling, pp. 223–245. Cambridge: Cambridge University Press.

30. Robertson JR (1985). Drug users in contact with general practice. *British Medical Journal,* **290**, 34–5.

31. Porter S & Ghodse AH (1996). Treatment of substance misuse problems in general practice. In *General Practice National Association of Fundholding Practices Yearbook*, pp. 318–21. Thornton Heath: Scorpio Publishing.

32. Department of Health, The Scottish Office Department of Health, Welsh Office, Department of Health and Social Services, Northern Ireland (1999). *Drug Misuse and Dependence: Guidelines on Clinical Management.* London: HMSO.

33. Royal College of Psychiatrists and Association of Police Surgeons (2000). *Substance Misuse Detainees in Police Custody: Guidelines for Clinical Management*, 2nd edn. Report of a Medical Working Group. (Council report CR81.) London: Royal College of Psychiatrists.

34. Driver and Vehicle Licensing Agency (2001). *For Medical Practitioners. At A Glance Guide to the Current Medical Standards of Fitness to Drive.* Swansea: DVLA.

Chapter 10

1. WHO Expert Committee on Drug Dependence (1998). *Thirtieth Report.* Geneva: WHO.

2. US Department of Health and Human Services (1996). *Treatment Works.* Rockville, MD: DHHS.

3. Rounsaville BJ, Tierney T, Crit-Cristoph K, Weissman MW & Kleber HD (1982). Predictors of outcome in treatment of opiate addicts: evidence for the multidimensional nature of addicts' problems. *Comprehensive Psychiatry,* **23**, 462–78.

4. Stimson G & Oppenheimer E (1982). *Heroin addiction. Treatment and Control in Britain*, pp. 229–52. London: Tavistock.

5. Cottrell D, Childs-Clarke A & Ghodse AH (1985). British opiate addicts: an 11-year follow-up. *British Journal of Psychiatry,* **146**, 448–50.

6. Rathod NH (1977). Follow-up study of injectors in a provincial town. *Drug and Alcohol Dependence,* **2**, 1–21.

7. Oppenheim GB, Wright JE, Buchanan J & Biggs L (1973). Outpatient treatment of narcotic addiction: who benefits? *British Journal of Addiction,* **68**, 37–44.

8. Thorley A (1981). Longitudinal studies of drug dependence. In *Drug Problems in Britain: A Review of Ten Years*, ed. G Edwards & C Busch, pp. 117–69. London: Academic Press.

9. Bewley TH, Ben-Arie O & James IP (1968). Morbidity and mortality from heroin dependence. 1. Survey of heroin addicts known to the Home Office. *British Medical Journal,* **i**, 725–6.

10. Ghodse AH, Sheehan M, Taylor C & Edwards G (1985). Deaths of drug addicts in the United Kingdom, 1967–1981. *British Medical Journal,* **290**, 425–8.

11. Engstrom A, Adamsson C, Allebeck P & Rydberg U. (1991). Mortality in patients with substance abuse: a follow-up in Stockholm County, 1973–84. *International Journal of*

Addiction, **89**, 851–7.

12. Oppenheimer E, Tobutt C, Taylor C & Andrew T (1994). Death and survival in a cohort of heroin addicts from London clinics: a 22-year follow-up study. *Addiction,* **89**, 1299–308.

13. Ghodse H, Oyefeso A & Kilpatrick B (1998). Mortality of drug addicts in the United Kingdom (1967–93). *International Journal of Epidemiology,* **27**, 473–8.

14. Caplehorn JRM, Stella M, Dalton YN, et al. (1994). Retention in methadone maintenance and heroin addicts' risk of death. *Addiction,* **89**, 203–7.

15. International Narcotics Control Board (1991). *Narcotic Drugs. Estimated World Requirements for 1993. Statistics for 1991.* Vienna: United Nations.

16. Ghodse AH, Sheehan M, Stevens, Taylor C & Edwards G (1978). Mortality among addicts in Greater London. *British Medical Journal,* **ii**, 1742–4.

17. Oyefeso A, Valmana H, Clancy C, et al. (2000). Fatal antidepressant overdose among drug abusers and non-drug abusers *Acta Psychiatrica Scandinavica,* **102**, 295–9.

18. Gossop M, Marsden J, Stewart D & Rolfe A (1999). *The National Treatment Outcome Research Study: Changes in Substance Use, Health and Crime. Fourth Bulletin.* London: Department of Health.

19. National Institute on Drug Abuse (1990). *Drug Abuse Treatment Outcome Studies, Background.* (http://www.datos.org/background.html#DARP and TOPs findings.)

20. Marsch LA (1998). The efficacy of methadone maintenance interventions in reducing illicit opiate use, HIV risk behavior and criminality: a meta-analysis. *Addiction,* **93**, 515–32.

21. Hubbard, RI, Craddock G, Flynn P et al. (1997). Overview of 1-year outcomes in the Drug Abuse Treatment Outcomes Study (DATOS). *Psychology of Addictive Behaviour,* **11**, 261–78.

22. Charney DA, Paraherakis AM & Gill KJ (2000). The treatment of sedative-hypnotic dependence: evaluating clinical predictors of outcome. *Journal of Clinical Psychiatry,* **61**(3), 190–5.

23. Broome KM, Flynn PM & Simpson DD (1999). Psychiatric comorbidity measures as predictors of retention in drug abuse treatment programs. *Health Services Research,* **334**, 791–806.

24. Hartnoll RL, Mitcheson MC, Battersby A, *et al.* (1980). Evaluation of heroin maintenance in a controlled trial. *Archives of General Psychiatry,* **37**, 877–84.

25. Mott J (1981). Criminal involvement and penal response. In *Drug Problems in Britain; a Review of Ten Years,* ed. G Edwards & C Busch. London: Academic Press.

26. Rydell CP, Caulkins JP & Everingham S (1996). Enforcement of treatment, modelling the relative efficacy of alternatives for controlling cocaine. *Operations Research,* **44**, 687–95.

27. Flynn PM, Kristiansen PL, Porto JV & Hubbard RL (1999). Costs and benefits of treatment for cocaine addiction in DATOS. *Drug and Alcohol Dependence,* **57**, 167–74.

28. Healey A, Knapp M, Astin J et al. (1998). Economic burden of drug dependency. Social costs incurred by drug users at intake to the National Treatment Outcome Research Study. *British Journal of Psychiatry,* **173**, 160–5.

29. Gerstein DR, Johnson RA, Harwood HJ, et al. (1994). Evaluating recovery services: the California drug and alcohol treatment assessment (CALDATA). Sacramento, CA: Department of Alcohol and Drug Programs.

Chapter 11

1. United Nations Office for Drug Control and Crime Prevention (2000). *World Drug Report 2000.* Oxford: Oxford University Press.

2. *Official Records of the United Nations Conference for the Adoption of a Convention against Illicit Traffic in Narcotic Drugs and Psychotropic Substances, Vienna, 25 November – 20 December 1988*, vol. I. New York: United Nations (Sales no. E94.XI.5).

3. International Narcotics Control Board (1999). *Report of the International Narcotics Control Board 1999.* New York: United Nations (Sales no. E.00.XI.1).

4. International Narcotics Control Board (2000). *Report of the International Narcotics Control Board 2000.* New York: United Nations (Sales no. E.01.XI. 1).

5. Ghodse H (1999). Guiding principles of drug demand reduction: an international response. *British Journal of Psychiatry*, **175**, 310–12.

6. Ghodse H (1995). International Policies on addiction. Strategy for development and cooperation. *British Journal of Psychiatry*, **166**, 145–8.

7. United Nations International Drug Control Programme (1997). *World Drug Report 1997.* New York: Oxford University Press.

8. International Narcotics Control Board (1997). *Report of the International Narcotics Control Board 1997.* New York: United Nations.

9. Ghodse H & Khan I (1988). *Psychoactive Drugs: Improving Prescribing Practices.* Geneva: WHO.

10. Falkowski J & Ghodse AH (1989). Undergraduate medical school training in psychoactive drugs and rational prescribing in the United Kingdom. *British Journal of Addictions*, **84**, 1539–42.

11. World Health Organization (1988). *Ethical Criteria for Medicinal Drug Promotion.* Geneva: WHO.

12. World Health Organization (1983). *The Use of Essential Drugs.* Report of a WHO Expert Committee. (Technical report series 685.) Geneva: WHO.

13. Falkowski J, Ghodse AH, Dickinson R & Khan I (1989). An international survey of the educational activities of schools of pharmacy on psychoactive drugs. *Bulletin of the World Health Organization*, **67**, 561–4.

14. Dorn N (1981). Social analyses of drugs in health education and the media. In *Drug Problems in Britain: A Review of Ten Years*, ed. G Edwards & C Busch, pp. 281–304. London: Academic Press.

15. Bell CS & Battjes R (eds.) (1985). *Prevention Research: Deterring Drug Abuse Among Children and Adolescents.* (NIDA research monograph 63.) Rockville, MD: Department of Health & Human Services.

16. Boys A, Marsden J, Fountain J, Griffiths P, Stillwell G & Strang J (1999). What influences young people's use of drugs? A qualitative study of decision making. *Drugs: Education, Prevention and Policy*, **6**, 373–87.

17. National Institute on Drug Abuse (1997). *Drug Abuse Prevention for At-Risk Individuals.* Rockville, MD: US National Institutes of Health.

18. Pittman DJ (1994). Substance misuse prevention, health promotion, and health education. *Current Opinion in Psychiatry*, **7**, 269–73.

19. World Health Organization (1993). *Health Promotion in the Work Place: Alcohol and Drug Abuse.* Report of a WHO Expert Committee. (Technical report series 833.) Geneva: WHO.

20. National Institute on Drug Abuse (1998). *Assessing Drug Abuse Within and Across Communities.* (NIH publication 98–3614.) Rockville, MD: Department of Health and Human Services.

21. Room R & Paglia A (1998). *Preventing Substance Use: Problems Among Youth: A Literature Review and Recommendations.* (Research document series 142.) Toronto: Addiction Research Foundation.

22. Tyrer P & Murphy S (1987). The place of benzodiazepines in psychiatric practice. *British Journal of Psychiatry*, **151**, 719–23.

23. World Health Organization (1989). *WHO Expert Committee on Drug Dependence: Twenty-Fifth Report.* (Technical report series 775.) Geneva: WHO.

24. Shufman EN, Porat S, Witztum E, et al. (1994). The efficacy of naltrexone in preventing reabuse of heroin after detoxification. *Biological Psychiatry*, **35**, 935–45.

25. Schuster CR (1992). Drug abuse research and HIV/AIDS: a national perspective from the US. *British Journal of Addiction*, **87**, 355–61.

26. London M (2001). Prevention of substance misuse. *Current Opinion in Psychiatry*, **14**, 207–11.

Chapter 12

1. International Opium Convention 1912. League of Nations, Treaty Series, vol. VIII, p. 187.

2. Bayer I & Ghodse H (1999). Evolution of international drug control 1945–1995. *Bulletin on Narcotics*, **LI** (1 and 2), 1–17.

3. International Opium Convention 1925. League of Nations, Treaty series, vol. LXXXI, p. 317.

4. Convention for Limiting the Manufacture and Regulating the Distribution of Narcotic Drugs 1931. League of Nations, *Treaty series*, vol CXXXIX, p. 301.

5. Convention for the Suppression of the Illicit Traffic in Dangerous Drugs 1936. League of Nations, *Treaty series*, vol CXCVIII, p. 299.

6. Protocol amending the Agreements, Conventions and Protocols on Narcotic Drugs 1946. United Nations, *Treaty series*, vol. 12, p. 179.

7. Protocol Bringing under International Control Drugs Outside the Scope of the Convention of 13 July 1931 for Limiting the Manufacture and Regulating the Distribution of Narcotic Drugs as amended by the Protocol 1946. United Nations, *Treaty series*, vol. 44, p. 277.

8. Protocol for Limiting and Regulating the Cultivation of the Poppy Plant, the Production of, International and Wholesale Trade in and Use of Opium 1953. United Nations, *Treaty series*, vol. 456, p. 3.

9. Single Convention on Narcotic Drugs 1961. United Nations, *Treaty series*, vol. 520, no. 7515.

10. Protocol amending the Single Convention on Narcotic Drugs 1961 (1972). United Nations, *Treaty series*, vol. 976, no. 14152.

11. Convention on Psychotropic Substances (1971). United Nations, *Treaty series*, vol. 1019, no. 14956.

12. United Nations Convention against Illicit Traffic in Narcotic Drugs and Psychotropic Substances (1988). *Official Records of the United Nations Conference for the Adoption of a Convention against Illicit Traffic in Narcotic Drugs and Psychotropic Substances, Vienna, 25 November – 20 December 1988*, vol 1. New York: United Nations (Sales no. E.94.XI.5).

13. United Nations Commission on Narcotic Drugs (2001). 44th session. Vienna: United Nations.

14. International Narcotics Control Board (2002). Report of the International Narcotics Control Board for 2001. New York: United Nations.

15. United Nations General Assembly (1998). *Declaration of the Guiding Principles of Demand Reduction.* (A/S-20/11.) Vienna: United Nations.

16. Ghodse H (1999). Guiding principles of drug demand reduction: an international response. *British Journal of Psychiatry*, **175**, 310–12.

17. Political Declaration and Global Programme of Action (1990). (Feb A/Res/S-17/2.) New York: United Nations.

18. Bucknell P & Ghodse AH (1996). *Misuse of Drugs*, 3rd edn. London: Sweet and Maxwell.

19. United Nations Office for Drug Control and Crime Prevention (1997). World Drug Report. New York: Oxford University Press.

20. United Nations Office for Drug Control and Crime Prevention (2000). World Drug Report. Oxford: Oxford University Press.

21. Rexed B, Edmondson K, Khan I & Samson RJ (1984). *Guidelines for the Control of Narcotic and Psychotropic Substances in the Context of the International Treaties.* Geneva: WHO.

22. Ghodse H (1995). International policies on addiction. Strategy developments and co-operation. *British Journal of Psychiatry*, **166**, 145–8.

23. Cabinet Office (2000). *The United Kingdom Anti-Drug Co-ordinator's Second National Plan.* London: Cabinet Office.

Index

Numbers in italics indicate *tables* or *figures* .